ANCIENT REMEDIES

ANCIENT REMEDIES

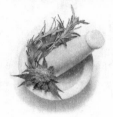

Secrets to Healing with Herbs,
Essential Oils, CBD, and the Most Powerful
Natural Medicine in History

DR. JOSH AXE

Little, Brown Spark
New York Boston London

Copyright © 2021 by Dr. Josh Axe

Hachette Book Group supports the right to free expression and the value of copyright. The purpose of copyright is to encourage writers and artists to produce the creative works that enrich our culture.

The scanning, uploading, and distribution of this book without permission is a theft of the author's intellectual property. If you would like permission to use material from the book (other than for review purposes), please contact permissions@hbgusa.com. Thank you for your support of the author's rights.

Little, Brown Spark
Hachette Book Group
1290 Avenue of the Americas, New York, NY 10104
littlebrownspark.com

First Edition: February 2021

Little, Brown Spark is an imprint of Little, Brown and Company, a division of Hachette Book Group, Inc. The Little, Brown Spark name and logo are trademarks of Hachette Book Group, Inc.

The publisher is not responsible for websites (or their content) that are not owned by the publisher.

The Hachette Speakers Bureau provides a wide range of authors for speaking events. To find out more, go to hachettespeakersbureau.com or call (866) 376-6591.

ISBN 978-0-316-49645-2 (hardcover) / 978-0-316-54177-0 (large print)
LCCN 2020943055

Printing 2, 2021

LSC-C

Printed in the United States of America

This book is dedicated to my beautiful, bold, and brilliant daughter, Arwyn; to my best friend, wife, and love of my life, Chelsea; and to my father God, for giving me the platform and favor to write this book. I am beyond blessed!

Contents

PART III

ANCIENT PRESCRIPTIONS

PART IV

RECIPES FOR ANCIENT NUTRITION

ANCIENT REMEDIES

Recognizing the Flaws of Pharmaceutical-Based Healthcare and Reclaiming Our Health

I was raised in a family that believed wholeheartedly in the power of Western medicine. My grandmother's conversations often began with the phrase "My doctor told me I should..." And she followed his advice to the letter. As a result, by the time she was sixty she was on fifteen medications and taking forty to sixty pills a day—so many that she carried her plastic pill container with her everywhere, pulling it out of her purse frequently to pop yet another small tablet or capsule into her mouth. In spite of her strict commitment to her doctor's advice, she was chronically unwell. Her health stood in sharp contrast to my grandfather's. He took zero medications until he was in his nineties—and he ran a full-time business, golfed, served the poor, and remained robust until he passed away at the age of ninety-six.

My mom shared my grandmother's faith in Western medicine, so when my siblings and I were growing up, we dutifully took meds for every sniffle and cough. I was raised in Troy, Ohio, and got sick pretty much every winter, often coughing through an annoying bout of bronchitis from early December to late February. Even though we now know that antibiotics are ineffective for bronchitis, which is caused by lingering inflammation in your bronchial tubes after an actual infection clears up, back then I essentially lived on the drugs for those chilly three months. Our doctor was a good man. He was only doing what he thought was right. But when I look back at all the unnecessary, ineffective, and harmful medications I ingested, I see that they contributed to the gut and liver issues I developed later — issues that healed only when I began using traditional remedies and food as medicine.

Although antibiotics can be lifesaving if you have a staph infection or bacterial pneumonia, for instance, it's best to reserve them for dire circumstances. These medications, designed to kill harmful bacteria, also wipe out the population of healthy, protective bacteria, known as probiotics, in your gut, putting you at risk for inflammatory bowel disease, heart disease, obesity, type 2 diabetes, anxiety, and depression. These medications we've all been led to believe are benign are actually quite dangerous. But you'd never know it by how frequently doctors prescribe them during outpatient visits — nearly 260 million prescriptions in 2017 alone.[1]

Our habitual reliance on prescription medications can be hard to change. In fact, it took a heartbreaking experience for me to finally begin to question the pill-for-every-ill mentality that pervades Western medicine. When I was thirteen, my mom was diagnosed with — and treated for — breast cancer. I'll never forget the shock of finding clumps of her sandy blond hair on our bathroom floor — a side effect of the toxic chemotherapy — or the months and years afterward, when I realized that while my mom's cancer was gone, she was far from well. Before her treatment, she was an energetic, athletic swim instructor and gym teacher, who juggled her substantial work and family responsibilities with apparent ease; after, she was chronically exhausted and depressed, she had hypothyroidism, and she struggled with bowel issues. I was still a kid, but even at that age, I found it hard to accept the idea that the only way to cure an illness was to take medications that left you more debilitated than you were before.

That's when the seed was planted: Maybe our kindly doctor didn't have all the answers. Maybe there were safer ways to heal disease.

Maybe that array of amber bottles in our medicine cabinet was actually part of the problem. And maybe I could, one day, find a more wholesome solution.

Those were radical ideas for me at the time. But looking back, I see how they began shaping my life—how they led me to question the medical and health status quo. For instance, I started connecting the dots between the foods I consumed and the way I felt. As a high school soccer player, I noticed that milk made me phlegmy, which was especially unappealing during practices. So I stopped drinking it. Not long after, I gave up soda—not because it made me feel bad, but because I read an article about it and learned that the beverages I guzzled every day contained zero nutritional value. So why was I—why was *everyone*—drinking them?

By the time I was in my early twenties, I'd committed myself to learning everything I could about healing. I was living in Florida, earning a chiropractic degree, and becoming more and more immersed in the study of nutrition, as well as Traditional Chinese Medicine (TCM), Ayurveda, and Biblical medicine.

I was avidly engaged in that mind-expanding mode when I received a life-changing phone call from my mom. The moment I heard her tearful voice, I knew it was bad. She told me she'd been diagnosed with cancer again. I felt sick with worry and fear, but I also knew there were strategies that might help—ones that wouldn't leave her debilitated afterward. I knew about the healing power of nutrition, and I'd begun learning about alternative healing modalities in TCM and other forms of ancient medicine. So I vowed to learn as much about cancer as I could.

The question I faced: Where should I focus my research? Since I was already painfully familiar with the side effects of the most commonly prescribed modern cancer treatments, the medical paradigm of the present seemed unlikely to provide hopeful solutions. So I looked to the past.

I wasn't sure what I'd find when I typed in the search term "ancient remedies for cancer." But I uncovered a trove of centuries-old wisdom that has been ignored—and sometimes intentionally maligned or buried—by the Western medical establishment. I learned that medicinal mushrooms have been used to treat cancer by traditional Chinese practitioners for years. I discovered research on epigallocatechin gallate (EGCG), an anti-cancer component in green tea. I was surprised again and again to read about the cancer-fighting benefits of herbs like ginseng, turmeric, and astragalus. As I compiled a list of safe, gentle, effective compounds that had been used for millennia, I felt like an explorer who had uncovered a map to buried treasure. Here was the path I'd been looking for. Here were the healing jewels that just might help my mom get well.

Based on my research on ancient healing, I completely overhauled my mom's diet, tossing out all the processed foods, sugars, and simple carbs that filled her cupboards and fridge, and replacing them with vegetables, berries, herbs, probiotic-rich foods, and bone broth. I taught her to eat healthy fats, like avocado, salmon, and olive oil, as well as a variety of mushrooms, like shiitake, cordyceps, and reishi, known as the "mushroom of immortality" in traditional Chinese medicine. We paired her healthy new diet with other healing modalities, like lymphatic massage, healing affirmations, prayer, and essential oils like frankincense and myrrh, ancient treatments that have been shown to relieve stress and anxiety, support immunity, and fight cancer. Instead of being crippled by toxic chemotherapy, she was supported by healing nutrients—and she began to feel better than she had in years.

Four months after we'd begun our regimen, she went for a CT scan. The images were a stunning affirmation of the path we'd chosen. Her tumor had shrunk to half its original size. She hadn't done any chemo or radiation, and yet her cancer was receding. We returned from that appointment feeling optimistic, hopeful, and even more determined to stay the course than we'd been before.

Nine months after that, our faith in ancient remedies received the best support we could have hoped for. My mom's lab work and CT images showed she was in almost complete remission—and she remains vibrant and healthy to this day. In her sixties, she runs 5K races, water-skis, and stays incredibly active. She continues to maintain the healthy diet and lifestyle approaches we devised after her diagnosis. And she says she feels better than she has in years.

Cancer is a challenging diagnosis. When you're facing a life-threatening illness, every choice should be weighed and decided upon with the help of trusted healthcare practitioners. But watching my mom get well was the final piece of evidence I needed to be certain that Western medicine didn't hold all the answers—and that looking to the past might be the best way to take care of our health in the future.

The seed for *Ancient Remedies* was planted in that pivotal moment when we learned that my mom's cancer had receded in the face of our gentle, holistic approach. In the intervening years, I've continued to learn as much as I can about TCM, as well as other ancient healing traditions, like the Indian Ayurvedic, ancient Middle Eastern, and Biblical approaches—and the more I've learned, the more shocked I've become. Why have we all been taking dangerous, costly pharmaceuticals when these safe, gentle, inexpensive treatments have been here all along? Why has Western medicine ignored plant-based therapies for so long? And those gnawing questions led to another pivotal one: What could I do to get this vital, buried medical information into the hands of the American public, who need it today more than ever?

The answer to that final question is the book you're holding in your hands. It's high time you understand that you don't need to take dangerous drugs for every ailment, that the Western medical system's profit-based approach isn't doing your health any favors, and that there are wonderfully effective alternative therapeutics that can heal your health issues and put you safely on the path to lifelong wellness. I'm thrilled to finally be able to introduce these wholesome, natural treatments to you so you can make the best health choices for you and your family.

In Part I, you'll learn how our medical system was hijacked by pharmaceutical companies, which put profits over people's health, and why the medications designed to make us well often create a cycle of sickness that's difficult to break. I also explain why ancient remedies are a smarter, safer choice, and lay out the basics of the ancient approach to curing disease, which lies in a single, simple strategy: Instead of treating symptoms, heal the root cause of the illness. You'll also learn how to use the tenets of ancient medicine to find a diet that's right for your body and how to combine foods in ways that make each healthy ingredient exponentially more beneficial.

In Part II, I provide insight into the fundamental foods and lifestyle habits that serve as the foundation for whole-body healing and health. You'll learn about the value of ancient spices and herbs—including CBD, a component of hemp!—essential oils, and healing mushrooms, as well as potent lifestyle changes like meditation, digital fasting, and various types of therapeutic movement, which can offer breakthrough healing.

Ancient healers not only believed in identifying the root cause of each patient's illness, but they also did years of meticulous research, cataloguing and studying which natural remedies, derived from plants, flowers, mushrooms, herbs, and spices, work best for which illness. Part III offers an immersive, easy-to-understand guide to this ancient knowledge. I explain an ancient way of looking at illness through the lens of TCM's Five Elements theory, which includes your organ systems, emotions, and lifestyle; provide eating plans to treat imbalance and ill health within each organ system; and offer ancient prescriptions for more than seventy common ailments that afflict far too many people in our country today, including digestive issues, hormonal havoc, immune dysfunction, neurological disorders, and autoimmune disease.

Finally, in Part IV, you'll find delicious, healthy recipes to help you put the dietary advice in this book into practice. By giving your organs, blood, and other tissues the simple, wholesome nutrients that have sustained humans for centuries, it's possible to not only prevent and cure disease, but also to transform your health, so you can live your best life.

As growing numbers of Americans fall ill after following their doctors' orders and taking dangerous pharmaceuticals, and more people question the wisdom of Western medicine, alternatives are desperately needed. I wrote *Ancient Remedies* to respond to that need. On every page, I offer a new way of thinking about health and healing—one based on the time-tested knowledge from ancient medical systems the Western establishment would rather you didn't know about. But by embracing these age-old approaches, you can, just as my mom did nearly twenty years ago, overcome chronic ailments, heal the root cause of your ill health, and reignite your inner spark. I'm grateful to you for picking up this book. In its pages you'll discover the tools you need to make the goal of lifelong health, strength, vigor, satisfaction, and joy a reality.

PART I

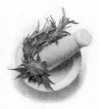

The Wisdom of Ancient Healing

CHAPTER 1

Ancient Medicine for a Modern World

How Pharmaceuticals Took Over Healthcare, and Why We Need to Reclaim It

It's surprising to think that the practice of Western medicine as we know it began less than two hundred years ago, when the American Medical Association was founded in 1847. The first pharmaceutical companies were formed around the same time, and in the intervening years, the two industries partnered to set unprecedented prices—and reap sky-high profits. The pharmaceutical era gave rise to an increasingly systematic and formulaic approach to healing—one that is focused on treating individual, superficial symptoms instead of addressing the true, underlying root cause of disease, and has forgotten that each human being is a complex, synergistic blend of body, mind, and spirit. In doing so, modern medicine turned its back on thousands of years of medical knowledge about how the body works holistically—and how best to support healing.

Ancient cultures around the world, including those in China, India, Greece, and the Middle East, created sophisticated medical systems at least four thousand years ago—and they're still in use today in many countries. In fact, interest in ancient remedies is surging, including in the United States. Here's why: Through years of trial and error, early physicians crafted gentle but powerful holistic therapies that relied on diet, herbs, essential oils, acupuncture, movement, and emotional strategies, like meditation, prayer, and spending time in nature. Their treatments were designed to heal the body on a deep level, curing disease from the inside out and elevating the mind and spirit to make you truly well—energetic, happy, robust, engaged. Today, these ancient approaches have been validated in hundreds of rigorous scientific studies. But most doctors in the United States still don't prescribe them.

Instead, they dole out pills. Have a fever? Take an antibiotic. High cholesterol? Use a statin. In pain? Pop an opioid. Feeling blue? Try an antidepressant. Seventy-four percent of doctor's visits end with a scribbled prescription.[1] It's so common, many of us never think to question modern healthcare's singular focus on medication. As a result, these lab-created drugs have stealthily taken over our lives.

The Kaiser Family Foundation recently reported that 50 percent of Americans aged thirty to forty-nine are currently taking prescription medication, as are 75 percent of those in their fifties, and nearly 90 percent of those sixty-five and older. More shocking, a third of people in their fifties—and more than half of those sixty-five and older—take *four or more* prescription drugs regularly.[2] Our culture has come to equate healing with drugs, so much so that many of us *expect* our doctors to give us medication, and we often feel disregarded or mistreated when we leave an appointment empty-handed.

Antibiotics are a tragic example. If you've ever had a chronic cough, or your child has had an ear infection, chances are your doctor prescribed one of these bacteria-killing drugs—and you might have been grateful to receive it. But here's the thing: We now know that these medications aren't effective at treating chronic coughs, ear infections, and many other common ailments for which they're routinely prescribed.

Worse, antibiotics can be far more dangerous than we've been led to believe. We've known for a long time that they wipe out billions of healthy bacteria in the gastrointestinal tract—microbes that play a vital role in helping us digest food, fight inflammation, and maintain a healthy mood and strong immune system. But did you know that taking antibiotics repeatedly might actually increase your risk of cancer? An analysis of a large medical records database, published in the *European Journal of Cancer,* found that the more courses of antibiotics a patient took in the prior year, the greater their risk of esophageal, gastric, pancreatic, lung, prostate, and breast cancers.[3] Healthcare professionals in the United States write roughly 260 million prescriptions for antibiotics every year.[4] Although the cancer risk from antibiotics is small, the drugs are jeopardizing millions of people's health.

As appalling, at least 30 percent of those millions of prescriptions are completely unnecessary, according to the Centers for Disease Control,[5] because they're prescribed for conditions that don't respond to antibiotics. (I believe that closer to 90 percent are unnecessary, since our bodies are capable of fighting most bacterial infections on their own; and if you need extra help, a number of herbs are effective antimicrobials, with few, if any, side effects.) Those needless rounds of medication not only harm the health of people who take them, but they also contribute to the development of antibiotic-resistant strains of lethal microbes. At least two million people in the US are infected with antibiotic-resistant bacteria every year, and twenty-three thousand die because the bacteria have learned to outwit even our most powerful medications.[6] Antibiotic resistance is one of the most urgent public health threats facing the world today. If you have a life-threatening infection, taking antibiotics makes sense. In all other instances, I agree with the sentiment of Francis Bacon, an early champion of the scientific revolution, who noted in the sixteenth century, "Sometimes the remedy is worse than the disease."

Antibiotics are the tip of the iceberg—and few people understand the true scope or seriousness of synthetic pills' risks. You probably don't know, for instance, that long-term use of *most* medications, both prescription and over-the-counter, can cause serious nutrient deficiencies. Proton pump inhibitors, which are routinely prescribed for acid reflux, limit the body's ability to absorb vitamins B12 and C as well as iron, calcium, magnesium, zinc, and beta-carotene.

They also raise your risk of dying from heart disease, chronic kidney disease, and gastrointestinal cancer.[7] Likewise, some diuretic drugs for high blood pressure deplete your body of calcium, magnesium, thiamin, zinc, potassium, folate, and iron.[8] These nutrients are absolutely essential for the healthy functioning of your brain, heart, and muscles. And those widely used types of drugs are just two examples, among dozens, of pharmaceuticals that can cause dire nutritional deficiencies. Check out this chart on commonly prescribed medications and the dangerous nutrient deficiencies they can cause.

	MEDICATION	NUTRIENTS DEPLETED
ANTACIDS	Pepcid, Zantac, Tums	Calcium, Folate, Iron, Phosphate, Vitamin B12, Zinc
ANTIBIOTICS	Penicillin, Amoxicillin, Tetracyclines, Cipro	Folate, Vitamin B1, B2, B6, B12, Calcium, Magnesium, Potassium, Zinc, Healthy Gut Bacteria
ANTI-ANXIETY	Valium, Xanax	Calcium, Melatonin
ANTI-DEPRESSANTS	Cymbalta, Lexapro, Paxil, Prozac, Zoloft	Folate, Vitamin B12
ANTI-DIABETIC	Metformin	Coenzyme Q10, Vitamin B12, Folate
ANTI-HYPERTENSIVES	ACE Inhibitors, Beta Blockers	CoQ10, Potassium, Zinc, Calcium, Magnesium, Vitamin B1
ANTI-INFLAMMATORY	Prednisone, Hydrocortone, Celestone	Vitamin C, Vitamin D, Folate, Calcium, Potassium, Selenium, Zinc
CONTRACEPTIVES	Norinyl, TriPhasil, Yasmin, & Others	Vitamins B2, B3, B6, B12, C, Healthy Gut Bacteria, Magnesium, Zinc
ESTROGEN	Estrace, Premarin, Prempro	Folate, Magnesium, Vitamins B1, B2, B5, B6, B12
NSAIDS	Aspirin, Acetaminophen, Motrin, Ibuprofen	Vitamin C, Folate, Glutathione, Iron, Potassium
STATIN CHOLESTEROL DRUGS	Lipitor, Crestor, Zocor, Mevacor	Coenzyme Q10, Calcium, Folate, Iron, Magnesium, Vitamins A, B12, D, E, K
THYROID MEDICATION	Synthroid, Levothyroxine, Levoxyl	Calcium, Iron, Phosphorus

You also may not know that adverse reactions to drugs—everything from allergic reactions to antibiotics (common in children) to hemorrhaging from blood thinners—send nearly six hundred thousand people to the emergency room every year,[9] 27 percent of whom fall so gravely ill that they're admitted to the hospital.[10] What's more, for every adverse drug reaction that leads to hospitalization, an estimated *thirty* minor cases are never brought to a doctor's attention.

The more meds you take, the greater the risk of an adverse reaction, which means that people over age sixty-five are particularly in danger. A 2019 report by the Lown Institute, an organization focused on exposing problems in healthcare, estimates that in the course of the coming decade, medication overload—the result of taking multiple prescription drugs at the same time—will cause the premature death of 150,000 older people in the United States.[11] On top of that, researchers at Johns Hopkins have reported that more than 250,000 people die in the United States every year due to medical errors. Think about that: Western medicine is literally killing hundreds of thousands of people.

I took an oath when I became a doctor, as all physicians do. That oath was "First do no harm." But how can any doctor be true to that oath if we rely exclusively on pharmaceuticals? As Sir William Osler, a revered Canadian physician in the 1800s, said, "The person who takes medicine must recover twice; once from the disease and once from the medicine."

What I've shared is just a glimpse of the vast pharmaceutical-fueled tragedy that's quietly unfolding across the country. But there's a deeper truth that makes our dependence on pharmaceuticals even worse: For years, Western medicine has disregarded, ignored, maligned, and sometimes intentionally buried information about safer ancient alternatives.

Take CBD, a non-euphoric substance in the ancient plant hemp (a variety of cannabis). It has been used for healing for thousands of years, but the US government outlawed its use for any purpose in 1970—putting it in a category with deadly drugs like heroin and, later, methamphetamines. Meanwhile, the government took out a patent on CBD and other so-called cannabinoids (chemicals found in the cannabis plant) in 2003—and is poised to rake in the money when drugs based on those compounds are created. In fact, in 2018, the Food and Drug Administration approved the first cannabis-based drug, Epidiolex, to treat intractable seizures in children. That same year, the government finally legalized hemp, so long as it contains less than 0.03 percent tetrahydrocannabinol (THC), the substance in cannabis that gets you high. That means that CBD from hemp—but not from other forms of cannabis—is legal on a federal level.

In other words, for nearly fifty years, the government prevented you and me and everyone else in the country from legally using CBD and other safe hemp-based substances, even though they knew these chemicals had medical benefits—and were secretly setting themselves up to profit from them.

If you feel as outraged by that as I do, you've come to the right place. I wrote *Ancient Remedies* to let you know that the pills that are making you sick aren't the only way to treat disease—and to share with you the very best of the ancient secrets from a variety of healing traditions around the world, including Traditional Chinese Medicine (TCM), Ayurvedic medicine, and Greek, Middle Eastern, and Biblical traditions. In these pages, I've gathered the true gems from these therapeutic treasure troves. You'll learn how to use medicinal herbs (including CBD and other cannabinoids), essential oils, healing movement, meditation, prayer, spending time in nature, acupuncture, and ancient ways of eating that are tailored to your personal needs.

While prescription meds come at a perilous cost, physically and financially, these ancient remedies are gentle but powerful, safe and effective when used properly, and affordable—or even free. Oliver Wendell Holmes Sr., one of the most renowned physicians of the nineteenth century, said, "I firmly believe that if the whole *materia medica* [medications], as now used, could be sunk to the bottom of the sea, it would be all the better for mankind—and all the worse for the fishes." When I think of the dangerous drugs doctors routinely dole out today, I wholeheartedly agree. If you're fed up with the big-pharma-driven status quo, and hungry for a natural, safe, and more effective approach, you'll find hope—and help—in *Ancient Remedies*.

Dangerous pharmaceuticals—and the safe alternatives no one wants you to know about

My criticism of Western medicine isn't intended to disparage all of the modern approach. If you're in a car accident or have a heart attack or brain aneurism or fall prey to a flesh-eating bacterial infection, there's no better place to be than an American hospital. But if you develop a chronic, preventable illness related to poor diet, stress, age, weight gain, or lack of exercise—the kinds of problems that routinely land most of us in a doctor's office—the pills your physician is likely to give you may not help. In fact, they'll almost certainly create another problem that actually makes your health worse.

Nearly every drug doctors prescribe has side effects, and some are severe. Take antidepressants. These drugs are among the most widely used pharmaceuticals ever. Some 15.5 million people in the US have been on an antidepressant for five years,[12] and 8.5 million have been on the drugs for a decade or more[13]—a risky experiment, seeing as clinical trials last only a couple of years, so there's zero safety data on long-term use.

The side effects we *do* know about are frightening. A 2017 meta-analysis published in *Psychotherapy and Psychosomatics* found that people taking antidepressants had a 14 percent higher risk of heart attacks and strokes and a 33 percent greater risk of death than those not on the drugs.[14] And many users experience problems like weight gain, insomnia, headaches, muscle pain, trouble with blood clotting, and reduced libido. Furthermore, weaning off the drugs isn't easy. With-drawal symptoms, like dizziness, fatigue, blurred vision, anxiety, cry-ing spells, and flu-like symptoms, are often so severe many users simply give up and go back on the medication.

For someone who is suicidal, or depressed or anxious to the degree that it seriously impairs their ability to function, the drugs may be helpful. But a study in the journal *Health Affairs* found that in 73 percent of appointments where antidepressants were prescribed, no official psychiatric diagnosis was reported.[15] In other words, millions of people with mild mood issues are putting their health unnecessarily at risk.

Those widely prescribed drugs stand in sharp contrast to the ancient remedies that can help with mood disorders. Take a look at these three time-tested ways of treating mood issues, and you'll see what I mean:

- *Herbs.* A number of ancient herbs, including saffron, ginseng, and chamomile, can ease depression, but the most thoroughly studied is St. John's wort, long used by TCM practitioners for treating mood disorders. A meta-analysis of twenty-seven clinical trials published in the *Journal of Affective Disorders* found that the herb is as effective as antidepressants for those with mild to moderate depression.[16] It's widely prescribed by doctors in Europe, but it's typically ignored, or written off as dangerous, by doctors in the United States. While you shouldn't use it at the same time as antidepressants, and it can interfere with some medications, like digoxin and contraceptive pills, the truth is it has few, if any, side effects.

- *Meditation.* Practiced since at least 4000 BC, meditation has now been the subject of hundreds of scientific studies, which have proven its benefits for relieving emotional issues. A rigorous literature review published in *JAMA Internal Medicine*, for instance, looked at forty-seven trials of meditation for dealing with a range of problems, including anxiety and depression, and found consistent, reliable reduction in symptoms across the studies.[17] Meditation works, in part, because it teaches you skills to counteract your dispirited or worried thinking. (I'll explain how to do one particularly beneficial form in chapter 9.) But over time, it also reshapes your brain by calming the amygdala, the fear center, and bulking up the parts devoted to attention. One study found actual brain growth in people who meditated thirty minutes a day for eight weeks.[18] What's more, there are no adverse side effects.

■ *Movement.* Yoga's use as a form of centering and calming the mind can be traced to eleventh-century India, and millions of people can attest to its mood-elevating power today. In recent studies, yoga has been shown to alleviate anxiety and depression in everyone from low-income and uninsured patients[19] to veterans suffering from PTSD[20] and women awaiting in vitro fertilization.[21] Instead of merely treating the symptoms of mood disorders, as medications do, yoga helps you learn to cope with your emotional challenges, so you can minimize, or even eliminate, the problem. Similarly, the traditional mind–body exercise known as tai chi, a form of slow, deliberate movement, dates back at least seven hundred years. A recent meta-analysis of thirty-seven randomized, controlled trials, published in the *International Journal of Behavioral Medicine*, found that it was an effective, safe way to ease depression, anxiety, and stress.[22] These ancient forms of gentle movement offer benefits that are similar to other contemporary forms of exercise, whether it's walking, running, cycling, or swimming, which have been shown to be as effective at treating mild to moderate mood problems as antidepressants.[23] Movement is helpful because it releases feel-good brain chemicals; promotes the growth of new neurons in the hippocampus, a brain region that shrinks with depression; and reduces stress, a primary contributor to mood disorders. And unlike antidepressants, which can cause health problems as a side effect, movement offers cardiovascular protection, builds healthy muscle tissue, and imbues practitioners with a can-do sense of self-worth.

Opioids are another example of a dangerous modern drug that could be replaced by safe, ancient alternatives. You undoubtedly know about the risks of opioids. By treating chronic pain (which afflicts an estimated 20 percent of adults in the United States[24]) with these pills, pharmaceutical companies and doctors have created an addiction crisis the likes of which our country has never seen. An estimated 41 percent of patients who are prescribed opiates for chronic pain misuse them or develop a dependency,[25] at which point they often switch to heroin or fentanyl, which are easier to get and even more dangerous. The toll of this tragedy is heartbreaking. More than 130 Americans die every day from an opioid overdose.[26] In 2017, sixty-three thousand lives were lost to drug overdoses, the majority to opiates[27] — a number that's roughly equivalent to the American casualties in the Vietnam and Iraq wars combined.

Three factors make the epidemic even more galling. First, pharmaceutical companies have always known how addictive the drugs are, but they convinced doctors that they were safe and sold them by the billions anyway. Second, opiates are no more effective at treating chronic pain than over-the-counter pain relievers, like acetaminophen and ibuprofen, according to a study in the *Journal of the American Medical Association*.[28] And third, a number of safe ancient remedies are as effective as opiates for treating pain, but doctors rarely, if ever, suggest them. Here's a sampling of some of the best:

■ *Acupuncture and acupressure.* Several meta-analyses conducted by Cochrane, the esteemed international nonprofit, have found that acupuncture is an effective way to cope with tension headaches and can help prevent migraines as well as, or better than, prescription medication.[29] Likewise, a meta-analysis of twenty-nine trials in the *Archives of Internal Medicine*, which looked at acupuncture for a range of conditions, including arthritis, musculoskeletal pain, and back and neck pain, found that it could reduce pain by 50 percent.[30]

■ *CBD oil.* The non-euphoric substance derived from the cannabis plant may help with arthritis pain by reducing inflammation, one of CBD's most notable effects. Although CBD research in people is relatively scant since the federal government has impeded its progress, animal studies have revealed that it may actually inhibit pain pathway signaling as well.[31]

■ *Herbal supplements.* Used for centuries in Chinese medicine, astragalus is a known anti-inflammatory, which probably accounts for the pain-relieving effects it has demonstrated in scientific studies on animals with osteoarthritis.[32] Likewise, another popular Chinese herb, schisandra, has been shown to ease gut pain in animal studies.[33] The herb dong quai contains ligustilide, a substance that has an anti-spasmodic effect, especially on uterine muscles,[34] which makes it a particularly helpful herb for premenstrual abdominal pain and cramping. Turmeric is also an effective treatment for pain, according to a review published in the *Journal of Medicinal Food*,[35] probably because it's so effective at reducing inflammation. Capsaicin, a substance found in cayenne, helps reduce the amount of substance P, a neuropeptide that tells your brain you're in pain.[36] Applied in a cream, it can be helpful for joint, muscle, and postsurgical pain. Finally, magnesium-rich Epsom salt is an effective painkiller for bone and joint pain and muscle soreness—and has been used for that reason for hundreds (maybe thousands) of years.

■ *Essential oils.* The scent of peppermint can reduce pain, particularly headache pain, according to a study in the *International Journal of Preventive Medicine*,[37] and frankincense oil applied topically has been shown to be helpful for knee osteoarthritis, according to research reported in *Nutrition Journal*.[38] Both can help manage inflammation. What's more, a meta-analysis in *Pain Research and Treatment* revealed that lavender oil aromatherapy can be helpful in relieving a variety of different types of pain,[39] probably thanks in part to the fact that it's relaxing, and pain causes the body to tense up.

■ *Tai chi, yoga, and meditation.* These ancient practices have been found to ease pain in people with a variety of conditions. A review published in *Scientific Reports*, for instance, looked at eighteen randomized, controlled trials of tai chi and found evidence that it can provide effective pain relief for those with osteoarthritis, low back pain, and osteoporosis.[40] Yoga has been shown to reduce pain and fatigue in patients with fibromyalgia,[41] knee osteoarthritis,[42] low back pain,[43] and neck pain.[44] Meditation, according to a review of thirty-eight studies, published in the *Annals of Behavioral Medicine*, not only reduces pain but also lifts depression and improves overall quality of life in pain sufferers.[45]

Healing without harm

It's clear to me that we've placed our faith in a medical industry that puts profits over people—one that is myopically focused on treating individual symptoms instead of seeing human health as a complex mix of physical, emotional, and spiritual wellness. Contrast that with ancient healers. For them, healing was a partnership. Without the benefit of microscopes or modern technology, they built a vast reservoir of knowledge based on careful physical examination, including listening to their patients' concerns and paying close attention to their emotional and spiritual well-being. Instead of targeting superficial symptoms, the therapeutics these early healers discovered, like acupuncture, meditation, herbs, and essential oils, work on a deep, holistic level, treating the root cause of disease and restoring the well-being of the body and mind as a whole. And physicians around the world continued to use them through the millennia not because they were profitable, but because they were safe and effective.

Western medicine still dismisses these ancient remedies as "alternative." But it's arrogant to marginalize thousands of years of wisdom. In fact, I believe that ancient treatments should be our go-to therapies for non-emergency health problems. And that happens to be the case in many places where people live the longest, including Japan, Hong Kong, and Singapore. Indeed, roughly four billion people around the world—or 80 percent of the population—rely on herbal medicine as a primary source of treatment.[46] Herbal remedies, as Yale neurologist Steven Novella has pointed out, "have been part of scientific medicine for decades, if not centuries." How can treatments that have stood the test of time be "alternative"?

The simple answer: They're not. Many contemporary drugs are derived from compounds found in herbs and other plants. More than two thousand years ago, Hippocrates prescribed the leaves of the willow plant for his patients with headaches and muscle pain. Fast-forward to the 1800s, when scientists discovered that those leaves contain salicylic acid, the active ingredient in aspirin. Similarly, in the seventeenth century, Jesuit missionaries in South Africa started using the bark of the cinchona tree to fight malaria, probably because the native population used it as a cure. Two hundred years later, scientists extracted quinine, a common modern malaria treatment, from the tree's bark.

Similarly, we think of mind-body wellness as a cutting-edge concept. But as early as 2000 BC, ancient Middle Eastern and Asian practitioners knew that our emotional, spiritual, and mental health affects our physical well-being, an idea that was also embraced by Hippocrates and other ancient Greek physicians—it is even mentioned in the Bible. In Proverbs 17:22, King Solomon says, "A joyful heart is good medicine, but a depressed and broken spirit dries up the bones."

And while fasting and using herbs might seem ultramodern, Hippocrates actually focused much of his practice on those very approaches. In fact, he documented more than two hundred healing herbs, and he taught that plant-based medicine could save lives. His philosophy was based on this core idea: "Everyone has a doctor in him or her; we just have to help it in its work. The natural healing force within each one of us is the greatest force in getting well. Our food should be our medicine. Our medicine should be our food."

Ancient Jewish texts and the Bible are filled with medical wisdom and health advice that's being "rediscovered" today as well. Prayer, meditation, essential oils, and fasting all have roots in early religious traditions. A passage in James 5:14 reads, "Is anyone among you sick? Let them call the elders of the church to pray over them and anoint them with oil in the name of the Lord." Holy anointing oil was a blend of myrrh, cinnamon, cassia, calamus, and olive—a combination that has potent healing properties. In the book of Leviticus, God tells the Israelites not to eat pork and shellfish, because they can contain toxins—concerns that have been confirmed by modern science.

Unlike the one-size-fits-all Western approach, ancient treatments are tailored to individuals in all their diversity and complexity. And that's how I believe we need to approach medicine going forward. Since you picked up this book, I assume you're interested in that idea as well—and I'm glad you're here.

An abundance of ancient wisdom awaits you in these pages. Some may be familiar to you, some completely foreign. Either way, the information will help you take control of your health and make more informed choices when faced with illness and disease. Every ancient remedy I endorse is effective for treating the ailments that plague modern culture and ruin too many people's health—and together, these time-tested treatments serve as a powerful antidote to our dangerous reliance on toxic, costly pharmaceuticals.

CHAPTER 2

Curing the Root Cause

Why Treating Symptoms Destroys Your Health — and Ancient Wisdom Heals

When I was a kid, every time I had a cold my mom gave me the same meal: canned chicken noodle soup and ginger ale. But you know what? It always took me a while to kick the virus. Maybe you had a similar experience when you were young. Given what I know now about healing, I understand why those foods didn't help me recover. The soup was filled with monosodium glutamate, white flour noodles, and other artificial, processed ingredients that cause inflammation in the body — the opposite of what your body needs to beat a virus — and the ginger ale was essentially carbonated high-fructose corn syrup with 40 grams of sugar per serving, another inflammatory substance.

But there is a valid reason my mom (and maybe yours) believed those foods were healing: In ancient Chinese and Jewish medicine, *homemade* chicken soup and ginger herb tea were cold-fighting staples. They're so effective they've been handed down through the millennia and even made their way into Western folk medicine. My grandmother gave those remedies to my mom when she was a child. And my wife, Chelsea, and I use them today to kick colds and other bugs with ease.

Those ancient remedies work because they target one of the

underlying causes of a cold: being too cold internally. That idea undoubtedly sounds odd if you were raised exclusively on the Western model. How can your body be cold? I admit, it's a different way of thinking about health and healing—and I'll explain this and other ancient concepts later in the chapter. For now, it's enough to know the basics: In TCM, if you're too cold on the inside, the cure is to eat warming foods, like ginger, garlic, oregano, cinnamon, cayenne pepper, and homemade chicken broth. Similarly, if your body has too much heat, you need to cool it down with foods like apples, grapefruit, cucumber, lettuce, celery, yogurt, eggs, and peppermint.

In ancient medicine, the goal of treatment is to restore balance to your internal environment and strengthen your organ systems (including your immune system), which accomplishes something Western pharmaceuticals don't: healing the underlying root cause of illness. Let's return to the example of viruses. You've probably heard of "germ theory"—the idea that many common illnesses are caused by contagious pathogens. Louis Pasteur, a French scientist, proved the theory in the 1900s. But it doesn't answer a critical question: Why does one person get sick and another remain healthy when they're exposed to the same microbes? The ancient answer is that toxicity and deficiencies due to poor diet, a sedentary lifestyle, smoking, and toxic stress, along with other negative emotions, weaken your organ systems and inhibit your immune system's ability to fight off pathogens. In other words, your underlying health makes you more susceptible not only to coming down with seasonal viruses but also to dying from them.

If it takes you a long time to recover from viral and bacterial infections, it's most likely a sign your immune system is weak. You can see this idea at play every cold and flu season, as well as during the Covid-19 pandemic, when people over the age of seventy or those diagnosed with immune deficiency were more severely affected, and more likely to die, than those who are young and healthy. The ancient truth is that healing doesn't come from a miracle drug, but from within your own body. If your immune system is strong and functioning optimally, you can fight off viruses and bacteria with relative ease. You might not even develop

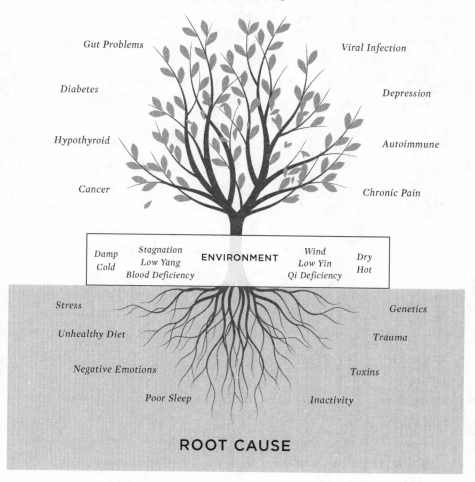

SYMPTOMS

Gut Problems

Viral Infection

Diabetes

Depression

Hypothyroid

Autoimmune

Cancer

Chronic Pain

| Damp Cold | Stagnation Low Yang Blood Deficiency | ENVIRONMENT | Wind Low Yin Qi Deficiency | Dry Hot |

Stress

Genetics

Unhealthy Diet

Trauma

Negative Emotions

Toxins

Poor Sleep

Inactivity

ROOT CAUSE

symptoms at all. One problem with relying on a new drug or vaccine to target a virus is there will always be another virus, which requires another medication or immunization. But if you build your immune system, which is designed to fight off all manner of foreign pathogens, you will not only protect yourself from dangerous bugs, but also reduce your risk of cancer, diabetes, and other chronic conditions. In other words, you'll improve your health overall. And here's what I find remarkable: Ancient remedies and lifestyle strategies can keep your immune system robust and, as a result, give you the protection you need to fight viruses and bacteria, even as you age.

Movement and meditation, both of which, as I've mentioned, have roots in ancient healing, have been shown to strengthen the immune system, as have probiotic foods, zinc, and vitamins A, C, and D—all plentiful in ancient diets. What's more, TCM has included strategies to protect the body from viral epidemics for thousands of years. The *Huangdi's Internal Classic*, written two thousand years ago, recommended immune-boosting herbs, a healthy diet, and other life-style approaches to increase qi (cellular energy) and strengthen the immune system in order to fend off rampaging pathogens.

Indeed, there's a whole world of ancient immune-boosting, virus-fighting herbs and essential oils that has long been ignored by Western medicine. Elderberry, echinacea, oregano, andrographis, astragalus, garlic, and turkey tail mushrooms all contain virus-fighting compounds that can help your body eradicate illness-causing pathogens. And they're remarkably effective. A paper published in the *Chinese Journal of Integrative Medicine* in April 2020 reported on seven studies looking at the performance of a TCM herbal formula during the 2003 severe acute respiratory syndrome (SARS) outbreak and the 2009 H1N1 flu pandemic.[1] The formula, which contains a variety of immune-strengthening herbs, including astragalus, atractylodes, licorice root, and others, provided protection to Chinese doctors and nurses during both outbreaks. In three studies on SARS, none of the participants who took the TCM formula contracted the deadly illness. Likewise, the infection rate of H1N1 was significantly lower among those who took the formula than it was among those who didn't. Similarly, there's pre-liminary research showing that substances in oranges (hesperidin), galangal (galangin), green tea (EGCG), and onions (quercetin) might suppress Covid-19 infection. I'm often asked why there aren't any large, randomized, controlled double-blind studies into the effectiveness of these remedies. Here's why: Those studies are expensive, and no big pharmaceutical company is going to fund them. But here's what we have in place of that evidence: Thousands of years of history of their use. (In chapter 6 you'll find an in-depth look at the antiviral properties of specific herbs, and chapter 8 delves into the most effective essential oils.)

Imagine a world where the government spent billions of dollars battling obesity, diabetes, and heart disease—factors that impair the immune system and, during the Covid-19 pandemic, doubled the risk of winding up in intensive care—and making sure everyone had a healthy diet of bone broth, citrus fruits, and an array of immunity-boosting vegetables. When the next contagious bug begins circulating, what if doctors handed out vitamin C, vitamin D, zinc, and an herbal formula with elderberry, echinacea, and astragalus? This type of care would dramatically bolster people's immune function.

In any case, these ancient dietary, herbal, and lifestyle approaches should be part of your stay-well arsenal during regular cold and flu seasons—and are especially important when a novel virus (one that your immune system has never encountered) is spreading like wildfire around the globe.

Think about how this ancient knowledge could change your everyday life when the next big superbug strikes. If you believe the Western paradigm—that we're essentially helpless without pharmaceutical intervention—you'll be overwhelmed by fear, which impairs your immune system. However, if you understand that keeping your organ systems and immune system strong gives you the power to fight off seasonal superbugs, you'll focus your energy on eating immune-boosting foods; reducing stress with strategies like meditation and regular exercise; and taking herbs and essential oils that fight viruses and fortify your immune system. I can tell you from working with thousands of patients over the years that the conventional medical mindset increases your risk of illness, while the empowering ancient medicine approach offers real protection—and leads to extraordinary health and longevity.

Tapping into your body's secret superpower: its ability to heal itself

Ancient healing is effective because it treats the two most common underlying causes of poor health: toxicity (from inflammatory foods, environmental toxins, and unhealthy emotions, like anger, worry, fear, loneliness, grudge-holding, resentment, and stress) and deficiencies (like vitamin and mineral deficits as well as lack of joy, hope, love, forgiveness, and connection).

Three Types of Medical Treatments

Conventional Medicine: drugs and surgery prescribed as a treatment to cover up symptoms

Integrative Medicine: general diet recommendations for everyone; supplements, exercise, and natural therapies to treat causes of symptoms

Ancient Medicine: personalized diet, herbal supplements, essential oils, exercise, holistic treatments, emotional health recommendations aimed at treating the root cause of the disease

While this is a departure from the current Western model, it couldn't be more needed. When I first opened my functional medical clinic in Nashville, I was shocked by how many patients came to see me after they had already been to three, four, six, or even more mainstream doctors. As I sat and talked with each of these patients, I heard the same basic story over and over: The cycle of starting a medication, developing side effects, then receiving another prescription or two to treat those secondary issues often continued for years—all the while, these people who had once been reasonably healthy, became increasingly debilitated, ill, and infirm. Just as disturbing, they started thinking of themselves as sickly—as people with chronic health problems that could be managed with medication but could never be cured. By the time they landed in my office, many had all but resigned themselves to a life of poor health.

During our first appointments, as I talked to them extensively about their lives and the histories of their symptoms, I was struck by the eerie similarities that emerged. In the majority of cases, the origin of a patient's health problems could be traced to a toxic lifestyle, an out-of-balance emotional life, or both. For instance, most were under a lot of stress, often due to factors like a divorce, an ill child or parent, financial concerns, or a crushing workload. Some had suffered trauma, either in childhood or adulthood, that still made them tear up years later. Many ate poorly, because they were always on the go, or they had too little time (or know-how) to cook, or the nearest market was a convenience store with no fruits or vegetables or fresh meat, fish, or chicken. A significant number didn't exercise, either because they sat at a desk all day, or had a long commute to and from work, or were uncomfortably overweight, or just had trouble getting into the habit.

When I started treating these patients with personalized dietary and lifestyle changes that have been used for centuries, as well as ancient herbs and essential oils, which reduce inflammation and bolster the functioning of key organs on a cellular level, they began to feel better. They lost weight, their energy rebounded, and they regained a sense of control over their lives.

What's more, with every appointment, I saw tangible—often dramatic—improvements. Over the course of a few years, more than fifty of my patients with type 2 diabetes were able to reverse their diagnosis. When they began moving more and eating more like our ancient ancestors—eliminating sugar and carbs and upping their intake of veggies, grass-fed beef, wild-caught fish, and healthy fats—their insulin production normalized and their blood sugar levels dropped, often to the point where they no longer needed medication. Similarly, dozens of patients with autoimmune disease, leaky gut syndrome, migraines, and clinical depression overcame their ailments and returned to good health.

And it wasn't just their bodies that healed. As their health turned around, these patients began seeing themselves in a different light. They no longer thought of themselves as sick people who would never be well; instead, they felt transformed into healthy people who occasionally got sick.

Ancient remedies aren't overnight cures or instant fixes—and that can be frustrating for those accustomed to a Western perspective.

When you feel poorly or learn that you have a health problem, it's natural to want to get better right away. Popping a pharmaceutical appeals to that desire for an instant fix. But our get-well-quick mindset overlooks an important truth: The body was designed to heal itself—to fight off bacteria and other viruses, knit together wounds, and kill off cells that have developed mutations. I believe that God put that healing power within each of us. But regardless of your beliefs, *your body heals itself.* Think about it: If you cut your hand, what happens? The skin weaves itself back together. Or how about when you get a cold virus? You spike a fever, feel crummy for a bit, then begin to get well. As Hippocrates said, "The natural healing force within each one of us is the greatest force in getting well."

Prescription (and even over-the-counter) drugs ignore and sometimes override the remarkable recuperative capacity hard-wired into our systems; they force the body to do things it wouldn't do naturally, which, not surprisingly, causes downstream problems. Ancient remedies, on the other hand, complement your internal restorative ability, gently coaxing and supporting your body to do what it does best: heal itself.

Just as a tree thrives with exposure to sun, rain, and rich soil, your body is strengthened by positive emotions, nourishing food, and a wholesome balance of activity and rest. And here's the truly remarkable thing: None of that requires a drug. By replacing inflammation-promoting foods with regenerative foods, by turning toxic emotions into positive ones, by moving more and working through past trauma, you have the capacity to bounce back from almost anything.

How identifying the underlying cause can help you find a cure

In 2012, Stephanie, a busy mom and healthcare provider with a thriving practice, came to my functional medicine clinic complaining of fatigue and thinning hair. As we chatted, she mentioned that she'd been diagnosed with hypothyroidism a couple of years earlier—another classic outcome of being too "cold" internally. Her Western medical doctor had prescribed Synthroid, a synthetic thyroid hormone medication that can cause hair loss, mood swings, fatigue, tremors, and headaches. It didn't help. So Stephanie saw a naturopathic doctor, who recommended that she reduce her sugar intake, eat more veggies, and take vitamin B12 and selenium as well as a probiotic to promote gut health. When she still didn't bounce back, she made an appointment with me.

I explained that from the Chinese medicine perspective, hypothyroidism is caused by two underlying problems: low qi (or vital energy) and low yang (I'll explain what this means in more detail later, but yang is related to energizing hormones like cortisol and adrenaline) — both of which can be traced to overtaxed adrenal glands. Your adrenals are sort of like your body's battery. Located on top of both kidneys, these tiny glands produce hormones, like cortisol, that help your body respond to stress, and also regulate blood pressure, metabolism, and other vital functions. When you're bombarded by stress, your adrenals are perpetually turned on, which eventually causes them to stop functioning optimally. In other words, low thyroid is the most obvious symptom of a deeper, underlying imbalance.

To restore Stephanie's internal equilibrium, I suggested she eat dark-colored, qi-building foods like cherries, figs, brown rice, miso soup, and bone broth, as well as yang-building foods like grass-fed beef, walnuts, cinnamon, fenugreek, and rosemary. To support her adrenals, I had her take ashwagandha and astragalus, herbs that help the body cope with stress.

Stephanie was a committed runner, but running doesn't build yang as well as strength training and interval training, so I asked her to switch to those workouts. What's more, she was drained emotionally, because she was working long hours and said yes to every volunteer opportunity at her child's school. To help her establish better boundaries, I suggested she practice saying no so she could create time for relaxation and downtime with her family, get more sleep, and recharge her body, mind, and spirit.

When I saw her three months later, her hair was thicker and she had more energy. Within another few months she'd gone off the thyroid

ADRENAL BODY BATTERY

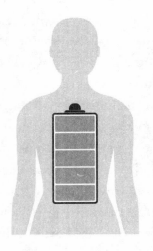 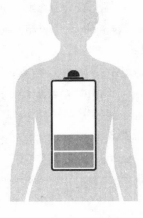

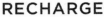

RECHARGE	DEPLETE
Faith	Stress
Hope	Fear
Prayer	Worry
Meditation	Low Self-Esteem
Spiritual Reading	Self-Comparison
Time in Nature	Overwork
8+ Hours of Sleep	Poor Sleep
Nutrient-Dense Foods	Unhealthy Diet
Light Exercise	Digital Devices
Deep Relationships	Toxic Relationships
Purpose	Lacking Identity

medication, and she was feeling great. She was surprised at how my simple suggestions had turned her health around, but I wasn't. Synthroid treats the symptoms of hypothyroidism, but it doesn't cure it—and neither did the healthy dietary changes the naturopath recommended.

Taking prescription medication is like taking the bulb out of your car's glowing check–engine light instead of having a mechanic look under the hood to identify the source of the problem. Ancient remedies, on the other hand, fix the engine so it can function optimally. These time-tested approaches to healing restore balance to your whole system—body, mind, and spirit.

While Western medicine rarely takes emotions into account, ancient healers respected the power our emotions have to both heal and harm our health. Intuitively, we all know this to be true. When you're worried or anxious, you might get an upset stomach. When a child has a nightmare, they often wet the bed. Why is that? It's because fear causes dysfunction in the kidneys and bladder. Anxiety affects the heart and brain, raising your blood pressure and clouding your thinking. And you've undoubtedly heard someone called an "angry drunk." People who drink to excess are more likely to become belligerent, because alcohol causes liver toxicity—and anger is related to the liver.

And grief can cause all manner of physical suffering, because it hampers the immune system. I had a patient who developed autoimmune disease after her daughter—her best friend—left for college. I encouraged her to schedule regular times to connect with her daughter, join a women's group, and adopt an immune-strengthening diet with plenty of chicken broth, garlic, and ginger. I also asked her to focus more on the future, whether that meant making fun plans or setting long-term goals for herself. Over the course of the next year, her health issues diminished drastically—and she felt happier and more at peace with her new stage of life.

When your body gets worn down by negative emotions, like worry, anger, or stress, you're more vulnerable to a host of illnesses and ailments. Some early Western practitioners were aware of this. In 1895, Daniel David Palmer, the founder of chiropractic medicine, said, "The human body gets sick as a result of excessive trauma or toxins or thoughts, or a combination of these agents."

Far earlier, ancient practitioners not only recognized the inextricable links between body, mind, and spirit, they viewed the body itself as a complex network of interconnected parts, rather than separate systems or organs. They understood that if one system of the body is out of whack, the rest will eventually be affected as well. As a result, they developed treatments designed to restore the whole system to health. Ancient Chinese practitioners, for instance, developed acupuncture (using tiny needles to treat the underlying cause of symptoms) and cupping, which involves the use of suction cups to increase blood flow to sore or injured muscles; both approaches are effective because they clear energy blockages and reestablish the healthy flow of qi throughout your body. They bring your entire system back into balance.

Conventional Western practitioners argue that since you can't find qi in the body, you can't explain how acupuncture works, and, as a result, it must be ineffective—despite the fact that studies show that acupuncture is an extremely effective treatment for numerous conditions. But they fail to acknowledge that we don't fully understand how or why many commonly prescribed medications "work," including antidepressants, lithium (a common treatment for bipolar disorder), and even the medicine cabinet staple acetaminophen. As Peter Imming, a German pharmaceutical chemist, told *The Scientist* website, "If we threw out all the drugs for which we do not know the molecular mechanisms, we wouldn't be left with a lot."[2]

What's more, ancient treatments have stood the test of time precisely because they *are* effective—and their effectiveness is more widely recognized today. For instance, in spite of the naysayers, acupuncture is increasingly covered by health insurance plans, and cupping is becoming popular among professional athletes, who say it helps keep them in top shape for competitive events.

My ancient remedies approach also utilizes treatments from Ayurveda. This four-thousand-year-old system of natural healing originated in India and is based on the premise that there are three doshas, or energies: Vata, Pitta, and Kapha. Ayurvedic healers believe that all disease and illness come from an imbalance in these three energies. Like TCM and ancient Middle Eastern medicine, it aims to cure the root cause of disease by healing one's thoughts, beliefs, and lifestyle habits with strategies like diet, stress reduction, and herbal remedies that bring the body into balance.

Traditional Western medicine sees illness only through the lens of measurable physical dysfunction, which reduces our bodies, and our suffering, to one-size-fits-all issues—as if we were all identical, with lives, emotions, physiological makeup, and DNA that are indistinguishable from one another. But the truth is that no two bodies or sets of circumstances are exactly the same. That's one reason I became such a strong proponent of ancient medicine. By striving to get at the root cause of your unique, personal problems, any treatment I recommend will be tailored to *you* and *your* needs and *your* life. And as ancient remedies gently heal and strengthen your body, they create improved equanimity, well-being, and overall health that can last for a lifetime.

Pinpointing the underlying cause, and cure, of disease

According to TCM, certain types of underlying imbalances are the root cause of all disease. Based on that fundamental belief, ancient Chinese physicians developed a comprehensive philosophy for understanding these imbalances. In this section, I will introduce you to this paradigm, along with the most common internal influences that can become unbalanced, including qi, blood, yin, yang, coldness, heat, dampness, dryness, stagnation, and wind. When I first heard these concepts, I thought they sounded a little strange. But after working with the TCM approach for years, I have learned how profoundly helpful this approach is for understanding health and illness, as well as healing diseases—even those that are, from the Western perspective, considered impossible to cure.

Here are twelve core diagnostic and healing concepts from ancient Chinese medicine, along with quick lists of foods that can bring more balance to your body if you have deficiencies or weaknesses in any of these areas. You'll hear more about these concepts in the coming chapters. Understanding them can revolutionize the way you think about your health. What's more, if you visit a holistic doctor who practices Chinese medicine (and I hope you do), the following information will give you some background and context so you have a better grasp of the approach.

Qi

Qi (pronounced "chee") is like your body's internal battery. A fundamental precept of traditional Chinese medicine, the word translates roughly to "life force" or "vital energy." Qi circulates throughout your body along pathways known as meridians, which connect all the organ systems. Acupuncture and acupressure help restore qi by treating specific meridian points throughout the body. Other ancient medical systems have similar concepts. In India, internal energy is called prana; in Japan it's known as ki; in Greece it's pneuma; and in parts of Africa it's known as ashe. In scientific terms, qi is similar to adenosine triphosphate (ATP), an energy-carrying chemical found in the cells of all living creatures. Like qi, ATP provides energy for everything from muscle contractions to nerve impulses. The organs most closely associated with qi are your adrenal glands, which produce energy-boosting hormones like adrenaline and cortisol. No matter the medical tradition, the underlying idea is this: When your internal battery is powered up, your body functions more efficiently, and you're better able to fight off cold and flu bugs that come your way. But like the battery in your phone, qi requires regular recharging. This vital, internal life force is fueled by healthy lifestyle habits, from emotional strategies like building self-esteem, finding your life purpose, and reducing fear to physical habits like getting plenty of sleep and practicing deep breathing exercises. Some signs of a qi deficiency include thyroid disorders, adrenal fatigue, irregular periods, infertility, weakness, anxiety, and susceptibility to infections.

■ *Qi-boosting foods:* Berries (especially goji berries), cherries, figs, green leafy vegetables, watercress, carrots, squash, pumpkin, maca, peas, lentils, beans, rice, quinoa, oats, chestnuts, coconut, miso, bone broth, grass-fed beef, pasture-raised chicken, wild-caught fish, free-range eggs, and all medicinal mushrooms, such as shiitake, reishi, and chaga.

■ *Qi-boosting herbs:* Rehmannia, ashwagandha, astragalus, rhodiola, fo-ti, schisandra, codonopsis, ginseng, cordyceps, reishi, licorice root, turmeric, fenugreek, and cinnamon.

■ *Qi-depleting foods:* Cold foods, like dairy-based ice cream, raw vegetables, and ice-cold drinks; refined sugar, hydrogenated oils, dried tropical fruit, alcohol, and excessive salt.

Blood

In TCM, blood is not only in charge of transporting oxygen and nutrients around the body, it is also responsible for warming, moisturizing, and nourishing our organs and is closely related to cardiac and mental health. According to TCM, blood houses our spirit, which is why the ancients were fond of saying things like "Love with all of your heart." Blood is created by the spleen and then moved throughout the body by the liver. With so many functions, it's no surprise that a lack of blood or undernourished blood can cause many health issues. This is called blood deficiency and can lead to anemia, fatigue, weakness, pale skin, light-headedness, poor memory, and insomnia.

■ *Blood-building foods:* Cherries, figs, goji berries, prunes, coconut, oats, beets, chard, kale, carrots, sweet potatoes, onions, spinach, pumpkin, eggs, liver, bone broth, grass-fed beef, turkey, venison, wild-caught salmon, sardines, walnuts, chickpeas, and ginger.

■ *Blood-building herbs:* Dong quai, peony, astragalus, cinnamon, parsley, and rehmannia.

■ *Blood-depleting foods:* Salads, raw fruit, raw vegetables, cucumber, excessive fruit, watermelon, tofu, dairy, refined sugar, chocolate, and ice-cold water.

Yin and Yang

Yin and yang are words you've undoubtedly heard. You might have even seen the symbol—a circle divided into two halves (one black, one white) by a curving line—that signifies the concept in Chinese medicine. But here's what that symbol means: Yin and yang represent the balance between the opposing forces of life—work and rest, for instance, or dark and light. Physically, it refers to the balance of hormones, with yin being calming "female" hormones, like estrogen, and yang being energizing "male" hormones, like testosterone. We associate yin and yang with Chinese medicine, but their foundational principles have far older roots. In fact, a number of historians believe that certain Eastern medicine philosophies started with Abraham, who is mentioned in several religious texts, including the Bible. Genesis 25:6 states, "To his sons...Abraham gave gifts and sent them eastward." Those gifts are thought to include medicine and healing practices, like incense made from herbs—and "eastward" meant India and Asia, where Ayurveda and Chinese Medicine began. And the concepts of yin and yang appear early in the book of Genesis, when God created Heaven and Earth, light and dark, night and day, male and female. Here are more examples of yin and yang:

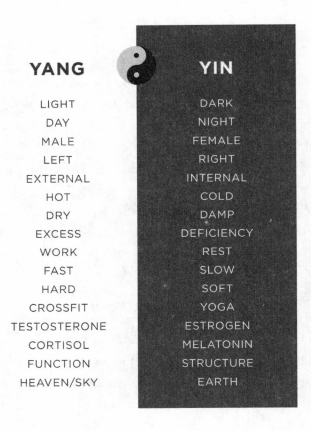

YANG	YIN
LIGHT	DARK
DAY	NIGHT
MALE	FEMALE
LEFT	RIGHT
EXTERNAL	INTERNAL
HOT	COLD
DRY	DAMP
EXCESS	DEFICIENCY
WORK	REST
FAST	SLOW
HARD	SOFT
CROSSFIT	YOGA
TESTOSTERONE	ESTROGEN
CORTISOL	MELATONIN
FUNCTION	STRUCTURE
HEAVEN/SKY	EARTH

From the Chinese perspective, in order to have strong qi, you need a wholesome balance of yin and yang. Signs of a yin deficiency include dry skin and hair, night sweats, excessive thirst, muscle aches, weakness (especially in the knees and lower back), poor memory, anxiety, irritability, restlessness, and poor sleep. A yang deficiency, on the other hand, can cause low energy, low sex drive, low testosterone, muscle weakness, cold feet and hands, or a cold that pervades the whole body.

■ *Yang-boosting foods:* Cherries, dates, garlic, raspberries, squash, carrots, pumpkin, grass-fed beef, lamb, trout, venison, chicken, fatty fish, eggs, sweet potatoes, oats, quinoa, black beans, kidney beans, root vegetables, hot peppers, shiitake mushrooms, hard cheeses, pistachios, walnuts, cocoa, and sea salt.

■ *Yang-boosting herbs:* Fenugreek, ginseng, codonopsis, cordyceps, black pepper, cinnamon, turmeric, rosemary, and deer antler.

■ *Yang-depleting foods:* Raw vegetables, salads, soy, refined sugar, ice cream, processed foods, and excessive salt.

For yin deficiency, see the dryness recommendations on page 48, since the patterns overlap.

Yin & Yang
FOOD BALANCE

ASPARAGUS	CITRUS	ROOT VEGETABLES	WALNUT
CUCUMBER	HONEY	CHERRIES	QUINOA
CELERY	POTATO	GARLIC	HARD CHEESE
TOMATO	SPELT	FENUGREEK	FATTY FISH
EGGPLANT	DAIRY	CINNAMON	BEEF
PEAR	DUCK	HOT PEPPERS	LAMB
TROPICAL FRUIT	TOFU	COCOA	EGGS
WATERMELON	HERBAL TEA	PISTACHIO	SEA SALT

YIN
Contracting & Cooling

YANG
Expansive & Warming

Cold and Heat

Cold and heat are two of the six "evils" or "pernicious influences" in Chinese medicine (the other four are detailed in the following two sections) that affect physical and emotional yin-yang balance and can lead to disease. Cold can invade your body from the environment or through a cold virus, but it can also be brought on by anxiety and fear. It manifests as fatigue, loose stools, poor digestion, slow metabolism, cold extremities, poor circulation, and getting sick easily. Traditional Chinese nutrition categorizes foods as hot or cold—based not only on their temperature but also on the way they affect the body— and uses them to balance the body's internal system. For instance, warming herbs and foods activate your immune system. When I first opened my clinic, an older man who lived in the country came to see me. He was sniffling and sneezing, and I said, "Hey, are you doing anything for that cold?" He replied, "I'm drinking hot toddies, with whiskey, cinnamon, and honey." I prefer alcohol-free treatments, but in theory, hot toddies make sense. Whiskey is the hottest type of liquor, and cinnamon is a warming herb. As I mentioned earlier in the chapter, foods' colors are significant, too. Ancient practitioners used chicken broth instead of beef broth to treat a cold because it's yellow— and yellow foods are powerful immune boosters known to strengthen the lungs and colon. Ginger and garlic are yellow as well.

■ *Warming foods:* Cherries, dates, peaches, bone broth, lamb, grass-fed beef, venison, chicken, squash, pumpkin, mustard greens, basil, garlic, dill, onions, rice, oatmeal, nut butter, pistachios, walnuts, pine nuts, butter, coffee, chocolate, and red wine.

■ *Warming herbs:* Cayenne pepper, black pepper, cinnamon, ginger, turmeric, holy basil, cloves, and oregano.

■ *Foods to avoid:* The cold and cool foods in the chart on page 45, especially excess fruit, cucumbers, dairy, raw foods, vegetables juices, and ice-cold water.

COLD	COOL	NEUTRAL	WARM	HOT
Cucumber	Asparagus	Artichoke	Brussels sprout	Hot pepper
Dandelion	Broccoli	Beet	Kale	Lamb
Rhubarb	Celery	Cabbage	Onion	Trout
Water chestnut	Eggplant	Cauliflower	Bell pepper	Cinnamon
Tomato	Radish	Olive	Pumpkin	Ginger
Banana	Spinach	Pea	Squash	Mustard
Cranberry	Amaranth	Potato	Black bean	Garlic
Lemon	Barley	Sweet potato	Oat	Horseradish
Lime	Buckwheat	Chickpea	Quinoa	Cayenne
Grapefruit	Apple	Kidney bean	Blackberry	Chile
Melon	Avocado	Lentil	Cherry	Hard alcohol
Mulberry	Blueberry	Corn	Date	
Watermelon	Kiwi	Rice	Peach	
Mung bean	Pear	Rye	Raspberry	
Yogurt	Strawberry	Fig	Beef	
Crab	Duck egg	Plum	Butter	
Tofu	Spirulina	Pomegranate	Bone broth	
Lemon peel	Peppermint	Chicken egg	Chicken	
Seaweed	Green tea	Milk	Salmon	
Sea salt	Beer	White fish	Pine nut	
		Tuna	Pumpkin seed	
		Almond	Walnut	
		Chia	Cacao	
		Flax	Coffee	
		Coconut	Miso	
		Sesame	Wine	
		Honey		

Excess "heat," on the other hand, is like running a car engine in a high gear with too little oil and coolant and substandard fuel. It accelerates wear and tear and leads to earlier engine failure. Similarly, eating a diet high in processed foods and sugar, burning the candle at both ends, and suffering from chronic stress cause heat in your body, which often corresponds to inflammation—an underlying driver of just about every chronic health condition you can think of. High blood pressure, rashes, fever, and insomnia are symptoms of excess heat as well.

Cooling foods: Apples, bananas, citrus fruit, kiwis, pears, melon, watermelon, coconut water, avocados, asparagus, celery, cucumbers, tomatoes, cabbage, green leafy vegetables, radishes, zucchini, cilantro, mung beans, water chestnuts, barley, millet, seaweed, raw fish, and yogurt.

Cooling herbs: Aloe vera, skullcap, peppermint, rose, fennel, mulberry, nettles, and andrographis.

Foods to avoid: Fried foods, spicy foods, lamb, red meat, nuts, hard alcohol, excessive oil, and warming herbs. Food prep matters, too. Eat more boiled, steamed, or raw foods than baked, deep-fried, roasted, or barbecued.

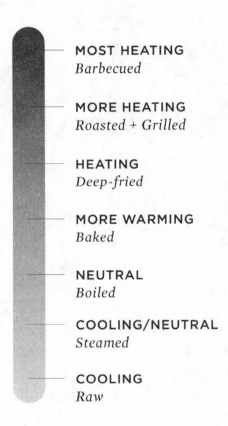

MOST HEATING
Barbecued

MORE HEATING
Roasted + Grilled

HEATING
Deep-fried

MORE WARMING
Baked

NEUTRAL
Boiled

COOLING/NEUTRAL
Steamed

COOLING
Raw

Dampness and Dryness

Dampness and dryness are also important yin-yang balance concepts—and they are the second pair of TCM's pernicious influences. A little bit of dampness in the body is normal; it moistens the digestive tract and mucus membranes. But if there is too much, it causes yeast to build up on your tongue and in your digestive tract. Here's one way of understanding what it means when your body is too damp:

Consider what happens when a basement floods. If it stays damp for too long, mold grows—a problem that, left untended, can be difficult to eradicate, and sometimes leaves the whole house uninhabitable. But if you make an effort to dry out the basement quickly, you prevent mold from growing. Dampness in your body can come from being too sedentary or having problems with the digestive system, especially the spleen, which controls your body's fluids. Excess dampness is characterized by phlegm, mucus, and candida overgrowth, conditions that, left untreated, can cause physical ailments. Phlegm in the lungs causes congestion and breathing problems; mucus in the digestive tract causes diarrhea; and candida overgrowth can cause fatigue, brain fog, joint pain, leaky gut, and poor digestion, among other things.

■ *Foods to reduce dampness:* Lemons, plums, pears, cherries, grapefruit, asparagus, celery, carrots, pumpkin, squash, peas, radishes, barley, corn, rice, oats, chickpeas, beans, walnuts, bone broth, chicken, grass-fed beef, tuna, wild-caught salmon, garlic, and onions.

■ *Herbs to reduce dampness:* Alisma, pau d'arco, poria, plantain, gentian, orange peel, oregano, cardamom, parsley, and thyme.

■ *Foods to avoid:* Foods that have a moist, almost phlegmy texture, like dairy, egg whites, tofu, oils, fats, bananas, and avocados, as well as refined sugar, wheat products, white flour products, dried fruit, pork, salads, raw vegetables, vegetable juices, and ice-cold water.

Excessive dryness, on the other hand, can be caused by dehydration, or a deeper issue, like a yin deficiency, which, as with heat, can come from pushing yourself too hard or sleeping too little and overstimulating your adrenals. The shifting hormones of menopause can also deplete yin, causing hot flashes and vaginal dryness. Dry eyes and sinuses, and the degeneration of the healthy mucosal lining of the gut, which can lead to gastrointestinal problems, are signs of yin-related dryness as well. Aging skin, constipation, chronic thirst, confusion, and poor memory are also symptoms of excess dryness.

■ *Foods to boost yin and reduce dryness:* Apples, mulberries, goji berries, mangoes, pears, pineapple, pomegranate, tropical fruit, watermelon, citrus, coconut, avocados, olives, asparagus, cucumbers, celery, tomatoes, eggplant, green beans, spinach, seaweed, peas, potatoes, sweet potatoes, yams, rice, spelt, fermented soybeans, tofu, sesame tahini, mushrooms, wild-caught fish, eggs, duck, bone broth, yogurt, dairy, honey, and herbal tea.

■ *Herbs to boost yin and moisture:* Slippery elm, marshmallow, CBD hemp, mullein, evening primrose, black cohosh, dong quai, and rehmannia.

■ *Foods to avoid:* Spicy foods, fried foods, refined sugar, lamb, pistachios, and hard alcohol.

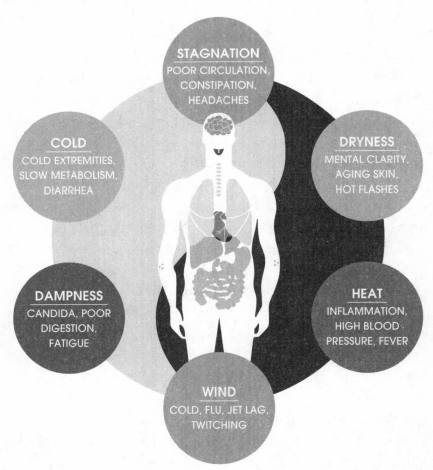

Stagnation and Wind

Stagnation and wind is the final pair of pernicious influences. Just like it sounds, stagnation is characterized by a sense of stuck-ness or lack of internal movement—so it includes problems like bruises that heal slowly, constipation, and cold hands and feet, a sign of poor circulation. Pain—both emotional and physical—is an indication of stagnation as well. Chinese medicine practitioners like to say, "If there is free flow, there is no pain; if there is no free flow, there is pain." Qi stagnation can result in headaches or discomfort after eating as well as emotional problems like anger or depression, while blood stagnation is often the underlying problem in conditions like premenstrual pain, endometriosis, or heart issues. One of the best ways to release stagnation is with movement. Acupuncture can be extraordinarily helpful as well, since it opens the energy channels throughout the body.

- *Foods to get qi moving:* Citrus fruit, peaches, plums, artichokes, asparagus, beets, broccoli, cauliflower, carrots, celery, radishes, onion, garlic, squash, mustard greens, watercress, turnips, sauerkraut, miso, garlic, fennel, horseradish, and apple cider vinegar.
- *Herbs to get qi moving:* Bupleurum, milk thistle, turmeric, cypress, citrus peel, sandalwood, cardamom, and dandelion.
- *Foods to avoid:* Fried foods, fatty foods, oils, dairy, cheese, butter, sugar, spicy foods, red meat, lard, beer, hard alcohol, processed foods, and artificial preservatives.

Wind is characterized by too much movement in the body. Think of it as being invaded by an unwelcome agent, like a virus, parasite, bacteria, or too much cold or heat. The flu and other viruses are wind-related illnesses, and wind invades the lungs and immune system first. But it can also manifest as everything from eye twitches, shaky hands, muscle cramps, and pain that moves around the body, to neurological illnesses like Parkinson's or migraines. Wind is often caused by unhealthy lifestyle habits, like too much alcohol and stress, which weaken the lungs and immune system.

■ *Foods to expel wind:* Plums, pears, cherries, grapefruit, coconut, asparagus, watercress, broccoli, celery, carrots, pumpkin, squash, radishes, rice, oats, flax, pine nuts, chickpeas, beans, bone broth, liver, chicken, tuna, salmon, garlic, and onion.

■ *Herbs to expel wind:* Cilantro, coriander, sage, peppermint, ginger, oregano, cardamom, parsley, and thyme.

■ *Foods to avoid:* Dairy, egg whites, refined sugar, fried foods, fatty foods, beef, wheat products, white flour products, bananas, dried fruit, tofu, pork, salads, raw vegetables, vegetable juices, and ice-cold water.

Demystifying common TCM diagnostic tools

Thousands of years ago, TCM practitioners didn't have the benefit of modern technology that allows us to peer inside the body. So in order to identify what type of imbalance a patient had, they devised other ingenious strategies, like looking at the tongue, feeling the pulse, and examining the facial complexion. Based on those diagnostic tools, they would recommend a personalized diet, specific herbs, lifestyle practices, and often perform a treatment, like acupuncture. Here's a deeper look at the three main diagnostic tools of TCM:

■ Tongue diagnosis is, as it sounds, a way of understanding the root cause of your condition by examining your tongue. So don't be shocked if a TCM physician asks you to stick out your tongue without saying "Ahhh." Just as modern doctors listen to your heart and lungs, Chinese medical practitioners believe the appearance of the tongue holds important clues to your health. They look at four factors: color, shape, coating, and moisture. The tongue's color points to the condition of the blood, qi, yin, yang, fluids, and yin-related organs like the heart, lungs, spleen, liver, and kidneys. Its shape can also provide clues

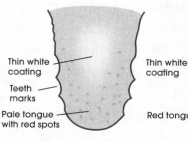

Thin white coating

Teeth marks

Pale tongue with red spots

Qi deficiency
Fatigue, digestion problems, loose stool, over-thinking, and worrying

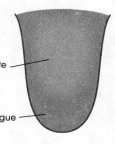

Thin white coating

Red tongue

Heat
Feel hot, sweat easily, thirst, constipated, irritable, skin problems, inflammation

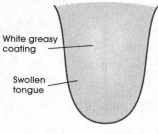

White greasy coating

Swollen tongue

Damp retention
Bloated, gas, candida, lethargic, phlegm, loose stool

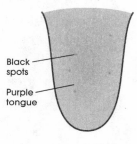

Black spots

Purple tongue

Blood stasis
Cold limbs, varicose veins, bruising, headaches, liver spots, poor skin

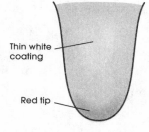

Thin white coating

Red tip

Qi stagnation
Poor sleeping, depression, irritability, constipation, PMS, mood swings

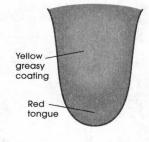

Yellow greasy coating

Red tongue

Damp heat
Skin problems, UTI, acne, eczema, joint pain

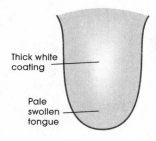

Thick white coating

Pale swollen tongue

Yang deficiency
Feeling cold, back pain, infertility, low thyroid, impotence, weakness, tendency to panic

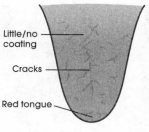

Little/no coating

Cracks

Red tongue

Yin deficiency
Insomnia, hot flashes, restlessness, sweat at night, irritable, ringing in the ears, menopause

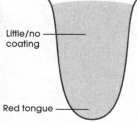

Little/no coating

Red tongue

Blood deficiency
Dizziness, fatigue, anemia, palpitations, poor concentration and memory, gynecological problems

to the health of the blood, qi, yin, yang, and bodily fluids. The coating is related to yang organs, like the small and large intestines, stomach, bladder, and gallbladder, and can give doctors a sense of where the problem lies. And the moisture of the tongue indicates the relative dampness or dryness of the body in general.

What's more, each area of the tongue is connected to particular organs. The tip relates to the heart. Just behind that is an area linked to the lungs. The center of your tongue corresponds with your spleen and stomach. The area behind the center is linked to the intestines. And behind that, the very back of the tongue is connected to the bladder and uterus. The root of the tongue corresponds to the kidneys. The sides of the top of the tongue are linked to the gallbladder, and the outer edges are linked to the liver. For instance, if you have blood stagnation, your tongue might have a purplish hue with dark spots. Someone who has too much heat might have a red-tipped tongue with a thin yellow coating in the middle. See the illustration on page 51 for other examples.

Chinese Medicine Map of the Tongue

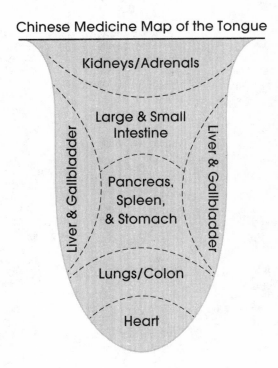

■ Taking your pulse allows TCM practitioners to feel what's going on inside your body. They're feeling not only for the speed of your pulse but also its depth, evenness, and quality. Pulse depth and strength reflects your level of qi, and pulse quality—whether it's choppy or flowing—can offer clues about myriad health issues. What's more, different sections of the pulse correlate to different organs. By taking my wife's pulse, my dear friend and Chinese medicine mentor Gil Ben-Ami was able to tell that Chelsea was pregnant two weeks before it was detected by a pregnancy test.

■ Face mapping, also known as *mien shiang*, stems from the ancient TCM belief that your skin reflects the state of your health—so a TCM practitioner may scrutinize your complexion as well. According to

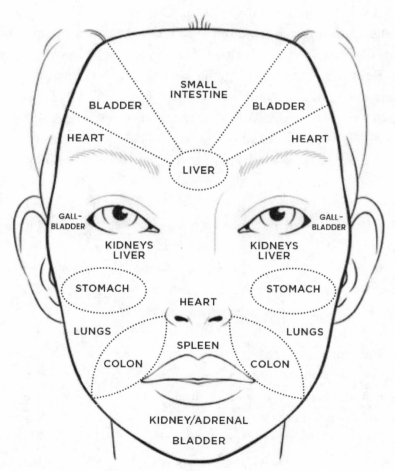

TCM, each part of your face corresponds to a different organ. Pimples or redness on your forehead might indicate issues with your small intestine or digestive problems, while rosy cheeks may mean you have stomach inflammation, since the cheeks correspond with the stomach, spleen, and respiratory system.

If you feel a little confused, don't worry. These ideas are unfamiliar to most people in the United States at the moment. But within ten years, I believe they will become far more mainstream, because ancient medicine is in the midst of a long-overdue resurgence. The 2019 version of the World Health Organization's International Statistical Classification of Diseases and Related Health Problems, which categorizes thousands of diagnoses and has a powerful influence over the healthcare agendas in dozens of countries, features details about traditional medicine, including Chinese medicine. Similarly, scientists from leading universities in the United States and Europe, including UCLA, Duke, and Oxford, are exploring the efficacy of traditional treatments for illnesses like diabetes and cancer—research that will begin to reveal how and why these approaches can be effective.

Meanwhile, growing numbers of people are becoming disenchanted with Western medicine and are increasingly captivated by ancient remedies. Sales of age-old herbal remedies are soaring. During the Covid-19 pandemic, stores struggled to keep ancient antivirals, like elderberry and oregano oil, in stock. And meditation and yoga are so popular they're no longer considered alternative. Dozens of apps, thousands of classes, and millions of people have already endorsed these profoundly beneficial practices.

This growing interest gives me hope that we're in the midst of a medical renaissance. As more and more of us recognize the pitfalls of treating superficial symptoms, we can begin to restore the healthcare system's ability to see disease as multifactorial—and treat patients as whole human beings. In any case, I believe it's time for everyone to understand what these treatments have to offer, and I hope that by the time you finish this book, you're as excited about their promise as I am.

CHAPTER 3

Eat Right for Your Ancient Element

A Personalized Approach to Understanding Yourself—and Using Food as Medicine

You are unlike anyone else on the planet. In other words, you're one in 7.5 billion. It's pretty amazing, when you think about it. While all human beings are far more alike than different, each of us has distinct traits that make us one of a kind—our fingerprints, of course, but also our bodies' genomes, the cellular operating instructions that make each of us who we are. In fact, in 2015, a consortium of scientists released the results of the 1000 Genomes Project, which concluded that there are four to five million differences between one person's genome and that of anyone else.[1]

Even so, most contemporary health and diet advice remains one-size-fits-all—a strategy that clearly doesn't work. If you've ever unsuccessfully tried a diet or health protocol that worked for a friend or colleague, you know what I mean. In some ways, these failures are worse than never trying at all, because in their wake you often blame yourself. You beat yourself up. You think you have no willpower or you're weak or flawed in some deep, fundamental way.

I can't tell you the number of patients who have come to me over the years, looking distressed and ashamed, and said, "What's wrong with me? Why is everyone else successful with this approach and I'm not?" Well, I'm here to tell you the same thing I tell my patients: *There's nothing wrong with you.* It's not you who has failed. It's the cookie-cutter approach.

That's especially true when it comes to diet. While conventional wisdom holds that there's one dietary pattern that is healthy for everyone, the truth is there is no single perfect diet. Let me say that again: There is no single perfect diet. Remember, our bodies are as unique as our individual fingerprints and our genomes, which means we respond to food (and drugs and exercise and stress and lack of sleep) in different ways, too. As a result, for you to achieve optimal health, you need a customized approach to eating that suits your unique makeup.

There's a lot of talk about personalized medicine these days. Hundreds of Western scientists are looking at using our unique genetic codes to understand individual differences in how we metabolize drugs or have a predisposition to a certain illness. The sad truth is that this may just lead to more unnecessary treatments—cases in which people are prescribed drugs preventatively, before they've even developed any condition. This approach gets at the root of Western medicine's fatal flaw: It believes that short of taking a drug, there is nothing you can do to treat or prevent an illness.

That philosophy couldn't be more wrong. Ancient practitioners recognized that our bodies have a natural capacity to heal, and that with the support of appropriate herbs, foods, and exercises, the body will in most cases heal itself. So TCM practitioners developed a system for understanding individual patients' emotional, physical, and spiritual health—one that would help them identify each individual's vulnerabilities and weak spots and make diet and lifestyle recommendations to prevent and heal disease based on those unique characteristics. This system, known as the five elements of ancient medicine, offers remarkable insights into your whole being—your physical traits, body type, emotional tendencies, and dominant organs, as well as diet tweaks and lifestyle strategies that can be particularly beneficial to you.

I think of the five elements of ancient medicine as the original form of personalized medicine. This paradigm offers a customized approach to diet and health—one that, based on my experience with hundreds of patients, can be especially helpful for people who have tried and failed to lose weight and get healthy in the past. I'm excited to share it with you because it can help you better understand and care for your unique body, mind, and health.

Why the five elements can offer unique insights into your health

Have you ever taken a personality profile test like the Enneagram, the Myers-Briggs Type Indicator, or the DISC (Dominance, Influence, Compliance, Steadiness)? If so, you know how valuable these tools can be in helping you understand more about yourself—your strengths, your weaknesses, your skills, your passions. Well, the five elements structure is like the ancient prototype for these tests, and to this day it remains the most comprehensive.

Ancient healers knew that every one of us has a deep connection with the earth and its elements, and they used five essential features of nature—fire, earth, wood, metal, and water—to explain the complex traits of our bodies and minds. They believed that these five qualities from the natural world exist within every human being—not literally, of course, but metaphorically. According to the theory, every human being is a unique composite of all five elemental categories, but typically one or two elements—known as one's "dominant elements"—best represent how a person thinks and feels, as well as what helps them thrive physically and emotionally, and what can thwart their efforts to get healthy.

Just as you might fit, to varying degrees, into several different Enneagram or DISC categories, the five elements can manifest in a variety of combinations. You might be dominant in fire and earth, for instance, but still have traces of wood, metal, and water. And your particular blend describes who you are—whether you're prone to impatience (a trait of people strong in the wood element), or you're incredibly well organized (like metal element types), or you're more introspective (as those strong in the water element tend to be).

When I began using the five elements approach in my functional medicine practice, I saw over and over again how beneficial it could be for understanding individual differences in emotional and physical health and helping to guide treatment choices as well as lifestyle and diet recommendations. For instance, when I was actively seeing patients, a friend, Nancy, came to my office. She was thirty-three and had been struggling with infertility for five years. She had also had several miscarriages. That pattern—having difficulty both conceiving and carrying a baby—told me that she was struggling in her water and earth elements. The water element relates to conception as well as the adrenal and reproductive organs, while earth is connected to carrying a baby as well as the pancreas and spleen.

Nancy was eating a paleo diet that was high in fat, nuts, and seeds, and low in carbs—a diet that can be super healthy for certain individuals. But healthy fats and nuts and seeds can increase stress on your spleen and liver, and when you're having trouble conceiving you want to nourish all your organs and treat them gently. Worse, she was incredibly stressed about her inability to get—and stay—pregnant, and her anxiety and fear were overtaxing her adrenal glands.

My advice for her was simple: To nurture her earth element, I recommended that she and her husband create a cozy environment in their home. As much as possible, I wanted them to read, snuggle under blankets, sit by the fire, and drink herbal tea. I also suggested that they stop actively trying to get pregnant and just have intercourse when they felt like it. To heal Nancy's adrenals, I suggested she take stress-easing herbs, like astragalus, rehmannia, and ashwagandha. Diet-wise, I suggested she cut back on the fats, nuts, and seeds and add some nourishing sweetness (she'd been strictly avoiding all carbohydrates) to her diet by eating pumpkin, butternut squash, sweet potatoes, and cinnamon.

Six months later Nancy called me. She was pregnant. Soon after, she had a healthy baby, and not long ago she and her husband had their second child. By seeing her pregnancy difficulties through the lens of the five elements, I was able to offer her advice that targeted the emotional and physical issues underlying her fertility problems—and ultimately help her and her husband fulfill their dream of starting a family.

Conception is just one of hundreds of health goals the five elements paradigm can help you achieve, which is why I believe it's important for you to understand more about it and discover where you fit in the five elements system.

Which element are you?

While the five elements model offers a new way of thinking about well-being in general, finding your dominant elements will give you specific insight into yourself and yield new strategies for taking care of your health. Each element has its own characteristics, strengths, and weaknesses. None is better or more important than another.

Take this quick quiz to identify your ancient element. For each item, choose the one answer that best describes you. When you're finished, tally the number of a's, b's, c's, d's, and e's, then read about the emotional characteristics of the ancient element or two you most resemble, along with lifestyle habits and activities that can keep you happily balanced. You may find that, instead of being dominant in one or two elements, you straddle multiple domains.

I tend to...

    a. be the peacekeeper in friends' or family members' disagreements
    b. be independent and self-sufficient
    c. be super social and the life of the party

d. be reliable — I'm someone people can count on to get things done the right way

e. be forward-thinking and visionary, and make plans and decisions quickly

I would rather...

a. work in a group than on my own

b. think things through by myself instead of consulting with a friend or colleague

c. be open, real, and vulnerable than put up a façade

d. abide strictly by the rules — even if it means missing out on something fun

e. be the first in my friend group to try a new restaurant rather than learn about it from someone else

I struggle with...

a. worry, and I don't like change

b. trusting other people

c. being overly passionate and dramatic

d. being critical and perfectionistic

e. working too hard, and I'm prone to frustration when things take too long

My idea of fun is...

a. gathering my whole family for a home-cooked meal

b. curling up with a good book

c. going to a party or connecting with other people in a meaningful way

d. fighting for a just cause; my principles are important, and often come before pleasure (but I do like to have a good time)

e. starting new projects, creating a vision board, and goal-setting

I rarely...

   a. put my needs ahead of someone else's
   b. brag about my accomplishments, even on social media
   c. feel pessimistic or down
   d. have days when I'm not disciplined and productive
   e. am shy about voicing my opinion

I'm particularly good at...

   a. supporting other people in fulfilling their dreams and encouraging them
   b. seeing the bigger picture in most situations
   c. understanding other people's emotions and feeling empathy
   d. maintaining focus, staying on task, and working hard to make sure things are done right
   e. seeing what needs to be done, envisioning a plan, and taking action

Physically, I have...

   a. a shortish thick-set or curvy body with strong legs, as well as a short neck, a squarish or oval face, and full lips
   b. a long torso with shorter legs, an oval or heart-shaped face with big eyes, a large forehead, and a dark complexion
   c. a slightly plump body, a pointy nose and chin, and a reddish complexion
   d. a strong, muscular body, a rectangular or round face, thin lips, prominent cheekbones, and a pale complexion, especially compared to others in my family
   e. a tree-like body with broad shoulders and a narrow waist, as well as a long, thin face, thin nose, and long fingers

Scoring:

Mostly a's: You're an earth type, which means you're nurturing and tend to be a stabilizing force in the world. You tend to be on the short side, with short fingers and neck and a squarish face. People like Oprah Winfrey, Fred Rogers, Dwayne Johnson, and Adam Sandler exemplify this type—thoughtful, responsible, compassionate, grounded, practical, and cheerful. Relationships are key for earth elements. You crave a sense of connection above all else and tend to focus your attention on others rather than yourself, which makes you a good listener, friend, parent, and spouse. It's important to you to create a safe, cozy home where everyone feels loved and cared for, and you're happiest when your relationships and the world at large feels harmonious. Through your compassion and empathy, you bring balance to people around you, whether it's helping to solve disputes or maintaining the status quo. You like doing things for others and enjoy feeling needed. The earth element is closely connected with being a mother. In fact, when women become pregnant and start mothering, their earth element tends to become more pronounced as they love, nurture, and care for their children.

Earth types do best when life is stable and predictable. Change can throw you off, making you feel unbalanced and triggering serious bouts of worry, which is your most defining emotional challenge. When something unexpected happens—you lose your job or someone you love dies or there's conflict in your relationships—it's easy for you to get caught up in circular, ruminative thinking. That type of toxic worry can derail you. If you get stuck in that mindset for too long, your qi can stagnate, putting you at risk for digestive disorders and weight gain. Another challenge for earth types: making too many commitments. People who need support will be drawn to your empathy—your defining positive emotion. But providing all that emotional support can be exhausting, and when you get tired you can become resentful and start wondering why you're the one doing all the giving. You'll be happier and healthier if you learn to set boundaries and say no when you feel your emotional tank running low. Setting boundaries can bolster your sense of self-worth as well, which is important since your tendency to give, give, give may stem from a deep-seated sense of being unworthy. To stay balanced and strong, spend time with people who are upbeat and supportive (you thrive when you have a community of loyal, caring friends); do things that bring you joy, whether it's exercising outside (nature can be particularly calming and reassuring to you) or working on an art or craft project; and accept help from others. That last one might not come naturally, but remember: the nurturer needs nurturing, too. The earth element is linked to the spleen and digestive system, which means you're prone to gut problems, bloating, and food allergies. Using gut-friendly herbs and foods, staying away from sugar, reducing stress, and keeping yourself centered and grounded will help you thrive.

Mostly b's: You're a water type, with a round face, thick eyebrows, big eyes, and a slightly more rounded body. Just as all life comes from water, you have the gift of giving birth to creative ideas, thanks to your ability to think outside the box. Your best ideas are most likely to bloom in solitude, which you probably crave. Like many innovators in science, the arts, or business—think Bill Gates, Robert Downey Jr., Alicia Keys, Ed Sheeran, and Emily Dickinson (who didn't leave her family's property for the last twenty years of her life)—you're a non-conformist who would prefer to live life on your own terms. You have a strong need to be in charge of your own time and schedule—to flow at your own rate, as water does—and may prefer to move more slowly than most. You're generally calm and peaceful—your most defining positive emotions. Similarly, you're probably on the quiet, introverted, and contemplative side—all wonderful gifts in our extrovert-obsessed world—and you prefer deep, meaningful conversations with a close friend or two to parties and lighthearted, social banter. Wisdom is a water trait, and people probably look to you for guidance, since you're a deep thinker. You flourish when you find a small tribe of people who enjoy solving the problems of the world, too.

But you need to watch out for becoming too withdrawn and aloof.

For instance, you might find yourself being in a group of people and still feeling lonely, left out, or different, and that sense of alienation can bring out your fearful side, your most challenging negative emotion. Likewise, the fluid-related organs, the kidney and bladder, are dominant in your life—and a sign they're out of balance is fear. Be warned: If you allow fear to take over and wall yourself off from others, it can mushroom into suspicion and distrust and even paranoia. Your tendency to keep your private thoughts and feelings to yourself can make your sense of "otherness" worse, inadvertently creating a rift with those who are close to you. So make an effort to open up in close relationships. Find friends who value your quiet creativity and innate wisdom, and balance spending time with them with nourishing alone time. You're prone to exhaustion, so avoid stress as best you can by adopting daily relaxing lifestyle habits like yoga or swimming (both have a waterlike flow, so they're particularly restorative), taking warm baths or showers, or walking—particularly near a lake, river, stream, or ocean. The organs related to water are the kidneys, adrenals, and bladder, so you may be prone to swelling and urinary tract infections; to stay healthy, drink plenty of fluids and build downtime in your day so you can go with the flow and limit stress.

Mostly c's: You're a fire type—and you have the spark that marks this lively element, as well as flamelike physical characteristics, with a pointier nose, chin, and head, narrow hips, and slightly rounder center. You're passionate, charismatic, warm, lively, and sociable, like Muhammad Ali, Salma Hayek, Cameron Diaz, or Ellen DeGeneres. In other words, you're fun to be around. And thanks to your natural enthusiasm, you're adept at rallying people to a cause. When you get excited about a project, you can spur others to action. Joy is the emotion most closely associated with the fire element, which makes people want to be around you. You tend to light up a room. You're a pleasure seeker, so late nights, adventurous activities, cities, crowds, and new experiences fuel you—but you also love making deep emotional connections with others. You love to talk—and speak eloquently. You're in touch with your emotions and need to be able to share them. Not surprisingly, the heart is associated with the fire element. You do best when you have a strong community of friends.

Like all flames, however, if you scatter in too many directions you have a tendency to burn out. For instance, you may love getting involved with many projects at once, but struggle to stick with them through the less exciting phases and fail to see them through to the end—which means you run the risk of letting people down, including yourself. In order to get things done, you need to rein in your tendency to get distracted and continually remind yourself what excited you about the project in the first place. Stress can be particularly problematic for you, causing you to panic and focus on worst-case scenarios. Underneath your usually joyful demeanor lurks a tendency to feel anxious, depressed, lonely, and restless—all signs your heart is out of balance. To stay grounded and healthy, avoid becoming overheated (you run hot, so heat can exhaust you); adopt stress-relief tactics that suit your personality, like dancing, cardiovascular exercise, walking meditation (sitting might be too challenging), or power yoga; indulge your innate need for adventure, whether it's by taking a rock-climbing class or going on a philanthropic mission to a developing country; get plenty of sleep and try to stick with a regular sleeping and eating routine; keep a journal, where you can download your daily thoughts; and maintain a strong connection with a few key friends you know you can turn to when you're feeling anxious and out of sorts. Since fire is related to the heart, you're most prone to circulatory problems; staying physically active, eating a healthy diet, and curbing stress will be especially beneficial.

Mostly d's: You're a metal type, which means you're strong, period. Like metal, you're thin, with thin lips and skin, particularly on the back of your hands, and you may have a rectangular face and pale skin. You have qualities we all wish we possessed in our distraction-filled world: focus, discipline, organization, precision, attention to detail. In today's language, you're Type A—think Margaret Thatcher, Angelina Jolie, LeBron James, or Arnold Schwarzenegger. You feel personally responsible not only for getting things right (whether it's reorganizing the garage or creating a presentation for work), but also for doing the right thing. Those qualities give you a unique ability to create order out of chaos—an invaluable gift. Colleagues and friends know they can count on you to not only get the job done, but to do it well. In the larger scheme, you crave a sense of purpose and want to feel like your work has meaning, so you're drawn to humanitarian and environmental projects—and you probably have a deep sense of spirituality, lofty principles, and a strong sense of right and wrong. The metal element is what gives any person a sense of justice, righteousness, and determination.

That said, be careful that your need to do things correctly doesn't alienate people close to you. Taken too far, that tendency can become perfectionistic, rigid, and judgmental, which can put you at risk for depression (perfectionism is a key cause). You have a tendency to dwell on the past, so it's easy for you to be thrown off balance by grief, regret, or shame over things that have happened. When you feel the tug of that downward spiral, it's a sign your lungs, your dominant organ, are out of balance. To keep your lofty goals and desire for order and accuracy at a healthy level, get in the habit of doing daily diaphragmatic breathing exercises, which calms the nervous system and helps you keep things in perspective. Also, consider trying qi gong. This ancient practice combines slow, flowing movements with deep rhythmic breathing (which will appeal to your controlled, methodical side), along with mindfulness (which will bolster your self-awareness and help you recognize when you're going overboard). Yoga, with its focus on mindfulness, can be beneficial, too. Gaining moment-by-moment awareness will help you stay calm, humble, and accepting of the people in your life, flaws and all. Metal is associated with the lungs, so you're prone to respiratory issues, like asthma, and will benefit more than most people from aerobic exercise and avoiding smoke, smog, and other airborne toxins.

Mostly e's: You're a wood type—like a tree, you're rooted in the earth but reaching for the sun, with the clear vision and goal-oriented drive that makes you a natural leader. You're even shaped like a tree, with long fingers, a long face, a long trunk, broad shoulders, and a narrower waist. People like Taylor Swift, Steve Jobs, Richard Branson, and Michael Jordan are strong in the wood element. You're a doer—adept at transforming ideas into reality. In fact, instead of shying away from challenges, you seek them out and push yourself to the limit to accomplish them. You understand strategy, see the bigger picture, have a knack for finding solutions, and work as well with others as by yourself, which makes you an asset to any group, team, or company. You don't like dilly-dallying, so you're the person who keeps ideas and projects moving forward. You also have a curious mind and you love learning new things and growing as a person, which makes you fascinating to be around. At your best, you're filled with hope, faith, and optimism—your strongest positive emotions. Some people may find you intimidating because you're decisive, direct (to the point of bluntness), determined, self-assured, and don't mind arguing to get your point across. But you're actually kind and fair-minded, so long as you keep yourself healthy.

The wood element is related to the liver, and if your liver is out of balance you can become resistant to change, an inflexibility that can lead to anger, your biggest emotional challenge. You have a strong desire to feel like a winner, so when projects stall, you have a tendency to become frustrated and stressed out. You're also prone to overdo it in a variety of areas, including work, shopping, and drinking. Underneath your drive to get things done can lie a simmering impatience that flares into anger when you're tired, stressed, overworked, or underappreciated. As a result, it's important for you to have supportive people in your life who acknowledge and appreciate your efforts. In addition, to stay in balance, you need to build restorative activities into your daily schedule. Take a walk outside among the trees (as a wood type, you have a particular affinity for them), do yoga (tree pose may be particularly calming), plant a garden (watching other things take root and grow is deeply healing for you), and force yourself to laze around the house. Just sit and listen to music or read a book or look out the window. Slowing down is difficult for you, which is precisely why it's important that you do so to maintain your equilibrium. The organ most related to the wood element is the liver, so cleanses that rid the body of toxins can be particularly helpful for you.

Each element is associated with particular traits. Here are the most common.

FIRE

ANXIETY, DEPRESSION,
LONELY, JEALOUS
JOYFUL, LOVE, GRATEFUL,
PASSION

EARTH

WORRY, LOW SELF-WORTH,
OBSESSED, OVERWHELMED
HAPPINESS, HARMONY,
SECURITY, COMFORT

WATER

FEAR, EXHAUSTION,
INADEQUATE, UNACCEPTED
PEACE, CONFIDENCE,
WISDOM, SELF-ESTEEM

WOOD

ANGER, GUILT,
FRUSTRATION, RAGE
HOPE, FAITH, OPTIMISM,
CREATIVITY

METAL

GRIEF, HURT, REGRET,
JUDGING, UNFORGIVING
CHEERFUL, HUMBLE,
FORGIVING, SIGNIFICANCE

Your guide to eating right for your element

See how the five-elements philosophy can give you insight into your strengths and weaknesses? I find it fascinating—and extraordinarily helpful in terms of self-awareness. But the paradigm also provides health guidance, particularly personalized food suggestions that are tailor-made for your body. In fact, if your diet is out of balance with your ancient element, your food choices may actually be undermining your health.

To be clear, the five elements approach isn't a full-fledged diet in itself. (In chapter 4 you'll find a more comprehensive, general guide to the ancient diet—and, as I mentioned, chapters 11 and 12 contain diet information for treating specific health conditions.) But if you understand this approach, you can tilt your everyday choices toward the foods that help provide balance for people dominant in your element.

Each of the elements corresponds with a taste—sour, salty, bitter, pungent, or sweet—and according to TCM, it's the taste and temperature of a food that determines its action in the body. (Remember: In this context, temperature doesn't refer to whether a given dish is served hot or cold; it is a measure of the food's effect on the body after digestion.) Likewise, each element corresponds to an organ in the body and a season of the year, and during each element's season, it's particularly important to nourish the corresponding organ.

While it's beneficial to understand your dominant element, you need to have a grasp of all of them, since they all exist within you to some degree and, depending on the season and your personal health goals, you may want to strengthen a certain element, even if it's not one of your dominant elements. Just as all your organs matter to your overall health, so do all the elements. Moreover, the five elements interact and flow into one another, much as the seasons flow from one to the next—they're sometimes referred to as the five phases or five movements to capture this idea—so supporting one bolsters the others. In the five elements paradigm, wood gives birth to fire, fire to earth, earth to metal, metal to water, and water to wood. Inside your body, their interactions can serve to promote or restrain one another, thereby bolstering health or disease. The goal: creating balance and harmony among the five elements.

Here are the essential things to know about each of the five elements and diet.

	FIRE	EARTH	METAL	WATER	WOOD
ORGAN SYSTEMS	Nervous System, Small Intestine, Heart	Pancreas, Spleen, Stomach	Lungs, Large Intestine, Skin	Kidney, Adrenals, Bladder	Liver, Gallbladder
FUNCTION	Metabolism	Digestion	Immunity	Hormonal	Detoxification
POSITIVE EMOTION	Joyful, Passionate, Grateful	Happy, Nurturing, Harmony	Cheerful, Humble, Justice	Wisdom, Peaceful, Confident	Leadership, Hopeful, Creative
OUT OF BALANCE	Jealous, Dramatic	Worry, Anxiety	Anxious, OCD	Withdrawn, Fearful	Frustrated, Angry
SEASON	Summer	Early Fall	Autumn	Winter	Spring
ENVIRONMENT	Heat	Dampness	Dryness	Cold	Wind
BODY TYPE	Pointed Features, Small Hands, Quick, Energetic	Large Round Features, Strong Legs	Triangular Features, Strong Voice	Round Features, Enjoys Fluid Movements	Tall, Slender, Strong Bones & Joints
PERSONALITY	Loves Attention, Talkative, Sensitive	Friendly, Calm, Generous, Caring	Meticulous, Strong-Willed, Focused	Loyal, Wise, Small Inner Circle	Leader, Hard Worker, Planner
TISSUE	Blood Vessels	Muscles	Skin	Bone	Tendons
COLORS	Red	Yellow	White	Blue	Green
TASTES	Bitter	Sweet	Pungent	Salty	Sour

Wood

Organs: Liver and gallbladder. The liver stores blood, aids the heart in moving blood, is responsible for keeping your energy flowing, and has an effect on your tendons and joints. The gallbladder stores bile and helps balance your emotions. Emotions like frustration, depression, and anger often correspond to liver problems, and indecisiveness and uncertainty can be linked to a deficiency in the gallbladder.

Health problems associated with the wood element: Orthopedic and muscle issues, because wood is related to sinew; vision problems, because wood is related to the eye; tooth and jaw problems (like temporomandibular joint disorder, or TMJ); premenstrual syndrome; migraines; and addiction.

Flavor: Sour. Adding tart foods to your diet will strengthen your wood element. Here are some good options: green apples, lemons, limes, grapefruit, pomegranates, kiwis, sauerkraut, and apple cider vinegar. Regardless of your element, sour foods are often used to treat illnesses associated with leaking, like sweating, bleeding, and diarrhea, and they benefit digestive absorption. Remember, with sour foods a little goes a long way. A single serving of sauerkraut and a quarter lemon in your water is about all the liver can handle—although in the spring it can take a little more and in the fall a little less.

Color: Green. Eating green foods nourishes the wood element, so make sure you get plenty of leafy greens, broccoli, avocados, asparagus, spirulina, parsley, basil, and mung beans, all of which help support the liver, gallbladder, muscles, and joints.

Season: Spring. This is the season to take special care of your liver and gallbladder—to do a fast or cleanse—and to eat light foods, like fresh greens, fruit, and pungent herbs and spices like cilantro, parsley, peppermint, fennel, rosemary, sage, and turmeric, which are attuned to the energetic growth of the season. Avoid foods that stress the liver, including fried foods, dairy, sugar, and large amounts of fat and alcohol. This is also the time of year for personal growth. Spend time visualizing things you want to achieve, setting goals, and creating a plan for a healthy and successful future.

WOOD ELEMENT
HEALTHY CHARACTERISTICS

Clear goals and vision
Strategic planners
Good decision makers
Encouraging

(continued)

SYMPTOMS OF IMBALANCE

Tendency to overwork

Addictive personality traits

PMS or headaches

Trouble digesting fats

SUGGESTIONS FOR BETTER HEALTH

Use herbs like bupleurum, milk thistle, and vitex for women.

Use oils of CBD, lavender, and chamomile to relax.

Schedule time to relax and not work.

Take a walk outside in nature among the trees and do yoga.

Avoid sugar, spicy foods, and fatty foods.

Fire

Organs: Heart and mind and small intestine. The heart is the home of your spirit, according to TCM, and it oversees the blood, but it is also intimately linked with your mind and sympathetic nervous system. In acupuncture, the heart meridian affects both the brain and the heart. Symptoms of a heart-mind imbalance include difficulty concentrating, stumbling over your words when you speak, depression, memory lapses, and poor circulation. The small intestine absorbs fluids and separates the nutrients in our food from the waste. It sorts the pure from the impure physically—and also helps separate and get rid of emotional toxins, while hanging onto nourishing emotions.

Health problems associated with fire element: Insomnia, high blood pressure, chest pain and other heart-related issues, headaches, and depression.

Flavor: Bitter. The bitter flavor enters the heart and small intestine and causes the energy of the body to drop. Bitterness reduces excess, which is why it helps balance out the intense energy of the fire element. Bitter foods include artichokes, arugula, coffee, cacao, romaine lettuce, asparagus, celery, rye, and many herbs and spices, including cinnamon, dandelion, dill, and turmeric. No matter your dominant element, bitter foods are helpful for reducing fevers or drying up dampness—if you have a cold or allergies, for instance.

Color: Red. Rosy-toned foods are good for your heart, small intestine, and brain, so be sure your diet includes some of these foods: beets, goji berries, tomatoes, strawberries, red beans, red bell peppers, and grass-fed beef.

Season: Summer. Your diet should be as light and bright as the season, with vividly colored, lightly cooked fruits and vegetables. Although it's tempting to increase your consumption of icy beverages and frozen treats like ice cream, don't overdo it; when you have too much cold food in this steamy season you can weaken your digestive organs. Try to stick with cooling foods like salads and watery fruits (like watermelon, cucumber, lemons, and limes). Avoid heavy foods like eggs, meat, nuts, and grains, which will drain your energy and drag you down. This is the time of year to get outside and do some cardio, go swimming, and spend time in your community building friendships.

FIRE ELEMENT

HEALTHY CHARACTERISTICS

Passionate
Energetic
Social
Joyful

SYMPTOMS OF IMBALANCE

Anxiety
Heart problems
Trouble sleeping
Overly dramatic

(continued)

> ## SUGGESTIONS FOR BALANCE
>
> Use herbs for heart and nervous system, including hawthorn, red sage, and CBD.
>
> Eat red foods, like beets and bison, and green leafy vegetables.
>
> Take a walk outside in the sunshine.
>
> Schedule some adventure in your life.

Earth

Organs: Spleen, pancreas, and stomach. Your spleen is responsible for recycling old red blood cells and fighting some bacteria, and your pancreas and stomach are integral parts of the digestive process, including the distribution of nutrients from food. Signs of spleen or pancreas imbalance include fatigue and feelings of physical and emotional stuck-ness, which can include symptoms like bloating, loose stools, and lack of appetite.

Health problems associated with earth element: Gastrointestinal problems, like irritable bowel and leaky gut syndrome; and hormonal issues, like adrenal fatigue.

Flavor: Sweet. This is the most ubiquitous flavor. Nearly every food has at least a little sweetness to it. Foods that are considered "full sweet" include meat, beans, nuts, starchy veggies, and dairy. Most fruits and sweeteners, like honey and maple syrup, fall into the category of "empty sweets," but that doesn't mean they're all "empty calories": empty sweets are cleansing and cooling and are unhealthy only in excess. Added sugar and artificial sweeteners, on the other hand, can damage the kidney, bones, and even spleen, the very organ the sweet flavor is meant to support, so do your best to avoid them.

Color: Orange and yellow. These colors are good for your digestive system and spleen, so be sure to eat things like pumpkin, sweet potatoes, corn, butternut squash, yellow and orange bell peppers, oats, egg yolks, pineapple, walnuts, and honey.

Season: Late summer/early fall. Often overlooked, late summer has an essence all its own. In TCM, it marks the seasonal transition from yang to yin, between the outward growth seasons of spring and summer and the inward, more withdrawn seasons of fall and winter. This is a time for finding inner harmony, so it's a good time to take up meditation and prayer, if you haven't already. It's also a good idea to eat foods that harmonize your system, like corn, cabbage, chickpeas, squash, potatoes, rice, apricots, and cantaloupe.

EARTH ELEMENT
HEALTHY CHARACTERISTICS

Nurturing and caring
Loyal friends
Brings peace and harmony
Fun and happy

SYMPTOMS OF IMBALANCE

Excessive/unnecessary worrying
Lack of identity, direction, and clarity in life
Overcommitting and feeling overwhelmed
Digestive problems including bloating, gas, or upset stomach
Cravings for sweets

SUGGESTIONS FOR BALANCE

Use herbs for digestion, including astragalus, licorice, cinnamon, and
   turmeric.
Eat warming, bland foods, like soup, sweet potatoes, pumpkin, and beef.
Spend time connecting with friends who are a positive influence.
Work on creating boundaries and practice saying no.

Metal

Organs: Lungs and large intestine. Your lungs are the main organ involved in breathing, but they also regulate water metabolism and help take in qi from the air, mix it with qi acquired from food, and distribute this vital energy throughout the body. Meanwhile, the large intestine absorbs water and excretes waste. An imbalance in the lungs can manifest as sadness.

Health problems associated with metal element: Lung problems, like asthma; skin issues, like acne; and gastrointestinal problems.

Flavor: Pungent. This flavor disperses stagnation and stuck, phlegmy energy in the lungs and large intestine. It stimulates circulation of both energy and blood and aids digestion. Hot chiles are good for protecting the lungs, as are miso, garlic, turnips, ginger, horseradish, and radishes.

Color: White and pale yellow. High-fiber foods in these categories, like oats, grains, and fruit pulp, are important for cleansing the lungs and colon. Other good whitish foods include pears, apples, cauliflower, chicken bone broth, rice, onions, and almonds.

Season: Autumn. This is the time for moving inward, both emotionally and physically—to find shelter at home and store up food and energy for the coming chill. In autumn, nature is in the process of contracting as well, as grass and leaves turn from a moist, vivid green to a desiccated brown. It's a time to eat sour foods and heartier flavors—things like sauerkraut, leeks, vinegar, cheese, yogurt, sourdough bread, and olives—and focus more on cooking, which engages the sense of smell and is intimately linked to the lungs. This is a time of year to prepare your body for healing. If you have past hurts, devote some time and energy to addressing them. Forgive others and spend time meditating on gratitude and focusing on serving and loving yourself, your family, and your friends.

METAL ELEMENT

HEALTHY CHARACTERISTICS

Very disciplined

Organized and structured

Good problem solvers

Seek justice for oppressed

SYMPTOMS OF IMBALANCE

Stricken with grief or depression
Overly critical or judgmental
Prone to problems of colon, lungs, and skin
Excessive sweating

SUGGESTIONS FOR BALANCE

Take herbs for immunity, including ginger, echinacea, and garlic.
Take probiotics.
Avoid mucus-producing foods, like dairy and wheat.
Do deep breathing exercise like qi gong and diaphragmatic breaths
    during exercise.

Water

Organs: Kidneys, adrenal glands, and bladder. Kidneys are where the body stores jing, the "kidney essence" (in the Western world this equates to your DNA and longevity). Jing is one of Chinese medicine's Three Treasures. The other two are qi and shen, which is related to your spirit in terms of knowing your purpose in life. The kidneys and bladder are both part of the urinary tract. Your kidneys filter blood, removing waste and extra water to make urine, which your bladder helps excrete. Your adrenals are responsible for hormonal balance and your body's fight-or-flight response. An imbalance in this system may show up in your emotional life as fear.

Health problems associated with water element: Urinary and prostate problems, kidney and bladder infections, and diseases or issues related to the sex organs.

Flavor: Salty. Foods high in sodium, like sea salt, soy sauce, miso, and seaweeds, help store heat deep in the body, but use them in moderation. An excess of salty foods weakens the kidneys, adrenals, and bladder, and can negatively affect the heart as well. Although the water element is primarily associated with salt, it also responds well to bitter foods, like endive, asparagus, quinoa, celery, and watercress.

Color: Black and dark blue. Foods in these colors nourish your kidneys, adrenals, and bladder, so water types should consume plenty of black beans, blueberries, blackberries, black rice, eggplant, black sesame seeds, black or dark purple grapes, raisins, and black tea.

Season: Winter. This is the time to seek inner warmth, to rest, and to preserve your physical energy. Kidneys and adrenals are the organs most affected by winter, but you can support them by eating steamed greens, which strengthen the kidneys, and hearty soups, whole grains, and roasted nuts, which cater to our need for sustenance and warmth at this time of year. This is a contemplative season, so it's a good time for meditation or prayer, as well as deep breathing exercises and reading to gain knowledge.

WATER ELEMENT

HEALTHY CHARACTERISTICS

Gives wisdom and sound advice

Courageous

Determined

Sense of purpose

SYMPTOMS OF IMBALANCE

Withdrawing and avoiding others

Fear and anxiety

Fertility or libido problems

SUGGESTIONS FOR BALANCE

Balance taking time for yourself and socializing.

Meditate, read, and pray.

Avoid stress and relieve stress with exercises like yoga or swimming.

Strengthen adrenals and reproductive organs with adaptogenic herbs and mushrooms.

By now, you should have a sense of how the five elements paradigm can help you understand your health, just as it allowed ancient physicians to understand the source of their patients' ailments and treat them accordingly. The approach can be as useful today as it was back then. It can offer insight into your own behavior, and if you apply the five elements to friends and loved ones, it can even allow you to see them and their behavior from a new, more empathetic perspective.

The five elements system can also guide you toward the foods that may be particularly supportive for you. But your body isn't static. It's constantly changing, so your nutritional needs vary, too. As a result, you'll find additional diet advice in upcoming chapters. By utilizing a combination of these strategies, you can make the wisest and most beneficial food choices for your individual needs in any given moment. Here's how to prioritize these highly effective ancient approaches:

Priority #1: Eat to cure the root cause of illness. For instance, if your body is damp internally and the dampness is causing candida and digestive issues, you need to consume foods and herbs that are drying, like celery, pumpkin, cardamom, and thyme. In chapters 11 and 12, you'll find dietary information that will help you address these underlying patterns of imbalance as well as specific illnesses, so you can restore the healthy harmony of your system.

Priority #2: Eat seasonally. Consuming foods in season helps your body adapt to changing weather conditions, as you'll learn in chapter 4. Spring, for instance, is windy, and it's the season when your liver is particularly active, so it's the right time to eat more sour and green foods.

Priority #3: Eat for your element. The diet guidance you've just read in this chapter is based on your element and its inherent strengths and weaknesses. If you're an earth element, for instance, and you're caught in a cycle of excessive worry, you'll want to consume herbs like astragalus and cinnamon to counteract the cortisol and keep your digestive system healthy.

I have personally found the five elements framework—including the nutritional support—to be meaningful, applicable, and beneficial. I rely on it daily to stay emotionally and physically healthy. I hope it enriches and enhances your life as well.

CHAPTER 4

The Ancient Way of Eating

How Food Pairings, Age-Old Meal Habits, and Eating Dirt Can Benefit Your Health

Did you know there's a reason you find curry powder or garam masala in many Indian foods or eat wasabi and ginger with sushi in Japan? Yes, they taste good. But ancient cultures created these meals to bring balance to your body. For instance, many classic Indian dishes feature dampening foods, like goat, cow, or coconut milk. To offset the dampness, they incorporate warming/drying ingredients, like black pepper, paprika, and curry powder (a mixture of ground spices, including turmeric, coriander, and cumin) or garam masala (a blend of nutmeg, clove, cinnamon, coriander, and cumin). Likewise, raw fish, rice, and seaweed are cooling, so to bring harmony to the meal—and, therefore, to your body—sushi dishes are served with warming foods, like wasabi and ginger.

In the United States, this type of ancient wisdom has been lost. Western medicine is so single-mindedly focused on pharmaceuticals that doctors receive little, if any, nutrition training in medical school. As a result, most physicians no longer understand the simple reality that foods are essential to healing, which means that when you visit your MD, you probably won't get any advice on improving your diet. And if you do, it might be dead wrong.

That lapse is one of the most infuriating—and troubling—aspects of modern medicine. But by turning to ancient wisdom, we can fill the gap and vastly improve the nutritional quality and balance of our meals. A number of millennia-old strategies can help. One is combining foods that work synergistically, thereby amplifying their benefits. Another is adopting ancient mealtime habits that can optimize your body's ability to utilize nutrition. And a third is, well, eating dirt. (Later in the chapter, you'll learn why that's one of the healthiest things you can do.) In this chapter, I'll explain how to utilize these strategies, and share a slew of ancient diet secrets that can elevate your eating habits right now.

Combine foods to foster greater internal balance

Ancient practitioners, particularly in the Middle East, China, and India, understood the value of "food combining," an idea that is finally being rediscovered today. A study published in *Planta Medica* found that when you consume turmeric by itself, you absorb very little of the beneficial compounds, including curcumin, into your bloodstream. But when turmeric is combined with piperine, an extract from black pepper, absorption soars by 154 percent.[1]

The scientific community congratulated itself for this finding, but it's a principle that has existed in Ayurvedic medicine for more than three thousand years. The Ayurvedic recipe for golden milk is turmeric plus a warming spice blend called trikatu, which includes black pepper, long pepper, and ginger, mixed with ghee, a type of wholesome clarified butter. Indian healers knew that consuming turmeric along with warming herbs improves its absorption into the bloodstream. And by adding healthy fat from ghee, they increased turmeric's absorption. And turmeric and piperine aren't the only healthful duo out there. Combining the right foods helps you maximize the nutritional value of your meals. The following chart will show you how different food pairings will help you absorb more nutrients.

Combine...	With...	Because...
Vegetables	Healthy fats (avocado, ghee, eggs)	Fat helps your body absorb more phytochemicals from vegetables, like lycopene from tomatoes, beta-carotene from carrots, and lutein from dark green veggies, as well as the fat-soluble vitamins A, D, E, and K.
Iron-rich foods (oatmeal, spinach)	Vitamin C foods (strawberries, citrus fruits)	Vitamin C can increase the absorption of plant-based iron.
Calcium-rich foods (salmon, tuna, egg yolks, milk, broccoli)	Vitamin D foods (salmon, tuna, mackerel, beef liver)	Vitamin D enhances the absorption of calcium in your intestines.
Rice	Beans	The protein in beans helps regulate the carbs in rice, preventing blood sugar spikes.
Healthy fats (avocado, ghee, eggs)	Bitter herbs (parsley and cilantro)	Bitter herbs help release bile from the liver so you can better digest fat.
Carbs	Cinnamon, ginger, cloves, rosemary, sage, and turmeric	These herbs and spices prevent carb-related spikes in blood sugar.
Dairy and eggs	Bitter herbs (peppermint, cardamom, orange peel, fennel, garlic, ginger, and turmeric)	Bitter herbs improve digestion by balancing the dampness of dairy and eggs.

Ancient dietary lessons you won't learn from your doctor

Doctors of old had a deep respect for food and the nourishment and protection it provides for your body, and new studies are confirming that ancient dietary theories can offer the kind of healing that is missing from our meals today. Maimonides, a twelfth-century Jewish physician and philosopher, offered some of the best general advice about eating I've ever read. The author of ten medical books, which combined health instructions from the Torah with ancient medical records from the Greek physicians Hippocrates and Galen, Maimonides offered advice that can guide you to a healthier way of eating. Here are my five favorite pieces of his wisdom:

■ *Eat until you're three-quarters full.* Overeating makes you feel sluggish and sick. Your body can digest only so much food at once, and when food isn't fully digested it causes poor nutrient absorption, gas, and bloating. From the TCM perspective, stuffing yourself causes stagnation, which leads to a number of health problems.

■ *Don't eat until you're warm—and move afterward to promote digestion.* Doing light exercise before you eat is an ancient concept. It gets your body warm and prepares it for digestion. A study published in *World Journal of Gastroenterology*, for instance, showed that a daily schedule of walking and aerobics improves gastric motility and digestion overall.[2] And movement after a meal is helpful, too. A study published in the journal *Medicine* found that walking after a meal, and eating at least three hours before you go to bed, improves digestion and decreases the risk of stomach cancer.[3] When Chelsea and I took a trip to Italy, we walked constantly—before and after eating—and noticed how easily we digested our food, even after a hearty Italian meal.

■ *Consume fruit by itself.* Ayurvedic and Chinese medicine both suggest this. Here's why it makes sense: Your body uses different enzymes to break down fruit than it does to digest meat and grains. Berries are easier to digest with other foods, but you're better off eating other fruits by themselves.

■ *Sleep eight hours—and wake up slightly before sunrise.* This allows your body's internal clock to stay in sync with the circadian rhythms of nature, which bolsters the functions of your body as a whole, including digestion. Maimonides also had advice on sleeping positions that can aid digestion. At the beginning of the night, he said, you should sleep on your left side to get more blood to your small intestine and liver, both of which are involved in digestion. If you awaken in the middle of the night, flip over and spend the latter part of your sleep cycle on your right side, to get blood to your heart and stomach, which prepares you for the day ahead.

   ■ *Eat according to the season.* As I mentioned in chapter 3, ancient Chinese philosophy holds that you should shift your food intake so you're eating foods that are fresh and ripe during each season. (However, if you have an underlying health problem, prioritize the more prescriptive diet advice in chapters 11 and 12.) Seasonal fare gives your body what it needs with the changing weather and temperature. In the summer, for instance, you should opt for cooling foods, like cucumber, melon, and salads with little seasoning. In the spring, consume pickled foods, like vinegar and fermented foods, to help your liver detoxify your body. Spring also tends to be warm and wet, so you want to stay away from dairy and other damp foods. Instead, stick with drying foods, like celery, turnips, and asparagus. In the winter, go for pungent foods that are balanced with sour—things like cooked veggies, parsnips, sweet potatoes, horseradish, garlic, onions, and olives. In the fall, fuel yourself with warming foods and spices, like lamb, pistachio, mustard, ginger, and cinnamon, and balance the chilly dryness of the season with moistening foods, like persimmons.

   In addition to those dietary lessons from Maimonides, here are four other age-old tidbits of eating-related advice that Chelsea and I live by:

   ■ *Savor your meals.* Turn off the TV, stash your phone, set the table, and gather with family and friends for home-cooked meals. Watching TV, scrolling on your phone, or working while eating activates your sympathetic nervous system, which interferes with digestion. It's also important to have fun with your food. Chelsea and I are big-time foodies. We like to play with ingredients and come up with delicious, nutrient-dense creations. One of our favorites is pizza night, featuring our homemade pizza with cauliflower crust, organic tomato sauce, fresh basil, mushrooms, and buffalo mozzarella. We savor every bite!

- *Chew!* Sounds obvious, right? But it's incredible how often I find myself eating while zipping from one place to another—and barely tasting the food. But digestion actually begins in your mouth, with a substance in your saliva known as amylase. There's an old saying, "The stomach has no teeth." Chewing breaks down food before it hits your gastrointestinal tract, maximizing your ability to extract its nutrients.[4] What's more, chewing allows you to enjoy food's flavor, which helps you feel more sated and may reduce your calorie intake.[5]

- *Eat with gratitude and joy.* Throughout the Middle East and Mediterranean, meals are celebrated as a time for nourishment and bonding. Before we eat, Chelsea and I always give thanks to God for the blessing of our food, our families, and all the good things in our lives. From the Biblical and Chinese perspective, the more we appreciate our food, the more nourishment it provides. Food is life-giving fuel that powers every cell in our bodies, from our muscles to our brains, and gives us energy to think, laugh, play, work, and love. That's a lot to be grateful for!

- *Heal your body with tea and soup.* In ancient times, herbal tea, as well as soups made with broth, vegetables, herbs, and rice, were the go-to foods for healing. Ancient cultures typically consumed tea one to three times a day for protective benefits. Chelsea and I have made a habit of starting our day with a cup of tea with a squeeze of fresh lemon. We love doing tea blends, but some of our favorite solo teas include green tea, which reduces inflammation and cholesterol and is a potent antioxidant; oolong tea, which is great for anti-aging and can reduce stress, blood pressure, and blood sugar levels; reishi mushroom tea, which has anti-cancer properties and boosts the immune system; tulsi herb tea, which can combat respiratory ailments and ease arthritis-related joint pain; ginger tea, which relieves nausea, strengthens immunity, and promotes healthy blood circulation; turmeric tea, which is a potent anti-inflammatory and can reduce arthritis pain, boost immune function, and ease irritable bowel symptoms; and chamomile tea, which can promote relaxation and reduce inflammation and blood sugar.

Avoid these three modern products that bear no resemblance to ancient food

Several food items have become so prevalent in our current packaged-food paradigm that people no longer think about the fact that these foods have no roots in the ancient world. Because they weren't a part of ancient diets, these foods shouldn't be part of yours, either. Here's what to avoid:

■ *Sugar and sugar substitutes.* Sugar is naturally found in certain foods, like fruits, vegetables, and dairy, but those foods also contain enzymes, fiber, vitamins, minerals, and antioxidants that slow their digestion, so your blood doesn't get a huge hit of sugar all at once. But that bag of white crystals in your pantry? Or those packaged cereals, cookies, flavored yogurts, sodas, and fruit drinks? They're *toxic.* As John Yudkin, a University of London nutritionist whose 1972 book *Pure, White, and Deadly* was the first to sound the alarm about sugar, said, "If only a small fraction of what we know about the effects of sugar were to be revealed in relation to any other material used as a food additive, that material would promptly be banned." Sugar increases blood pressure and chronic inflammation, causes weight gain (in part, by tricking your body into turning off its appetite-control system), and damages your cardiovascular system. In one fifteen-year study by Harvard researchers, people who got 17 to 21 percent of their calories from added sugar had a 38 percent higher risk of dying from cardiovascular disease than those who consumed 8 percent of their calories from added sugar.[6] And artificial sweeteners are no better. For a hit of sweet, stick with the sweeteners ancients used, like local honey, dates, maple syrup, and molasses. (My desserts in the recipe section call for sweeteners that have been used since the beginning of time.)

■ *Processed oils.* I call them the seven deadly oils: corn, cottonseed, canola, soybean, refined sunflower, safflower, and vegetable. Many are genetically modified Frankenfoods. What's more, hydrogenated oils, found in potato chips, packaged cookies, crackers, and snacks, fried food, coffee creamers, microwave popcorn, and margarine, contain dangerous trans fats, which increase inflammation as well as heart attack and stroke risk, and impair blood sugar control. A *New England Journal of Medicine* study of eighty-five thousand women found that those who consumed the highest amounts of trans fats were at significantly higher risk of developing diabetes. Opt for these oils instead: coconut oil, olive oil, avocado oil, flaxseed oil, ghee, or wild organic animal fat (beef tallow and chicken fat).

■ *Refined grains.* Today's wheat is a far cry from the stuff the ancients ate—it's higher in gluten and carbs and far less nutrient dense. I recommend staying away from most breads and other grain products. Instead, eat rice, congee, oats, and other gluten-free grains. (Sourdough bread is fine, too, since it's fermented.) When the ancients prepared grain for food, it was sprouted, then either fermented or made into congee, a rice dish made by boiling rice in water for twelve to twenty-four hours until it breaks down into a sort of porridge. The Chinese have used congee as a medicinal food since 206 BC. They believe it warms and heals the digestive system, enhances energy circulation (especially if you eat it in the morning), and improves sleep. I prefer congee made from brown rice, but you can make it from corn, quinoa, millet, and most other grains. If you're paleo or keto, try cauliflower congee. And add seasonal ingredients, like mushrooms, seaweed, or mulberries in the winter; celery, green pepper, kiwi, or lemon in the spring; strawberry, apple, tomato, carrot, or beet in the summer; squash, pumpkin, yam, banana, mango, or pineapple in the late summer; and onion, water chestnut, white radish, or cauliflower in the fall.

Protect your gut the way the ancients did: eat dirt (or the next best thing)

Trillions of microorganisms live in your gastrointestinal tract. They help support immune function, enhance nutrient absorption, aid in the synthesis of key brain neurotransmitters (which has been shown to bolster mood), and promote the healthy functioning of your body as a whole. But in order for these microorganisms to protect your health, you need a wholesome balance of good and bad bacteria. When bad bacteria become too abundant (antibiotics are one common cause, as I pointed out in chapter 1), your risk of developing gastrointestinal problems, which can undermine your health as a whole, increases dramatically. But ancient cultures didn't have that problem. They were able to achieve a healthy balance of gut bacteria naturally because their diets contained plenty of probiotics: the beneficial bacteria you get from food.

Before the introduction of refrigeration in the early twentieth century, people got probiotics by eating fresh food from healthy soil that was teeming with bacteria. In addition, for millennia, various cultures around the world stored food by burying it in the ground or putting it in a dirt cellar. They gardened and farmed, and their children played outside—then they'd all come inside and eat.

They literally ate dirt. Sound unhealthy? It's not. Dirt contains soil-based organisms (SBOs), microbes that keep plants healthy and well nourished and help prevent them from becoming contaminated by yeast, fungi, and molds. Without SBOs, plants wither and die. And guess what? These soil-based microorganisms are equally vital for us. (My book, *Eat Dirt*, explains this concept in detail.) In fact, more than eight hundred scientific studies have looked at SBOs and found that they can help relieve allergies, asthma, irritable bowel syndrome, ulcerative colitis, flatulence, nausea, indigestion, nutrient malabsorption, nutrient deficiencies, autoimmune disease, inflammatory disease, and bacterial, fungal, and viral infections.

Even in this age of refrigeration and sanitation, you can find ways to introduce more healthful bacteria into your diet. Here are four of my favorites.

■ *Eat fermented foods.* Before refrigeration, people ate tons of fermented foods. Fermentation not only preserves veggies, fruits, and dairy products, it also promotes the growth of natural bacteria. When you eat fermented food, these helpful microbes inhabit your intestines, where they serve as a first line of defense against harmful bacteria and toxins. Sauerkraut, or fermented cabbage, is a great example. It has nearly one hundred times more lactobacilli, the beneficial bacteria that makes plain yogurt so healthy, than raw cabbage.[7] Much of the sauerkraut that's available in stores now isn't naturally fermented, so it doesn't contain valuable probiotics. But you can still find the good stuff at natural food stores—or make your own. I encourage you to try Asian fermented foods, too, like kimchi, natto, and miso. Research has found that kimchi lowers the risk of heart disease, diabetes, and metabolic syndrome.[8] Natto is made from fermented soybeans that contain *Bacillus subtilis*, a potent probiotic that bolsters the immune system,[9] supports cardiovascular health,[10] and increases circulating levels of vitamin K2,[11] which promotes bone density. Miso (fermented soybeans), a salty staple of the Japanese diet for centuries, has long been used to relieve fatigue, regulate digestion, decrease cholesterol,[12] prevent cancer, and lower blood pressure.[13] Miso is one of my favorite probiotic-rich foods, especially during flu season. It helps strengthen the immune system and the lungs. When it comes to respiratory issues, consuming a classic miso soup is one of the most powerful remedies on the planet. Another healthful fermented food is full-fat kefir, a beverage made from the milk of cows, goats, or sheep. Kefir is one of the most microbe-rich foods in the world, with up to thirty-four different strains of bacteria in each serving—and a staple of my diet. Plain goat's milk and sheep's milk kefir are the healthiest kinds, but coconut kefir is a good option too, especially for vegans. Just avoid versions with added sugar. Likewise, full-fat yogurt contains two super healthy probiotics—lactobacillus and bifidobacterium—and often an array of others. Opt for plain, organic, grass-fed yogurt. Goat's milk and sheep's milk yogurt are my preference, because they contain more nutrients and are less likely to cause digestive issues than cow's milk products. (Goat and sheep milk contain A2 casein, a type of protein that is easier to digest than the A1 casein found in cow's milk.) If you struggle with dampness or candida, avoid dairy for at least a few months as the condition clears; eat coconut kefir and fermented vegetables instead.

■ *Consume raw honey and bee pollen.* Seasonal allergies are on the rise—and one way to combat them is with these two natural beauties. A study on rodents published in *Pharmaceutical Biology* found that a mixture of raw honey and bee pollen offered a significant reduction in inflammation and strengthened immune function.[14] And case studies have shown that an oral regimen of bee pollen can significantly reduce seasonal allergies. When consumed, the microbes in local honey and pollen take up residence in your gut, where they help your immune system adjust to seasonal allergens. Manuka honey, produced in New Zealand by bees that pollinate manuka trees, is one of the most beneficial types of honey—for reasons unrelated to allergies. It has antibacterial properties and has been shown to combat *Clostridium difficile*,[15] a bacterium that causes dangerous gastrointestinal infections; it also inhibits cell division in antibiotic-resistant *Staphylococcus aureus*.[16]

■ *Adopt a dog.* In addition to playing fetch, guess what dogs like to do? Romp around in the dirt. And they bring those diverse, dirt-based microbes into your home, so you get them on your hands—which often go into your mouth. And that's a good thing, because it exposes you to those protective SBOs. Another pet benefit: Exposing infants to dogs or cats in their first year protects them from developing allergies to animals, according to a study in *Clinical and Experimental Allergy*.[17]

■ *Take an SBO probiotic supplement.* Soil-based organisms are missing from our overly clean diets—but we need them. A supplement is an easy way to ensure you get enough. Look for ones that contain *Lactobacillus plantarum*, *Bacillus clausii*, *Bacillus subtilis*, *Bacillus coagulans*, and *Saccharomyces boulardii*. These spore-forming bacteria are able to seed your gut with beneficial microbes, so the protective bacteria will thrive, support healthy digestion and bowel function, and strengthen immunity.

By adopting these ancient lifestyle and dietary strategies, you will make smarter food choices and get the most out of every meal—more nutrition, more satisfaction, more joy. In other words, you'll transform food into what it is meant to be: a source of true sustenance for the body, mind, and soul.

CHAPTER 5

Meals Are Medicine

The Ancestral Foods You Need to Add to Your Diet Right Now

Before the era of pharmaceuticals, food and herbs were the backbone of medicine. Maimonides, the twelfth-century Jewish physician whose wisdom I shared in chapter 4, said, "No disease that can be treated by diet should be treated with any other means." I believe he's right. We should look to our food not only to bring pleasure and to meet our basic nutritional needs, but also to protect our health and help us recover from illness.

Unfortunately, in the United States today, food is the furthest thing from medicinal. In fact, poor diet is a leading cause of many of the country's biggest killers, including heart disease, cancer, stroke, and diabetes. A 2019 study in *The Lancet* analyzed the diets of people in 195 countries and found that about 11 million deaths a year are linked to poor diet—more than are caused by smoking or roadway accidents.[1] Countries where people eat lots of vegetables, fruits, nuts, and healthy oils had the lowest rates of diet-related death and disease. Those with the highest rates were eating way too much sugar, processed meats, sodium (which is high in processed foods), and trans fats. Of the 195 countries included in the report, the United States ranked forty-third, well below Japan, Israel, France, Spain, and other countries.

Today, roughly 77 percent of the American diet consists of processed foods.[2] These packaged products typically have been dried, milled, canned, mixed, or frozen—and they're usually supplemented with dangerous amounts of sugar, sodium, and unpronounceable additives to boot. Not surprisingly, research has found that the more processed foods people consume, the lower their intake of wholesome, nutritious ingredients, like protein, fiber, vitamins A, C, D, and E, zinc, potassium, phosphorus, magnesium, and calcium.[3] In my mind, processed foods are the nutritional equivalent of dangerous pharmaceuticals—products that are marketed as safe and beneficial but actually undermine, and sometimes destroy, your health.

Ancient cultures had no processed foods, so they were more intimately familiar with the effects of real food on the human body—and they recognized, and revered, its healing potential. They intentionally crafted medicine from vegetables, broths, and berries—elderberry syrup was a favorite immune booster and virus fighter—and consumed a slew of healthy straight-from-nature edibles that we've largely forgotten about today. They even recognized that certain foods, thanks to their shape and color, hold obvious clues about the specific ways they can enhance your health. Fortunately, this wisdom hasn't been totally lost. I've gathered what I think is the best of it here. Embracing these ancient remedies and overlooked foods and philosophies will give you a unique opportunity to protect your health—and, if you get sick, to restore it.

The ancient superfoods that need to be in your pantry—and on your plate

In 1902, Thomas Edison predicted a return to the food-is-medicine mindset—a return we're finally starting to see today—when he said, "The doctor of the future will give no medication, but will interest his patients in the care of the human frame, in diet and in the cause and prevention of disease." In the years since Edison uttered those words, our diets have undergone a transformation he couldn't have predicted: Packaged and processed foods have taken over our lives. Many foods that were common in ancient diets around the world gradually disappeared, or were simply ignored, as these convenient, nonperishable items began to dominate our diets.

Now that we understand the dangers of packaged products, it's time to return to those long-lost ancient foods. Some are so essential for your overall health that I tell everyone to add them to their diets ASAP. Here are the top eight foods on my start-eating-these-now (or eat *more* of them) list:

■ *Bone broth.* Made by simmering the bones and ligaments of beef, chicken, fish, and lamb, this nourishing food was a staple for our ancestors, who used every part of an animal as sustenance. But until recently it was almost completely absent from our modern diet. The cooking process triggers the release of healing compounds found within the animal tissue, like collagen, and its amino acids, proline, hydroxyproline, glycine, and glutamine, which help preserve youthful skin and joints. (An added bonus for joints: Bone broth contains chondroitin, glucosamine, and hyaluronic acid, compounds that reduce inflammation and ease arthritis pain.) Getting collagen in your diet is critical, since your skin, hair, nails, bones, discs, ligaments, tendons, connective tissue, gut lining, and blood vessels are all made up largely of collagen. In fact, there is more collagen in your bones than calcium and all other minerals combined! Just as you need to eat muscle-building protein to gain lean muscle, you need to consume collagen to protect these vital tissues. A twenty-four-week study found that athletes who took collagen daily experienced a significant reduction in joint pain.[4] And in a recent randomized, placebo-controlled trial, German researchers found that taking collagen daily improved skin hydration, elasticity, texture, and density.[5] What's more, researchers from University of Nebraska Medical Center found that the amino acids in chicken broth significantly reduced inflammation—one reason it's beneficial for upper respiratory tract infections.[6] Bone broth also contains vital minerals—like calcium, magnesium, phosphorus, and sulfur—all in a form your body can easily absorb. It's healthy for the gut, too, because it promotes the growth of good bacteria, fights sensitivities to wheat and dairy, and reduces inflammation in the digestive tract. And because bone broth contains glutathione, a potent antioxidant, it helps control the healthy regulation of cell proliferation and death. If you don't want to make bone broth on your own, you can buy ready-made versions at the store or make it from a bone broth protein powder. I put one scoop of bone broth protein powder in my ancient superfoods smoothie every morning, and I also take a multi-collagen protein supplement daily. As a result, I get 30 to 40 milligrams of collagen each day, amounting to 20 to 30 percent of my daily dietary protein intake. That's a healthy goal for everyone.

■ *Organ meats.* A basic tenet of TCM is that organ meats from animals support the same organs in your body. And we now know that's true: Organ meats optimize the function of your organs and promote their repair. Ancient cultures intuitively knew that organ meats were some of the most nutrient-rich foods on the planet—far higher in nutrients than the muscle meats we're used to eating. For instance, beef liver contains fifty times as much vitamin B12 as steak. We've gotten away from eating organ meats, often called glandulars, but there are dozens of reasons to add them to your diet. Liver, for instance, is enormously healthy and full of an array of B vitamins, vitamin A, selenium, and folate. Venison, beef, and chicken liver are more nutrient-dense than spinach or kale—and they give your body key nutrients to support the detoxification of your own liver. Other organ meats from cow, lamb, goat, deer, bison, chicken, and duck are nutritious, too. Heart meat has copious amounts of CoQ10, an antioxidant that is useful for preventing and treating high blood pressure and heart disease. Kidney is loaded with selenium and other key nutrients that support adrenal and thyroid health. Spleen, pancreas, thyroid, thymus, and brain are all excellent options as well. The good news: If you have trouble eating organ meats, you can now get the profound benefits of their nutrients in supplement form. I take three grams of a liver capsule supplement that comes from buffalo or venison every day.

■ *Healthy fats.* For years, Western medicine demonized fat as enemy number one for cardiovascular health. But some of the healthiest cultures around the world have eaten high-fat diets for millennia, and their hearts, arteries, brains, and bodies have remained robust. In the Mediterranean and Middle East, for instance, olives and olive oil have long been dietary staples. In South America, avocados have always played a role in daily diets. Coconut is a mainstay in tropical climates, like the Caribbean, and India has been using ghee, or clarified butter, for centuries. Finally, in the past ten years, mainstream American culture has begun to recognize the health value of these high-fat foods. One study published in the *New England Journal of Medicine* compared subjects eating a Mediterranean diet (high in healthy fats) with others eating a low-fat or low-carb diet. The result? Those on the high-fat plan lost the most weight—probably because fat is satisfying to eat and slower to digest, so it keeps you full longer—and slashed their levels of bad cholesterol,[7] a finding that's likely due to the fact that monounsaturated fatty acids have a healthy effect on cholesterol and reduce heart disease risk.[8] What's more, fat is essential for your overall health. You need it to absorb fat-soluble vitamins, like A, D, E, and K, and it's a requirement for maintaining energy levels, building strong cell membranes, and replenishing healthy skin. Plus, eating a variety of high-fat foods can bolster brain function.[9] While you need to steer clear of highly processed fats, like refined vegetable oils, processed meats, and packaged snacks (think: chips, crackers, and cookies)—all of which are legitimately terrible for your heart—I encourage you to embrace ancient fats. Virgin coconut oil is one of my favorites. It contains medium-chain triglycerides (MCTs), which are quicker to burn than other types of fats, making them a great source of fuel. And unlike long-chain fatty acids found in other plant-based oils, MCTs are easy to digest, are not readily stored as fat, and have antimicrobial and antifungal properties. Olive and extra virgin olive oil—staples of the uber-healthy ancient Mediterranean diet—are packed with antioxidants and have the ability to reduce cholesterol and blood pressure,[10] relieve pain,[11] and work as a probiotic, increasing the numbers of good bacteria in your gut.[12] Furthermore, foods like ghee; grass-fed butter; nuts and seeds; eggs; avocado; grass-fed organic beef; full-fat dairy (especially goat or sheep milk products); oily fish like salmon and sardines (packed with super-healthy omega-3 fatty acids); and other coconut-based products can all be a boon for your health.

■ *Herbs and spices.* For millennia, people around the world recognized that these tiny edibles were nutritional powerhouses, but that wisdom was slowly lost. For instance, did you know that turmeric, cilantro, and cinnamon are more nutrient dense than broccoli, kale, and blueberries? Somewhere along the way, we relegated these healing foods to the realm of seasonings—something we sprinkle into recipes to add a bit of zip. Well, no more. A growing body of research has begun confirming what our forebears knew to be true: Herbs and spices are nature's most potent medicine. In chapter 6, I explain which herbs and spices are commonly used to make potent healing tinctures and teas. But some of the most powerful herbs are probably already stashed in your spice rack at home. Some standard favorites, like basil, cumin, coriander, parsley, thyme, rosemary, sage, ginger, garlic, oregano, and turmeric, are packed with polyphenols, plant compounds with potent antioxidant and anti-inflammatory effects. Rosemary is great for reducing inflammation, improving memory, reducing anxiety, enhancing sleep,[13] and even promoting hair growth. Thyme offers a variety of benefits thanks to its anticancer and antimicrobial properties, and in the Mediterranean, it has long been used to treat respiratory disorders. Indeed, recent studies have shown that it can improve underlying physiological issues in those with chronic obstructive pulmonary disease[14] and protect against oxidative damage to the DNA of both cancerous and healthy lung cells.[15] Garlic can reduce cholesterol and high blood pressure.[16] Sage can suppress the stress hormone cortisol, while increasing 5-HT, a neurotransmitter that's often low in those with depression.[17] Oregano is so effective at killing bacteria that I think of it as nature's antibiotic.[18] And the latest scientific studies have shown that ginger, a common folk remedy for nausea, is beneficial not only for relieving an upset stomach, but also for aiding digestion.[19] There's even preliminary evidence that the oils of some of these herbs hold potential for fighting cancer[20] and heart disease[21] and improving cognitive health.[22]

■ *Mushrooms.* Fantastic fungi have been part of healing traditions around the world for centuries, and by now we know quite a bit about their many benefits. Mushrooms contain a type of fiber called beta-glucans, which acts as the fungi's immune system. When you consume mushrooms, their immune system augments and supports your own. Mushrooms also contain ergothioneine, a potent antioxidant that can protect cardiovascular health and reduce the risk of metabolic syndrome. What's more, research shows that specific types of mushrooms confer unique benefits. Lion's mane mushrooms, for instance, can improve anxiety, cognitive function, and depression,[23] probably by enhancing the growth of axons and dendrites, the parts of brain cells that meet at the synapse (the space between cells), enhancing intercellular communication. Reishi mushrooms (known as the mushroom of immortality in Chinese medicine) and cordyceps mushrooms might help shrink tumors[24] and bolster the immune system.[25] Maitake, oyster, and button mushrooms have anticancer properties, too. Cremini mushrooms contain high quantities of vitamin B3, B2, and B5, giving them the potential to treat and prevent fatigue. Shiitakes, meanwhile, have a host of potential benefits, including fighting obesity, supporting immune function and cardiovascular health, and bolstering energy and brain function. Fortunately, many grocery stores carry a variety of mushrooms in the produce section. Sauté a mixture of mushrooms and serve them as a side dish, or add them to soups, stews, and omelets to supercharge your meals.

■ *Berries.* Since the beginning of time, humans have relied on a berry-heavy diet. A variety of berries are readily available in the wild, and early healers from around the world used them in ancient remedies. If I could eat only one category of fruit for the rest of my life it would be berries. Blueberries, raspberries, and blackberries are the most nutrient dense of all fruit. But there are lots of other ancient berries that are loaded with antioxidants and healthy nutrients, and I encourage you to add them to your diet. They're delicious fresh or dried, but can also be taken in supplement or powder form. Elderberry can be particularly helpful in this age of pandemic viruses. It not only bolsters immunity, but can also directly inhibit the flu virus's entry into—and replication within—human cells.[26] Goji berry (also known as wolfberry or lycium) is listed among the top 120 herbs in the *Shen Nong Ben Cao Jing*, the oldest book on Chinese herbs, which dates back to 200 BC. It has been used ever since to strengthen the body and prolong life. Indeed, a study published in the *Journal of Alternative and Complementary Medicine* found that when subjects drank goji berry juice every day for two weeks, they reported improvements in energy, athletic performance, quality of sleep, and ability to focus.[27] Other research has shown that goji berries can help manage blood sugar, improve sexual function, fight cancer by increasing T-cells, and support the immune system.[28] Likewise, triphala, a remedy blended from amla, bibhitaki and haritaki berries, has long been popular in the Middle East and India. In Ayurveda, it became known as the "king of medicines" because it heals the gut lining, improves digestion, reduces intestinal inflammation, and improves irritable bowel syndrome and inflammatory bowel disease. In laboratory and animal studies, it has been shown to treat infections, inflammation, gastrointestinal issues, high cholesterol, and even cancer.[29] Amla, also known as Indian gooseberry, is plenty healthy in its own right. A study in the *European Journal of Clinical Nutrition* found that study subjects who took an amla supplement for four weeks had significant decreases in cholesterol.[30] Other research has shown that it can reduce blood pressure, too.[31] Tart cherry can be helpful for reducing inflammation, including in those with arthritis; drinking tart cherry juice twice a day for three weeks reduced pain in arthritis sufferers, according to research in the *Journal of Food Studies*.[32] Currant (red and black), acai, camu camu, and maqui have also been used for centuries to reduce inflammation and keep people healthy—and are among my favorites as well. I add a tablespoon of goji berry powder to my collagen-boosting smoothie every morning because its high vitamin C content is critical for collagen formation.

▪ *Vegetables.* You might be surprised to learn that the recent wave of enthusiasm for plant-based diets has ancient roots. Vegetables have long been the most recommended foods in all of Chinese medicine—and for good reason. One of the largest studies on the effects of vegetables and fruit intake was published in the *Journal of the National Cancer Institute:* Compared with participants who ate less than 1.5 servings a day, those who consumed eight servings, on average, were 30 percent less likely to have a heart attack or stroke. The foods most associated with cardiovascular protection were leafy greens like spinach, Swiss chard, and kale; broccoli; cauliflower; cabbage; brussels sprouts; and bok choy.[33] Vegetable consumption is also associated with a reduced risk of cancer (including breast, mouth, throat, esophagus, stomach, and lung), diabetes, cataracts, and macular degeneration, and it helps protect gastrointestinal health because the high fiber content of vegetables helps food pass through the system more easily. TCM advises that you consume roasted, steamed, or sautéed vegetables in the fall and winter and a mix of raw and cooked vegetables in the summer and spring. If you have digestive issues, however, stick with cooked vegetables year-round, since they're easier to digest. I fill half my plate with vegetables—an array of different types, including asparagus, broccoli, cauliflower, cabbage, carrots, green beans, brussels sprouts, onions, spinach, and kale.

▪ *Seaweed and super greens.* Seaweed does far more than bring a briny crunch to food. Its high-fiber content promotes digestion, it fights free radicals, it lowers cholesterol,[34] and because it contains healthy quantities of iodine, it supports thyroid health. Some of my favorite seaweeds are wakame, ogo, nori, kombu, and hijiki. Spirulina, a type of blue-green algae, is a seaweed too, and it comes with seriously jaw-dropping benefits. It is helpful for detoxing heavy metals, including arsenic; has antimicrobial properties and may be particularly helpful against candida; fights cancer, according to more than seventy peer-reviewed scientific papers; bolsters energy; and reduces blood pressure and cholesterol. Chlorella is a green algae that, as its name implies, is loaded with chlorophyll (the substance that makes plants green), giving it a range of benefits. It can protect you from exposure to heavy metals by decreasing their absorption[35] and it bolsters immunity,[36] both of which can help protect you from cancer. It lowers blood sugar and cholesterol as well.[37] Moringa, a tropical plant, has gained a reputation for fighting inflammation. It's also a libido and immune system booster that has been used in Ayurvedic medicine for years to prevent or treat stomach ulcers, liver disease, kidney damage, digestive issues, and fungal and yeast infections, including candida. Cilantro's fresh flavor has become popular, but you probably didn't know that it also bolsters heart health by lowering cholesterol and blood sugar,[38] settles digestive upset, and protects against some strains of bacteria that cause food poisoning.[39] Parsley has similarly impressive benefits, including providing relief from bloating, improving digestion, reducing bad breath, protecting bones (thanks to its heavy dose of vitamin K), and potentially fighting cancer. In Chinese medicine, parsley is used as a treatment for hypertension, cardiac disease, and urinary tract infections as well. Wheat grass juice, which was a favorite among ancient Egyptians, who used it to support their health and vitality, can increase the absorption of electrolytes and vitamins C and E. It can also reduce free radical damage, reduce cancer risk, support the effects of chemotherapy,[40] and help lower cholesterol.

The ancient strategy that can guide you toward specific foods that are right for you

In the preceding chapters, I shared some of the most effective eating strategies from the ancient world. But there's another fascinating approach that can help you home in on specific foods that are best for *you*. Known as the doctrine of signatures, or "like supports like," the theory says that foods that look like a body part are beneficial for that body part. Paracelsus, a Swiss physician in the fifteenth century, explained it this way: "Nature marks each growth...according to its curative benefit." Take carrots. Slice one open, and you'll see that it actually looks like an eye. Today there are numerous medical studies that have proven that the nutrients in carrots, like beta-carotene and lutein, improve eye health.

The idea that nature holds clues for how to use food medicinally was hit upon, seemingly independently, by a variety of cultures around the world, from Asia to the Middle East. Pliny the Elder, the Roman naturalist who died in AD 79, was the first to mention it in the West—and the idea was picked up through the years by a number of well-known physicians and botanists. William Coles, a seventeenth-century botanist, wrote that God "stamped upon [edible plants] a distinct forme but also hath given them particular Signatures whereby a man may read the use of them." Although the idea is generally scoffed at in the West today, I believe he was right. Here are some super healthy foods that science has shown abide by the doctrine of signatures. You can also use this as a guide to the foods that can treat your health weaknesses.

■ *Carrots resemble eyes—and bolster vision.* These crunchy veggies are great sources of lutein and beta-carotene, antioxidants that support eye health and protect against age-related eye diseases like macular degeneration. What's more, beta-carotene converts into vitamin A, which helps you see in the dark.[41]

■ *Walnuts look like mini brains—and are the best nut for brain health.* Research in mice with Alzheimer's has shown that a walnut-heavy diet improves memory and learning,[42] and studies of aging people have shown that eating walnuts improves cognitive processing speed, mental flexibility, and memory.[43]

■ *Celery stalks look similar to bones—and protect bone health.* Celery contains silicon, which contributes to bone strength. It's also an excellent source of vitamin K, which works with calcium to build strong bones, and potassium, which neutralizes acids that erode bone calcium.

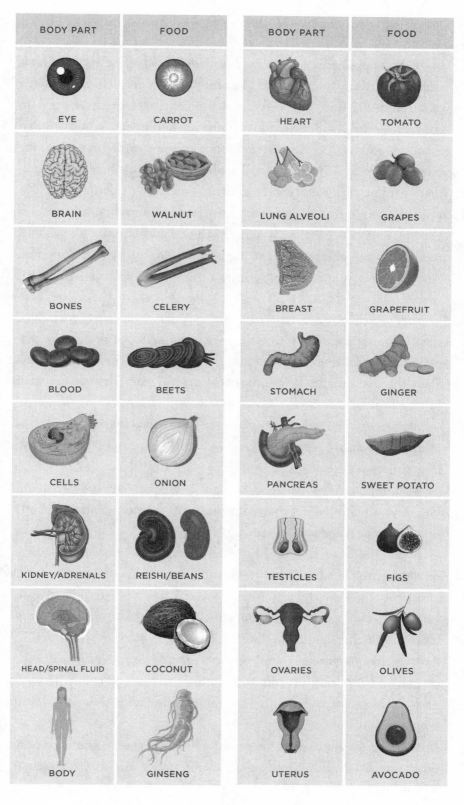

BODY PART	FOOD	BODY PART	FOOD
EYE	CARROT	HEART	TOMATO
BRAIN	WALNUT	LUNG ALVEOLI	GRAPES
BONES	CELERY	BREAST	GRAPEFRUIT
BLOOD	BEETS	STOMACH	GINGER
CELLS	ONION	PANCREAS	SWEET POTATO
KIDNEY/ADRENALS	REISHI/BEANS	TESTICLES	FIGS
HEAD/SPINAL FLUID	COCONUT	OVARIES	OLIVES
BODY	GINSENG	UTERUS	AVOCADO

■ *Beets are blood red—and can help with anemia, blood flow, and blood pressure.* Rich in iron, these red beauties can bolster hemoglobin, the red protein in blood that's responsible for oxygen transport. Beets also contain nitrates, which transform into nitric oxide, a substance that dilates blood vessels, lowering blood pressure and improving the body's ability to deliver oxygen-rich blood to tissues. Research shows that beet juice improves exercise stamina up to 16 percent.[44]

■ *Onions resemble cells—and protect them.* Onions contain vitamin C, which shields cells from damage caused by unstable free radical molecules, and potassium, which is required for normal cell function. And because they contain sulfur, onions can protect cells from cancer.

■ *Tomatoes look like heart chambers—and they're cardioprotective.* Slice open a tomato and you'll find heart-like chambers. Studies show that eating tomatoes reduces blood pressure, protects the heart from damage during a heart attack, improves survival rates in patients with heart failure, and reduces the risk of stroke.

■ *Grape clusters look like lung alveoli—and protect lungs.* Grapes contain anthocyanins, a type of flavonoid that's critical for maintaining lung function as you age.

■ *Ginger looks like a stomach—and is a potent antidote for nausea.* Gingerol, the ingredient that gives ginger its tangy taste, has the ability to prevent nausea and vomiting.

■ *Sweet potatoes are shaped like a pancreas—and promote its healthy functioning.* In TCM, sweet potatoes are used to support the spleen and pancreas. And even though they're "sweet," they contain slow-release carbs and the hormone adiponectin, which help promote healthy blood sugar, thereby helping the pancreas do its job.

■ *Reishi mushrooms resemble kidneys and adrenals—and support these glands.* In TCM, reishi is considered a tonic for qi, and studies show it promotes energy and stamina, even in those with fatigue-causing conditions like fibromyalgia.[45]

■ *Avocados look like a uterus—and support reproductive health.* Avocados contain a healthy dose of folic acid, a B vitamin that's crucial during pregnancy for the health of the baby and can reduce the risk of cervical dysplasia, a precancerous condition.

■ *Figs resemble testicles—and they benefit sperm.* They've long been used to enhance fertility, and recent research has confirmed that fig extract can improve sperm count and motility.[46]

■ *Olives look like ovaries—and protect reproductive health.* Healthy fats are critical for manufacturing the reproductive hormones necessary for conception, and they're good for maintaining general reproductive health in both men and women.

■ *Coconuts look like heads—and coconut oil is good for brain health.* Research shows that consuming medium-chain triglycerides, the type of fat in coconut oil, can improve brain function in people with mild forms of Alzheimer's.[47]

■ *Ginseng roots look like mini humans—and support whole-body health.* Ginseng is used to increase energy, improve cognition, reduce blood sugar and stress, promote relaxation, and enhance overall well-being.

■ *Organ meat and glandulars from animals support the same organ in people.* As I mentioned above, livers of beef and chicken, for instance, have extremely high levels of B vitamins, including vitamin B12, which promotes liver health. Animal hearts contain CoQ10 and iron, both of which support the human cardiovascular system. Muscle meat, like chicken breast and steak, supports healthy muscle tissue. Likewise, bone broth enhances our bone marrow, bones, ligaments, tendons, gut lining, and skin—all of which are made up of collagen.

I'm thrilled to be able to share these ancient secrets with you. They've been hidden too long. By eating more like the ancients did, you'll give your body the fuel it needs to fight viral and bacterial infections, power through your days with plenty of energy, and function at your highest level.

PART II

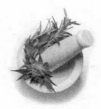

Your Ancient Pharmacy

CHAPTER 6

The Healing Value of Herbs, Spices, and Mushrooms

How to Use the Potent Medicine Available in Your Local Grocery Store

Recently, my father, who is seventy and lives in Florida, was waterskiing. (Yes, you read that right.) It was December, so the water was a chilly 60 degrees. Several days later, he was hospitalized with pneumonia. His physicians put him on high-dose antibiotics, but I didn't believe he needed them. So I flew to Florida and said, "Dad, we are going to get you out of here"—and I brought him to my home in Nashville.

I called Gil Ben-Ami and Dr. Anis Khalaf, two of my closest friends and colleagues, who have vast experience with ancient medicine. I often consult with them on serious or challenging cases. This time, we put together a program to expel the water from my dad's lungs and strengthen his immune system, since what he really needed was strong internal defenses to fight the bug causing his illness.

Dr. Anis gave him acupuncture treatments, and I treated him with cupping. We also had my dad consume a diet designed specifically to strengthen his immune system and lung function. It included chicken bone broth soup, baked pears with walnuts, and steamed asparagus, cauliflower, and radishes with tahini. At the same time, we had him take a combination of herbs, including astragalus, elderberry, echinacea, ginger, licorice, and garlic. Finally, we had him watch funny movies and consciously try to cultivate joy, because the metal element (remember, the lungs correspond with metal) can be hampered by sadness. And of course I prayed for him every day.

In just a few weeks, my dad was as good as new. When he went back to Florida, I told him he wasn't allowed to water-ski for a month, and I advised him to drink warming beverages and herbs before and after skiing in chilly conditions.

I realize that goes against everything Western medicine wants us to believe, which is that pharmaceuticals are the only way to cope with disease. But ancient doctors would have considered the pills and tablets inside those ever-present amber bottles toxic to the body. Early physicians relied on herbs, spices, mushrooms, organ meats, and essential oils—gentle, natural remedies that successfully treat a vast range of conditions by restoring balance to the body. Even today, throughout the Middle East, India, and Asia, herbal formulas and teas are used for healing—yet most of these treatments are still disregarded, demeaned, and even concealed by Western medicine. As a result, you've never heard of, much less used, some of the safest, least expensive, and most effective medicines available—including medications that can disable viruses and bolster your immune system.

Well, that's about to change. In this chapter and the three that follow, I provide an in-depth guide to these buried secrets, complete with practical information on what conditions they can treat, and the latest science supporting their effectiveness. When I began learning about these approaches, I was stunned that this alternate universe existed, and I was eager to begin practicing medicine in a way that was guided by millennia-old traditions. The intervening years have only made me more enthusiastic about these overlooked healing jewels. As you learn more about how these approaches work, and come to understand why these ancient remedies can transform your health in ways that toxic prescription meds never will, I believe that you'll begin to share my excitement.

Meet nature's most potent medicines — and learn how they can optimize your health

Like medications, herbs and mushrooms contain active ingredients, each of which makes these simple plants particularly good at targeting specific health problems. In chapter 4, I provided a quick overview of some well-known culinary herbs, spices, and mushrooms and the ways they can improve your health. Now I want to take a more in-depth look at some of the plants I've already mentioned — and introduce you to some of my favorite lesser-known remedies, along with how to use them. With any herbal supplement that has a range of dosages, start with the lowest to see how it makes you feel, then take more as needed. Here are eleven common health problems and the superstar herbs and mushrooms that can treat them:

The top immunity boosters and virus fighters

Your immune system is on duty round-the-clock, fighting bacteria and viruses, getting rid of dead or dying cells, clearing away mutated cells that could turn into cancer, and scanning for foreign substances. In other words, keeping it strong is one of the most important things you can do for your health — especially when new bugs come along, like the novel Covid-19 virus. To keep your internal defenses as robust as possible, add these potent herbs to your stay-well arsenal now.

- *Reishi.* Known as the "mushroom of immortality," this adaptogen strengthens adrenal qi, enhances longevity, and supports and strengthens immunity. In TCM, reishi is the most widely prescribed medicinal mushroom. I use it on a regular basis to keep my immune system strong, and it was one of the go-to supplements I had my mom take when she was fighting (and overcame) cancer, because it not only strengthens the immune system, but has also been shown to be specifically effective against cancer, especially tumors in the lung, breast, prostate, and bone.[1] Research shows that reishi increases the activity of natural killer cells.[2]

This mushroom actually needs antibacterial and antiviral compounds to survive, so it naturally contains significant quantities of these substances. Not surprisingly, studies show that this super fungus has the ability to fight a number of viruses, including herpes and influenza A—a strain that's common during most flu seasons. A paper published in the *British Journal of Sports Medicine* found that a reishi supplement improved the function of lymphocytes (one of the main types of immune cells) in athletes exposed to stressful conditions.[3] They're also high in triterpenes, which can reduce allergies and asthma. Reishi are available in capsule, powder, or tincture form. Check the package for the species name, *Ganoderma lucidum*. Use 2 to 9 grams a day.

■ *Elderberry.* Elderberry-based medicines date back to ancient Egypt, and Hippocrates described the plant as his "medicine chest" because it could mitigate such a huge array of health concerns. Thanks to its high content of anthocyanidins (plant pigments with potent antimicrobial properties), elderberries can be exceedingly helpful against viruses and bacteria. When used within the first forty-eight hours of the onset of cold or flu symptoms, for instance, an extract of elderberry may shorten the duration of the illness.[4] A study published in *Nutrients* found the extract can reduce cold duration and severity among air travelers.[5] There's also evidence that it can help treat bacterial sinusitis.[6] What's more, it can act as a natural diuretic, ease allergies, and help prevent cancer. Look for elderberry syrup, the most effective form of the herb, for treating viral and bacterial infections. Take according to package directions.

■ *Echinacea.* Native Americans used this botanical remedy to treat mumps and measles—and early settlers adopted the practice. Today, it's known best for its cold-slaying power. One study in *Lancet Infectious Diseases* found it reduces the risk of catching a cold by 58 percent.[7] And if you take it when your symptoms first appear, it can save you from coming down with a full-on cold, or at least limit its duration.[8] What's more, a 2015 study found that the herb was as effective as prescription Tamiflu for treating the flu.[9] Liquid forms of the supplement may be the most beneficial. For cold prevention, take 2,400 milligrams daily for four months during cold and flu season. To treat a cold, take 500 milligrams twice a day for 10 days.

■ *Andrographis.* This super-herb is used in both Ayurvedic medicine and TCM, and was referred to as "king of the bitters." Its bitter flavor activates the liver, which spurs blood circulation, reducing inflammation; it also helps eliminate dampness from the body, which aids the immune system. Alone, or as part of a multiherb product, andrographis has been shown to lessen the intensity of coughs and sore throats. A double blind, placebo-controlled trial published in *Phytomedicine* showed that an andrographis extract was 50 percent more effective than a placebo at treating a range of cold symptoms.[10] The herb's key ingredient, andrographolide, enhances several virus-fighting components of the immune system, including the activity of T cells (cells that help determine the immune system's response to foreign substances), natural killer cells (white blood cells that fight infections and cancer), and phagocytes (cells that protect the body by ingesting bacteria, viruses, and other foreign particles), which hamper virus replication and prevent viral illnesses from developing.[11] Look for a supplement that contains andrographolide; take 4 milligrams three times a day when you're fighting a cold or flu bug.

■ *Honorable mention:* Astragalus, thyme, oregano, sage, eucalyptus, myrrh, goldenseal, garlic, and turkey tail mushrooms.

The proven digestion supporters

The obvious symptoms of gut issues can be distressing enough on their own, but they also have negative ramifications on the rest of your health, especially your mood and your immunity. Here are three natural ways to support gut health.

■ *Astragalus.* Likely the number one prescribed herb in all of Chinese medicine, astragalus is, in my opinion, an herb all of us could benefit from using on a regular basis. It is incredibly effective at protecting and enhancing both digestion and immune function, which makes sense given that strengthening your gut health is one of the best ways to boost your immune system. The protective effects of astragalus are likely due to its high levels of flavonoids, polysaccharides (long chains of carbohydrate molecules), and saponins (a class of chemicals found in certain plants), which, according to a recent study in *Evidence-Based Complementary and Alternative Medicine*, can improve your cellular health.[12] As a result, it has a powerful impact on conditions like leaky gut syndrome, candida, hypothyroidism, IBD, autoimmune disease, colds, viruses, chronic inflammation, and cancer. And that's not all. A review paper published in *Aging and Disease* reported that astragalus is an effective anti-aging substance. It actually helps reverse the cellular aging process by increasing the activity of telomerase, an enzyme that prevents the shrinkage of telomeres, the caps at the end of each strand of DNA that protect chromosomes. As a result, it keeps us young.[13] Other research shows that astragalus reduces stress, fights inflammation, protects the brain as it ages, and fights cancer.[14] This herb acts as an adaptogen, and it is gentle, so it can be taken in low to moderate doses daily or used at higher doses to fight more severe illness. Take astragalus per package instructions; the most common dose is 500 to 2,000 milligrams daily.

■ *Ginger.* I bet you already know about the most common use of ginger: It helps treat nausea. One review of twelve studies found that ginger effectively decreased nausea in pregnant women.[15] Another study found that the same was true for chemotherapy patients.[16] This pungent root can also prevent the formation of stomach ulcers, possibly by decreasing levels of inflammatory proteins and blocking the activity of enzymes related to ulcer development.[17] One final benefit: Ginger supports digestive health (and may prevent gastrointestinal symptoms) by accelerating stomach emptying by as much as 25 percent, according to a study in *World Journal of Gastroenterology*.[18] Add thin slices to smoothies; grate it into soups, salads, and sauces; or juice it with other vegetables. Supplements and powders are also available. For nausea, use 1,000 to 2,500 milligrams.

■ *Triphala.* Made from the dried powder of three different fruits—amla, haritaki, and bibhitaki—this Ayurvedic formula is a natural laxative. It's gentler than most over-the-counter products and nourishes the digestive tract as it encourages elimination. It also naturally cleanses the colon, which has a positive effect on the nervous system, including symptoms like fatigue and anxiety. When it comes to elimination, amla supports intestinal repair and healing, haritaki strengthens the intestinal muscles to contract more efficiently, and bibhitaki cleanses. The combination can be healing. One animal study showed that triphala can reduce colitis in rats.[19] Triphala can also lower cholesterol and promote weight loss. If you're using triphala as a laxative, take it in the evening, about two hours after eating and at least thirty minutes before bed.

■ *Honorable mention:* Slippery elm, licorice, cardamom, fennel, and peppermint.

The anti-aging, beauty-enhancing superstars

The beauty industry is constantly touting the latest "it" ingredients, many of which come and go quickly. But these ancient plant-based treasures have stood the test of time. They will help you look—and feel—younger.

■ *Fo-ti.* In TCM, this anti-aging herb actually has its own legend: Hundreds of years ago, an ill man named Mr. He was forced to subsist on wild plants, including fo-ti, during a famine. Instead of suffering, his health improved. His skin became more youthful, his energy rebounded, and his graying hair returned to its original black. Today, fo-ti is known to be a potent anti-inflammatory that is used to treat acne and protect skin from aging. What's more, a study in the *Journal of Advanced Pharmaceutical Technology and Research* found that it activates a signaling pathway that is down-regulated in graying hair.[20] There's also evidence it can protect your memory. Look for fo-ti supplements that contain *Polygonum multiflorum*, the plant's Latin name. Take as directed—usually 560 milligrams two to three times a day— but don't overdo it. Although fo-ti has been used safely for hundreds of years, high doses of the herb may harm the liver.

■ *Schisandra.* Chinese emperors and Taoist masters were fans of schisandra, and in the 1960s Russian scientists discovered that it bolsters adrenal function and balances the negative effects of stress.[21] Historically, schisandra was used to heal liver disease, strengthen the immune system (especially to overcome conditions like mononucleosis and pneumonia), and balance blood sugar. Schisandra is one of the only foods in the world that has all five flavors—pungent, sweet, sour, bitter, and salty—which gives it the ability to bring balance to the entire body. As a result, it has long been a key ingredient in many TCM herbal formulas. More recent research has shown it can fight mental fatigue and exhaustion,[22] and it's a natural beauty tonic that can protect the skin from wind and sun exposure as well as toxins. Put powdered schisandra in a smoothie (use about 3 grams a day), take a supplement (1 to 3 grams daily, with a meal), or make it into a tea by steeping 1 to 3 grams in hot water for forty to sixty minutes before drinking.

■ *Matcha.* This wonder food has more antioxidants than blueberries and leafy greens. And since the powder form is made of ground tea leaves, its antioxidants are super concentrated, making it a potent anti-aging beverage. What's more, matcha's bright green color comes from its off-the-charts chlorophyll content—and guess what chlorophyll can do? Protect the skin from the damaging rays of the sun that cause wrinkles and age spots. It also contains epigallocatechin gallate (EGCG), which helps rejuvenate skin cells, promote skin strength, and prevent cancer. I drink a cup or two of matcha every day. You can also use it topically to moisturize and rejuvenate your skin. Just mix matcha powder with coconut oil and apply a light coating. Let it seep into your pores for ten minutes, then wash off.

■ *Honorable mention:* Goji berry, astragalus, royal jelly, and ginseng.

The best energy boosters and adrenal supporters

Lack of energy was one of the most common complaints I heard in my functional medicine clinic—and I came to rely on these three treatments to help patients regain their vitality.

■ *Rehmannia.* In TCM, this herb is the go-to choice for treating yin deficiency and fatigue, its hallmark symptom. It's also useful for treating qi deficiency and is the most prescribed herb in Asia for adrenal fatigue, hypothyroidism, and boosting stem cell production. There's scientific evidence that rehmannia is helpful for treating anemia,[23] strengthening bones, supporting heart health, nourishing blood, and reducing inflammation. The standard dosage is between 55 and 350 milligrams a day. (Don't take it if you're pregnant or breastfeeding or have chronic liver disease.)

■ *Panax ginseng (Asian and American).* Used in both Asia and North America for centuries, ginseng is known for improving physical endurance as well as mental focus—and it's often prescribed as a treatment for chronic fatigue as well. A 2018 literature review published in the *Journal of Alternative and Complementary Medicine* concluded that ginseng can indeed be effective in fighting fatigue.[24] Ginseng can be taken for ten to thirty days to treat infections like colds, flu, pneumonia, or any major immune weakness. It's also helpful as an energy-boosting long-term daily supplement for those over fifty-five. Take 500 milligrams twice a day.

■ *Cordyceps.* This medicinal mushroom is a longtime staple of holistic medicine, and it's known for its ability to optimize energy and combat the effects of aging and stress. It has been shown to significantly increase the amount of time rodents can swim, probably because it boosts the production of adenosine triphosphate (ATP), the main energy source for the body's cells.[25] Indeed, a study published in the *Journal of Alternative and Complementary Medicine* found that cordyceps supplementation improved exercise performance and contributed to overall wellness in older adults.[26] Take 1,000 to 3,000 milligrams a day to improve energy.

■ *Honorable mention:* Rhodiola (an herb with roots that are considered an adaptogen, a substance that helps deal with stress and balance hormones), eleuthero (also known as Siberian ginseng), and matcha green tea.

The brain-optimizing all stars

If you're like most people, keeping your mind sharp as you age is likely a top concern. Western medicine has little to offer on this front, but these three ancient remedies really work.

■ *Lion's mane.* This quirky-looking mushroom, which resembles the scruff of a lion, has long been popular in Chinese medicine for its ability to enhance brain function. Now, studies have revealed that this incredible fungus may offer hope for those with Alzheimer's and Parkinson's, because it supports the growth of brain cells' axons and dendrites, which in turn might slow or reverse brain degeneration. Animal studies have found that lion's mane can improve memory in those with and without Alzheimer's.[27] What's more, a double-blind, placebo-controlled trial in humans determined that it improves mild cognitive impairment[28] and may hinder the advancement of Parkinson's disease.[29] It's also great for anyone looking to improve focus, boost memory, and enhance the gut-brain connection to enhance mood. You can safely take 300 to 3,000 milligrams, one to three times a day, but start with a smaller dose to see how your body responds.

■ *Bacopa.* Ayurvedic healers have used this plant (also known as brahmi) to treat brain-related disorders for thousands of years, and new research is confirming its effectiveness. In one double-blind, placebo-controlled trial, Australian researchers found that people who took 300 milligrams of bacopa for twelve weeks showed improvement in learning and memory. They were also significantly faster at processing visual information than they had been pre-study, as well as compared to those in the placebo group.[30] A meta-analysis published in the *Journal of Ethnopharmacology* reviewed nine scientific studies and concluded that bacopa holds promise for improving cognition,[31] possibly because it increases brain chemicals that are involved in thinking, learning, and memory. The plant might also be helpful for anxiety, depression, ADHD, and schizophrenia. Effective dosages range from 300 to 450 milligrams per day.

■ *Ginkgo biloba*. Also known as maidenhair, ginkgo biloba is a potent anti-inflammatory and is one of the most widely investigated—and commonly used—herbs for improving brain health. Ginkgo contains flavonoids and terpenoids, antioxidants that may slow the progression of age-related cognitive decline. The herb may also be helpful in slowing Alzheimer's, according to a study in *Phytomedicine*.[32] People with dementia should use 40 milligrams three times a day, while healthy people who want to improve their cognitive function can use 120 to 600 milligrams daily. Look for ginkgo preparations that contain 24 to 32 percent flavonoids and 6 to 12 percent terpenoids.

■ *Honorable mention:* CBD oil, frankincense oil, rosemary, ginseng, rhodiola, and ashwagandha.

The ancient candida cures

The fungal infection known as candida is too often overlooked as an underlying cause of disease, but it can contribute to everything from oral thrush and sinus infections to fatigue and joint pain. These ancient treatments can combat the infection at its source.

■ *Pau d'arco*. A South American herb, pau d'arco is known as an inflammation fighter, with antiviral, antiparasitic and antifungal properties as well. It contains chemicals known as naphthoquinones, including lapachol and beta-lapachone, which can kill a variety of bacteria, viruses, and fungi. One study on lapachol found it was as effective as prescription drugs in fighting *Candida albicans*,[33] a major cause of fungal infections. Take 1 to 2 milliliters of a liquid extract three times a day or two to four 500-milligram pau d'arco capsules once or twice a day.

■ *Cinnamon*. If you use this common spice only in holiday recipes, you're missing out on one of the healthiest edibles on the planet. When researchers in Hong Kong tested the antioxidant capacity of twenty-six herbs and spices, cinnamon was in the top three, along with clove and oregano.[34] It's also an anti-inflammatory and a potent antifungal, and has been shown to lower cholesterol, blood pressure, and blood sugar. When Chinese researchers gave cinnamon oil to patients with *Candida albicans* in the gut, 72 percent cleared the fungus within fourteen days and the other 28 percent showed a significant reduction.[35] I sprinkle cinnamon into smoothies, coffee, oatmeal, and many recipes. To reap optimal benefits, use organic Ceylon cinnamon powder (which contains only trace amounts of coumarin, a substance that, in large quantities, can cause liver problems), cinnamon essential oil, or cinnamon pills or capsules. Take as directed.

■ *Garlic.* This potent plant is a true superfood, with more than 6,100 peer-reviewed studies attesting to its ability to fight a range of ailments, from heart disease to cancer. When you crush or chop a fresh clove, two substances—allicin and alliinase—combine to form agoene, a powerful antifungal. In a lab study published in the *Journal of Applied Microbiology*, researchers in the United Kingdom found that fresh garlic can inhibit the growth of *Candida albicans.*[36] What's more, it's an antibacterial and antiviral, and has been shown to be effective against the flu, colds, and viral pneumonia.[37] Take 2 to 5 grams (roughly one medium-size clove) of minced fresh garlic, or 600 to 900 milligrams of freeze-dried raw garlic, per day.

■ *Honorable mention:* Oregano, clove, and alisma (water plantain).

The natural inflammation tamers

Short-term inflammation—the pain and swelling after an injury, say—is healthy. But chronic inflammation is a scourge, and it's one of the root causes of most diseases that plague our modern culture, including cancer, Alzheimer's, arthritis, chronic pain, depression, heart disease, and autoimmune disease. If you're striving for optimal health, reducing inflammation should be near the top of your list. (CBD is one of the hottest inflammation-tamers around. I'll give you the lowdown in chapter 7.)

■ *Turmeric.* It's difficult to overestimate the inflammation-fighting power of turmeric, most of which is due to curcumin, its active ingredient. Turmeric works to fight inflammation by both nourishing and moving the blood, which speeds healing. A study in the journal *Oncogene* evaluated the efficacy of a number of anti-inflammatories, including aspirin and ibuprofen, and found that curcumin was more effective than either one.[38] Turmeric can also reduce depression, curb Alzheimer's, improve symptoms in those with arthritis, help manage diabetes, and kill cancer cells. Using turmeric in food is great, but just 3 percent of the powdered form is actually curcumin. To take advantage of its benefits, take 500 to 2,000 milligrams per day of a supplement that contains 95 percent curcumin.

■ *Boswellia.* This resin extracted from the frankincense tree is high in terpenes, the strong-smelling antioxidant phytochemicals in eucalyptus, basil, and peppermint. But it also contains a number of other substances that can slash inflammation, including AKBA, which targets inflammatory enzymes, and incensole acetate, which is particularly good at protecting neurons and fighting brain inflammation. Take 600 to 700 milligrams of a boswellia supplement (it should contain at least 37 percent boswellic acids or boswellin) several times a day. Or put a few drops of frankincense oil, which is made from boswellia, under your tongue every day.

■ *Chaga.* This mushroom has been used for thousands of years across Asia and in Siberia. It's known for boosting energy, strengthening immunity, and lowering inflammation. Chaga is an adaptogen, a unique category of healing plants that help stabilize your body's hormones and ease the effects of stress. Chaga mushrooms also have one of the highest oxygen radical absorbance capacity (ORAC) scores of any food, making them healthy in numerous ways. As for inflammation, laboratory and animal studies have found that these fungi can reduce the problem by preventing the production of inflammation-triggering cytokines. Chaga mushrooms are available as a tincture, capsule, tablet, or powder. You can also find mushroom coffee or tea that includes chaga. Use the products as directed.

■ *Honorable mention:* Galangal (a stem plant similar to ginger), ginger, rosemary, and skullcap.

The first-rate heart and blood protectors

Your heart and blood are life-giving. Protect them from disease with these two ancient herbs.

■ *Dong quai.* In TCM, this is one of the most recommended herbs for women. It's the number one herb for strengthening blood to fight anemia, a top five herb for balancing hormones, and it is known as female ginseng because of its ability to boost energy. This herb can also lower blood sugar, thereby helping to prevent diabetes. Research published in the journal *Food and Function* showed that mice who were given dong quai for four weeks had lower blood sugar levels and better insulin function.[39] Likewise, the same study showed that treating mice with dong quai for four weeks decreased their levels of total cholesterol as well as triglycerides—an outcome that can help prevent heart disease. And dong quai may be beneficial for those with high blood pressure, another heart disease risk factor. Take 2 to 4 grams of a supplement, divided into three doses, per day.

■ *Hawthorn.* Often called the "heart herb," hawthorn is prized for its ability to treat heart-related ailments, an ability that probably stems from its high antioxidant content. Studies have found that it can lower blood pressure, treat angina, reduce cholesterol, and treat patients with heart failure. In a paper published in *Preventive Cardiology* on herbs for the treatment of heart disease, the author, a researcher from George Washington University School of Medicine, highlighted hawthorn's benefits for those with congestive heart failure.[40] If you don't have a cardiovascular problem, there's no need to take it. If you do, take up to 1,800 milligrams a day for no more than twenty-four weeks. It may take up to twelve weeks for symptoms to improve. (Don't take hawthorn if you're pregnant or breastfeeding, and don't give it to children.)

■ *Honorable mention:* Peony, reishi, cinnamon, holy basil, turmeric, and green tea.

The age-old hormone balancers

Hormones govern everything from mood to menstrual cycles, fertility, and metabolism. Keeping them at healthy levels can help your body function optimally. Here are four herbs that shine in this realm.

- *Ashwagandha.* A potent adaptogen, this herb is great at balancing hormones. If you have low thyroid (hypothyroidism), ashwagandha can normalize it. If you have high blood sugar or high cholesterol, ashwagandha can lower it. It has the same balancing effect on stress, anxiety, and depression—all of which are controlled by hormones. Take 300 to 500 milligrams per day of a supplement that contains 5 to 10 percent withanolides (naturally occurring hormones). Many supplement instructions suggest taking between 1,000 and 1,500 milligrams per day, but work your way up to that.

- *Vitex.* One of the most popular herbal remedies for PMS and cramps, vitex helped decrease PMS-related complaints in 93 percent of study subjects according to a paper published in the *Journal of Women's Health and Gender-Based Medicine.*[41] Vitex (also known as chasteberry) can also improve fertility. In one double-blind, placebo-controlled trial, researchers from Stanford University School of Medicine gave fifty-three women who had tried unsuccessfully to conceive for six to thirty-six months an herbal blend containing vitex, as well as green tea, vitamins, and minerals, while forty women received a placebo. The menstrual cycles of the women taking the vitex blend normalized, and fourteen of the women (26 percent) became pregnant within three months, while another three conceived after six months. On the other hand, only four of the women in the placebo group got pregnant.[42] There's also evidence that vitex treats endometriosis, amenorrhea, and menopause symptoms and supports healthy milk production in breastfeeding women. It can also inhibit the proliferation of prostate cancer cells in men. For PMS, take 400 milligrams a day before breakfast. For infertility and menopausal symptoms, take 160 to 240 milligrams a day. For endometriosis, take 400 milligrams a day.

■ *Fenugreek.* This herb, which increases sexual arousal and testosterone levels, is used to treat hernias, erectile dysfunction, and male pattern baldness. When Australian researchers gave thirty healthy men a fenugreek supplement, they found a positive effect on their sexual arousal, energy, and stamina. They also found that the supplement helped participants maintain normal testosterone levels.[43] The herb also seems to support healthy milk flow in breastfeeding women who are experiencing low milk supply. Take 600 milligrams of fenugreek seed extract every day.

■ *Black cohosh.* This herbal remedy contains phytoestrogens—plant-based estrogens—and, as a result, is known for its ability to treat hormonal issues, including the symptoms of menopause. Indeed, a recent study in eighty postmenopausal women with hot flashes found that over eight weeks, black cohosh was able to significantly reduce the severity and frequency.[44] The herb can reduce hot flashes in breast cancer survivors as well. What's more, it can improve your sleep during menopause, according to a randomized, double-blind, placebo-controlled trial published in *Climacteric.*[45] Getting plenty of rest is also vital to balancing hormones naturally. Take 160 to 200 milligrams a day.

■ *Honorable mention:* Clary sage, wild yam for women, and ginseng and epimedium (also known as horny goat weed, used to treat erectile dysfunction) for men.

The super system-wide detoxifiers

Toxins, pesticides, preservatives, and additives all make their way into our bodies, and the liver is the organ responsible for clearing them out. These three herbs support the liver's ability to remove these unwanted contaminants.

■ *Milk thistle.* This herb, also known as silymarin, is used for everything from weight loss to skin health—but it's best known for providing natural support for the liver. Indeed, it's the most well-researched plant in the treatment of liver disease, like cirrhosis, jaundice, and hepatitis.[46] Milk thistle cleanses the liver by rebuilding liver cells, reducing damage, and promoting toxin removal, one of the liver's main functions. What's more, laboratory studies have shown that it suppresses cellular inflammation by activating cell repair pathways.[47] To detox the liver, take 150 milligrams one to three times a day. For ongoing liver support, take 50 to 150 milligrams daily.

▪ *Bupleurum.* In TCM, this herb has long been relied upon for liver detoxification, and new research helps explain why it's so effective. In a laboratory study, researchers from Bulgaria identified two potent antioxidants, narcissin, and rutin, in bupleurum and tested their effect on liver cells. What they found: Narcissin and rutin protect the liver on both the cellular and subcellular levels by limiting the damage caused by free radicals, unstable atoms that can damage cells, leading to illness and aging.[48] Bupleurum is available in pill or liquid form and is included in a number of liver formulas that also include other herbs like milk thistle and dandelion root. Take as directed.

▪ *Dandelion root.* Like bupleurum, dandelion root is rich in antioxidants, which probably helps account for its protective benefits to the liver. But research has revealed other promising liver-saving mechanisms associated with dandelion root. In a study published in the journal *Molecules*, researchers gave mice polysaccharides (long chains of carbohydrate molecules) extracted from dandelion root and found that the substance protected the rodents' livers from acetaminophen-induced liver injury.[49] What's more, dandelion root seems to increase the flow of bile, which is essential for breaking down fats. Most dandelion root supplements and extracts contain 500 to 1,500 milligrams per serving. As with any supplement, start with the lowest dose to see how it makes you feel.

▪ *Honorable mention:* Artichoke, cilantro, cypress, gentian (an herb known for its ability to help with digestive problems), turmeric, and seaweeds, like chlorella and spirulina.

The time-tested sleep-well solutions

Whether due to stress, menopause symptoms, anxiety, depression, or chronic pain, insomnia hits all of us at some point, leaving us wiped out and vulnerable to everything from weight gain to car accidents. Here are three plant-based remedies that can help you get a good night's sleep.

■ *Valerian*. Research shows that valerian reduces the time it takes to fall asleep and improves sleep quality. In one double-blind study, Swedish researchers found that a valerian-based supplement helped improve sleep in 89 percent of participants.[50] Another randomized, triple-blind trial in the journal *Menopause* found that valerian extract improved the quality of sleep.[51] Valerian bolsters sleep by increasing the brain's level of gamma-aminobutyric acid (GABA), a neurotransmitter that inhibits the central nervous system. Valerian has also been shown to calm anxiety. To improve sleep, take 1 teaspoon of a valerian tincture or fluid extract daily. It can take two weeks for the effect to take hold. Once sleep improves, keep taking valerian for two to six weeks.

■ *Chamomile*. You might already know that a cup of chamomile tea before bed can calm you down and set the stage for sleep. One reason for this is that it reduces anxiety. Indeed, a study trial of chamomile in people with moderate to severe anxiety found a meaningful reduction in anxiety symptoms over eight weeks, with a response rate similar to pharmaceutical treatments for anxiety.[52] Try a cup or two of chamomile tea before bed. For greater benefit, take between 220 and 1,600 milligrams of a chamomile supplement instead.

■ *CBD*. Cannabis has been used for relief for thousands of years, and cannabidiol (CBD), a non-euphoric component of cannabis, has experienced an enthusiastic resurgence in the past few years. There's a good reason for this: CBD is a potent anti-inflammatory that may help cut the risk for dozens of diseases. You'll learn more in chapter 7, but for now I'll touch on one important benefit: CBD can help you sleep because, among other things, it calms the central nervous system. In a study published in the *Permanente Journal*, researchers at the University of Colorado observed people with anxiety or poor sleep who were treated with CBD. Within the first month, nearly 80 percent of patients with anxiety showed reduced anxiety scores, and sleep scores improved in 67 percent.[53] Because CBD is relatively new, dosing isn't clear, but in the Colorado study, patients were given 25 to 75 milligram capsules of CBD every day. For anxiety, patients took it in the morning after breakfast. For insomnia, they took it every evening after dinner.

■ *Honorable mention:* Lavender, lemon balm, linden, passionflower, and poppy seed.

This should give you a good introduction to the many ways plant-based medicinals can improve your health. There are literally hundreds of options to choose from—many of which are barely known in the United States. In upcoming chapters, you'll learn more about how to use these ancient remedies to treat a variety of conditions—and improve your overall health.

CHAPTER 7

Cannabis: The Forbidden Herb

The Medication That Pharmaceutical Companies Want to Keep for Themselves

Several years ago, a sixty-year-old man named John came to see me at my functional medicine practice. His daughter, Amy, brought him in because she was worried about him. He had been on antidepressants and opioids for ten years to treat chronic back pain, she explained, but the medications had changed him. "He used to be fun and encouraging and engaged," she told me. "Now he's robotic and withdrawn."

I felt for them, and I was honest with them. Getting John off the medications wouldn't be easy, I said, and we'd need to do it very slowly, dropping the dosage by tiny increments. What's more, he'd need to participate in the process by adopting some dietary and lifestyle changes. He agreed to try.

I gave him dietary recommendations, including milk thistle, to start moving energy and blood through his body again because his liver had become sluggish from the antidepressants, a common side effect. I also suggested he use the scent of citrus essential oil to lift his mood and prescribed yoga and nature walks to support his liver. But none of it would work unless we could address his pain. And for that I recommended topical CBD (cannabidiol) oil. CBD, a non-euphoric substance in the cannabis plant, not only supports the movement and healthy flow of qi, but it is also an effective pain reliever that fights inflammation.

The process of getting John off the drugs took two painstaking years. But he eventually did it. Along the way, his personality slowly returned, and he was even able to play golf again, a sport he'd loved before his back problems started. When I chatted with him toward the end of the process, he told me the thing that helped the most was the CBD. It reduced his pain, he said, adding, "I think it saved my life. If it hadn't been for that, I'd still be on the drugs."

Chances are, you think of CBD as a modern phenomenon. But here's the truth: Humans have been using this remedy for healing for millennia. In 2900 BC, Chinese emperor Fu Hsi wrote a Chinese medicine textbook in which he observed that the popular substance *ma* (the Chinese word for cannabis) contains a blend of both yin and yang. Some 250 years later, Chinese emperor Shen Nung began explaining the healing properties of the herb, including pain relief, sleep, and reducing inflammation and anxiety.

CBD is what's known as a cannabinoid, the name for the therapeutic substances found in the cannabis plant. Research shows there are hundreds of cannabinoids. Some of them, including CBD, are found in hemp, a type of cannabis plant that has been used for thousands of years to make products like paper, clothing, rope, fabric, and building materials. In fact, the Gutenberg Bible, the world's first book printed on a moveable printing press, in 1454, is printed on paper made from hemp.

Today, by law, hemp doesn't contain any cannabinoids that have euphoric effects, as opposed to marijuana, a similar type of cannabis plant, which contains varying levels of tetrahydrocannabinol (THC), the cannabinoid chemical that can make someone feel high. As a result, the CBD oils and tinctures on the national market in the United States are made primarily from the leaves and flowers of the hemp plant.

References to the medical use of the cannabis plant have cropped up around the world throughout the ages, from India's ancient Ayurvedic medicine to records from Greece dating back nearly two thousand years. And this fact might really surprise you: For many years, cannabis was a commonly used medicine in the United States. In fact, in the 1800s, doctors considered it so safe that it was marketed to new moms to relieve babies' teething pain.

Then, in the 1930s and '40s, the United States government began stoking fears about the dangers of cannabis, and the United States and other countries banned the substance. In 1970, the United States government tightened cannabis restrictions even more drastically by passing the Controlled Substances Act, which classified the cannabis plant, along with all the cannabinoids it contains, including CBD, as a Schedule 1 substance—a category that also includes high-risk drugs, like heroin and methamphetamine.

The Controlled Substances Act also specified that drugs in this category have no known medical uses—including cannabis. That's like saying exercise has no medical value. And it's especially ironic, because just five years later a study in the *Journal of the National Cancer Institute* (which at the time was published by the government's National Cancer Institute), found that using cannabinoids to treat lab animals with lung cancer inhibited the tumors' growth.[1]

Fortunately, the legal status of cannabis is undergoing a transformation. As of this writing, thirty-three states and the District of Columbia have legalized medical cannabis (both marijuana and hemp). Meanwhile, as I mentioned in chapter 1, CBD derived from hemp, but not other forms of cannabis, is now legal on the federal level. Even so, research into CBD and other cannabinoids' medical uses has been badly hampered by the federal government's marijuana regulations.

That's a shame, because most studies that *have* been conducted show that CBD and other cannabinoids can be beneficial if they are used in the correct ratio and dosage to replace synthetic medications—and it's likely we've just scratched the surface of their potential. Preliminary research has bolstered the hopeful idea that CBD and other cannabinoids can shrink cancerous tumors, for instance.[2] Other studies show they may arrest Alzheimer's plaque formation[3] and slow the progress of concussion-related brain disease.[4] And a number of studies have demonstrated that CBD can reduce anxiety, improve digestion, curb nausea, aid sleep, boost brain health, and relieve chronic pain and inflammation. And, as I mentioned in chapter 1, in 2018 the US Food and Drug Administration approved the first-ever CBD-derived drug, Epidiolex, designed to treat children with intractable seizure disorders.

The majority of healthcare professionals support the legalization of medical cannabis,[5] and doctors across the country—including the Knox Docs (Rachel, Jessica, Janice, and David Knox), a family of four physicians pioneering the field of cannabinology—are helping patients understand how to use it safely and effectively. And two high-profile MDs—CNN's chief medical correspondent Dr. Sanjay Gupta and Dr. Mehmet Oz—have become vocal advocates for medical cannabis, partly due to compelling evidence showing that states where medical cannabis is legal saw a 20 percent decline in opioid-related overdose deaths from 1999 to 2010.[6] (In 1996, California was the first state to legalize medical cannabis, and the trend quickly spread.)

Furthermore, patients say cannabinoids work. In a survey published in *Drug and Alcohol Review*, 92 percent of medical cannabis patients said the substance alleviated their symptoms, including chronic pain, arthritis, migraines, and cancer.[7] Ironic, isn't it? A substance our own government still demonizes as dangerous is, at this very moment, safely providing extraordinary relief for millions of people.

I want to be clear. I'm not endorsing the use of recreational marijuana—or even long-term use of medical marijuana containing THC, the intoxicating component of the plant. But I believe that hemp-based CBD and other cannabinoids, like cannabigerol (CBG) and cannabinol (CBN), have enormous potential for improving your health—and they're an integral component of my ancient remedies program. As a result, it's important to me that you understand what cannabinoids are and why they work. With that in mind, the following sections explain the life-saving biological system that allows us to respond to cannabis, as well as the plant's most promising chemicals, and the research supporting its extensive—and remarkable—benefits.

Why cannabinoids have a multitude of health benefits

Embedded in your body is an ancient system of neurotransmitters and receptors known as the endocannabinoid system. It actually produces its own cannabis-like chemicals, known as endocannabinoids, which your body churns out as needed to keep you healthy. These natural endocannabinoid receptors are found all over your body—in your brain, skin, bones, organs, immune cells, glands, heart, blood vessels, gastrointestinal tract, and muscles.

As a result, the endocannabinoid system is woven into nearly every organ system within your body and works hand in hand with your nervous system and endocrine system. Not surprisingly, the endocannabinoid system has a hand in regulating a broad range of vital functions, including mood, memory, gut health, hormone balance, appetite, pain, inflammation, and immunity. But its overarching function is to maintain your body's homeostasis, or steady state—so your internal environment remains stable and runs smoothly, regardless of the external challenges it faces. Think of it as a body-wide motherboard. The endocannabinoid system continually monitors your body and mind, releasing chemicals as needed to maintain biological harmony.

Your body has two main types of endocannabinoid receptors: CB1 receptors are located in high concentrations in your brain and spinal cord, and they control your central nervous system and affect things like sleep, mood, stress, and memory. CB2 receptors are located in a variety of places, but there are high concentrations in your immune cells, which regulate inflammation—and keeping inflammation in check is one of the most important things you can do for your health, since it plays a role in nearly every modern disease, from heart disease to Alzheimer's.

And here's what's really amazing: Like a key in a lock, a number of cannabis molecules (known technically as phytocannabinoids, because they come from plants) plug into these receptors, where they unlock the healing effects of your body's natural endocannabinoids.

Endocannabinoid SYSTEM

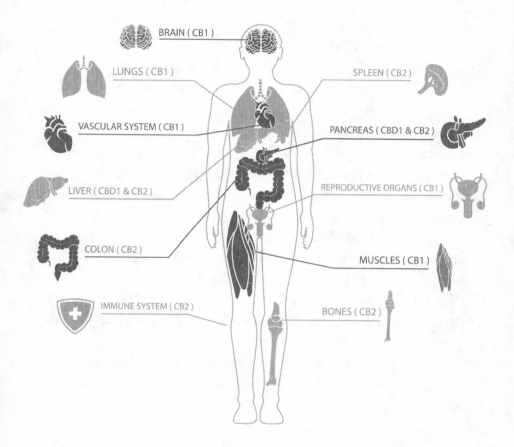

BRAIN (CB1)

LUNGS (CB1)

SPLEEN (CB2)

VASCULAR SYSTEM (CB1)

PANCREAS (CBD1 & CB2)

LIVER (CBD1 & CB2)

REPRODUCTIVE ORGANS (CB1)

COLON (CB2)

MUSCLES (CB1)

IMMUNE SYSTEM (CB2)

BONES (CB2)

Hemp 101

The hemp plant contains hundreds of individual compounds, including cannabinoids and terpenes. Although we hear a lot about CBD, the truth is that all cannabinoids work best when they're used in combination with one another and with terpenes, just as whole foods are healthier than single supplements. This phenomenon is known as the entourage effect. For instance, terpenes and flavonoids (healthy chemicals that give plants their color) can enhance CBD's therapeutic effects. A review of studies published in the *British Journal of Pharmacology* found that using terpenes and plant cannabinoids together may help with a range of problems, including cancer, anxiety, pain, inflammation, and epilepsy.[8]

Here's a quick cheat sheet for understanding these substances and how to use them.

■ *Cannabidiol (CBD).* In TCM, this cannabinoid is a moistening yin tonic that supports qi movement, calms the mind, and reduces inflammation. Found in high concentrations in hemp as well as in medical strains of cannabis that have been bred for high CBD levels, the substance can be helpful for anxiety,[9] nausea,[10] seizure disorders,[11] and arthritis pain.[12] In my practice and personal experience I have also seen it work effectively to improve sleep, help digestion, and balance hormones. The reason CBD is one of the most powerful medicinal compounds on the planet is that it puts your body in a relaxed state. It triggers the relaxing branch of your nervous system, known as the parasympathetic system, while decreasing the activity of the sympathetic branch, so it lowers cortisol and is great for combating stress.

What's more, CBD is a neuroprotective antioxidant more potent than vitamin C, so it safeguards the health of your brain. CBD doesn't fit into either the CB1 or CB2 endocannabinoid receptors, but it changes the way the receptors respond to THC and other cannabinoids, making their effects more beneficial. It also binds to TRPV1 receptors,[13] which are involved in the transmission and modulation of pain as well as the control of inflammation. CBD also seems to slow the rate at which your natural endocannabinoids are broken down, allowing them to linger in your system and, as a result, have a greater effect on your body. This feature of CBD can be incredibly helpful for those who have an "endocannabinoid deficiency," a possible underlying cause of irritable bowel syndrome, fibromyalgia, migraines, and other tough-to-treat conditions. Studies show that people with those illnesses have suboptimal endocannabinoid levels[14]—and cannabis eases their symptoms. One study published in *Pharmacotherapy* found that daily use of medical cannabis reduced pain and cut the frequency

PARASYMPATHETIC NERVES   SYMPATHETIC NERVES

Rest & Digest   *Fight or Flight*

Parasympathetic Nerves (Rest & Digest):
CONSTRICT PUPILS
STIMULATE SALIVA
CONSTRICT AIRWAYS
SLOW HEARTBEAT
STIMULATE DIGESTIVE FUNCTION
STIMULATE GALLBLADDER
STIMULATE NUTRIENT ABSORPTION & ELIMINATION
CONTRACT BLADDER

Sympathetic Nerves (Fight or Flight):
DILATE PUPILS
INHIBIT SALIVA
RELAX AIRWAYS
INCREASE HEARTBEAT
INHIBIT DIGESTION
INHIBIT GALLBLADDER
INHIBIT INTESTINES
SECRETE EPINEPHRINE & NOREPINEPHRINE
RELAX BLADDER

of migraine attacks by more than half.[15] Although more research is needed, it's possible that by slowing endocannabinoid metabolism, CBD-rich cannabis restores healthy cannabinoid levels in people with these mysterious, treatment-resistant conditions.

■ *Cannabigerol (CBG).* A lesser-known cannabinoid that's just starting to gain popularity, CBG is available only in trace amounts in most hemp strains, but it has terrific healing potential. Known as the mother of all cannabinoids, it's the first cannabinoid the plant produces and the precursor from which all other cannabinoids are synthesized. Like CBD, it's not intoxicating. It can bind to both CB1 and CB2 receptors as well as to the alpha-2 receptor in your brain stem and peripheral nerves,[16] where it mimics the parasympathetic nervous system by producing a calming effect. It also blocks the uptake of anandamide, one of your body's natural endocannabinoids—known as the "bliss molecule" because it bolsters feelings of pleasure. By allowing anandamide to linger in the system, CBG has the ability to improve mood. It also seems to be an effective anti-inflammatory and antibacterial (and may even work against antibiotic-resistant strains of staph).[17]

■ *Cannabinol (CBN).* Another lesser-known cannabinoid, CBN comes from the breakdown of aging THC molecules, so it's not found in living, growing plants. Studies show it may provide relief for chronic muscle pain disorders, including temporomandibular (jaw) pain and fibromyalgia.[18] It also seems to stimulate appetite, which can be helpful for people with cancer and AIDS and other chronic illnesses.[19] And preliminary research shows it may enhance sleep[20] and treat inflammatory diseases, like autoimmune disorders and inflammatory bowel disease.[21]

■ *THC.* The molecules of this intoxicating chemical are extremely similar to those in the "bliss molecule," anandamide. And just like anandamide, THC can plug into both CB1 and CB2 receptors. As a result, it has wide-ranging effects. Recent research shows that THC may help people with PTSD[22] and chronic pain.[23] A review published in the *British Journal of Clinical Pharmacology* looked at the results of eighteen high-quality trials using THC alone or in combination with other cannabinoids in people with chronic pain (including nerve-related pain and rheumatoid arthritis) and found that all but three showed the substance has significant pain-relieving effects.[24] That said, from the TCM perspective, heavy or regular THC use depletes qi—it drains your adrenals, takes a toll on your liver, and kills your libido. And research shows that frequent use of THC can increase the risk of psychosis,[25] impair memory,[26] and cause anatomical brain changes.[27] So it makes sense to use it only when it's really needed—for pain after surgery or to fight nausea during chemo, for instance. In most cases, it's best to stick with cannabis strains that have a ratio of at least 10:1 CBD to THC to minimize THC's side effects.

- *Terpenes.* There may be more than 120 of these chemicals in hemp, which give the plant its distinct odor. Terpenes are also found in high amounts in essential oils; in fact, they're responsible for giving essential oils their medicinal qualities. Although research is in its infancy, several terpenes found in cannabis seem to have protective health effects. Limonene, for instance, may improve mood and kill breast cancer cells.[28] Myrcene combats inflammation and is a sedative and muscle relaxant.[29] Pinene has anti-inflammatory and antibacterial properties, and it bolsters memory to boot.[30] Linalool can reduce anxiety and may help prevent seizures.[31]

For most health issues, the effective dosage of CBD is in the range of 10 to 40 milligrams daily. But for certain ailments that are best treated by combining CBD with low doses of THC, it's a bit different. Here are the recommended oral CBD oil doses.

Condition	Dosage
General Wellness	10–50 milligrams of CBD oil daily
Chronic pain	10–100 milligrams of CBD oil daily
Epilepsy	50–300 milligrams of CBD oil daily
Sleep disorders	40–160 milligrams of CBD oil daily
Schizophrenia	40–1,000 milligrams of CBD oil daily
Glaucoma	20–40 milligrams of CBD oil daily
Loss of appetite in cancer patients	2.5 milligrams oral THC, plus 1 milligram CBD oil for 6 weeks

Herbs, foods, and essential oils that mimic and support cannabinoids

The following common foods influence your endocannabinoid system and can work synergistically with cannabinoids to improve your health.

■ *Essential oils.* Rosemary, black pepper, lavender, cinnamon, clove, and copaiba oils are able to mimic some of the immune-related benefits of cannabinoids. The reason: They contain beta-caryophyllene, a terpene that engages CB2 endocannabinoid receptors, which are primarily found in the immune system.

■ *Holy basil.* This herb, also known as tulsi, contains beta-caryophyllene and other terpenes that lower cortisol and reduce stress.

■ *Echinacea.* A well-known cold fighter, echinacea contains N-acylethanolamines, which bind to and activate endocannabinoid receptors.

■ *Black truffles.* This delicacy contains anandamide, the "bliss molecule" and one of your body's natural endocannabinoids.

■ *Cacao.* Another delicious food that contains anandamide, cacao also deactivates a type of fatty acid that breaks down anandamide.

■ *Helichrysum.* Typically used as an essential oil, this flowering plant produces compounds that mimic CBG and cannabigerolic acid (CBGa).

■ *Omega-3 fats.* These healthy fats are involved in the synthesis of new endocannabinoids in the body and react with existing endocannabinoids to create a type of endocannabinoid that binds to receptors in your immune system.

■ *Maca.* Maca has long been known as an adaptogen, a substance that helps the body respond to stress. Research suggests that compounds in maca known as N-alkylamides mimic the biological action of cannabinoids.

The six conditions cannabinoids are especially good at treating

While their full range of benefits has yet to be realized, cannabinoids seem to hold real promise for a few conditions in particular. I've mentioned some of the research above, but the following six health issues are so common—and can have such devastating health effects—they're worth exploring in greater detail.

■ *Stress and anxiety.* Stress contributes to virtually every disease known to humans, but the endocannabinoid system is present in stress-responsive neural circuits, which strongly suggests it plays a critical role in regulating our response to stress. Indeed, studies show cannabis can help combat this modern scourge. A study in the *British Journal of Psychiatry* found that a 300-milligram dose of CBD was enough to curb anxiety in a public-speaking trial (but lower and higher doses weren't as effective).[32] A review of CBD for anxiety disorders, including generalized anxiety, panic disorder, and social anxiety, concluded that the evidence "strongly supports" it as a treatment.[33] And a first-of-its-kind study published in 2018 in the *Journal of Affective Disorders* looked at reports from nearly nine thousand sessions of people using medical cannabis (a combination of CBD and THC); it reduced stress and anxiety by an average of 58 percent.[34]

■ *Sleep.* Chronic insomnia afflicts 10 to 15 percent of people in the United States, and another 25 to 35 percent of us have occasional trouble sleeping, which can affect mood, decrease productivity, and increase vulnerability to accidents and illnesses. But many researchers believe that CBD and other cannabinoids can improve sleep, and a fascinating 2020 study in *Digestive Disease and Sciences* found this to be the case. The study looked at people with autoimmune hepatitis, a painful condition that often causes insomnia, who used CBD for relief. Eighty-seven percent said it improved their sleep, and 12 percent of those said CBD allowed them to get off their prescription sleep medication.[35]

■ *Pain.* Chronic pain is an intractable problem in the United States, one that is complicated by the fact that prescription pain drugs are dangerously addictive. But cannabinoids offer hope. There's evidence that cannabinoids can reduce opioid use[36] and overdose mortalities[37]—and the study of patients with autoimmune hepatitis I referred to in the sleep section above bears it out: 82 percent of participants said CBD offered significant pain relief, and 47 percent of those were able to go off their prescription pain meds as a result.[38]

■ *Inflammation.* Endocannabinoid receptors are found on immune cells, which means that cannabinoids play an important role in the immune system and one of the immune system's primary responses: inflammation. I already mentioned that CBD binds to TRPV1 receptors, which mediate inflammation and pain, and desensitizes them. And several studies show that cannabinoids suppress inflammatory responses by downregulating cytokine and chemokine production (two inflammatory chemicals).[39]

■ *Brain health.* Endocannabinoid receptors are abundant in the brain—one reason CBD and other cannabinoids seem to be so beneficial for mood disorders. But cannabinoids also seem to be healthy for the brain in general. In one study, CBD was able to prevent the development of social recognition deficit in mice with early-stage Alzheimer's disease, possibly slowing the disease's progression.[40]

■ *Gut health.* More than 1.5 million people in the United States have inflammatory bowel disease (like Crohn's disease or ulcerative colitis), and available medications aren't highly effective. Cannabis has been used for millennia to treat gut inflammation,[41] and contemporary research supports its use. A small study in Israel found that patients with Crohn's disease experienced significant symptom relief after using cannabis oil (with CBD and THC).[42] And there's evidence that CBD can also be beneficial for leaky gut[43] and colitis.[44]

While those conditions are the most well researched, there are a number of other ways in which cannabinoids may be beneficial for health. Here's a glimpse of the promising research we're likely to learn more about in the next few years.

■ *Anti-tumor effects.* In animal studies, CBD and other non-euphoric cannabinoids have demonstrated anti-tumor and cancer-fighting benefits, and may be effective in preventing the spread of breast, prostate, brain, colon, and lung cancer. Cannabinoids seem to have a variety of effects, from inhibiting the viability of tumor cells to limiting the activity of cancer stem cells, which are required for cancer's spread.[45]

■ *Acne treatment.* CBD targets the two primary pimple-causing pathways—inflammation and oil production—and other cannabinoids may offer similar benefits.[46]

■ *Diabetes treatment.* Research in mice found that treating them with CBD could prevent the development of diabetes. While 86 percent of the untreated mice developed the disease, just 30 percent of those treated with CBD did.[47]

■ *Heart health.* Recent research has linked CBD with a number of benefits for the heart and circulatory system, including the ability to lower blood pressure,[48] affect diabetes (as mentioned above), and reduce stress. In fact, the substance can actually cause the blood vessels to relax, which protects against vascular damage in those who eat a high-glucose diet.[49]

■ *Autoimmune disease.* Multiple studies have shown that CBD can calm an overactive immune system and reduce inflammation, the root causes of autoimmune disease. For instance, a recent study published in *Frontiers in Immunology* found that CBD can ameliorate autoimmune encephalomyelitis (a mouse model of multiple sclerosis) in mice.[50]

I'll provide more information in upcoming chapters on CBD and other cannabinoids. But now that you understand the research on these ancient substances, I hope you will share my enthusiasm for their ability to enhance health and healing in a variety of realms—and find safe, effective ways to use them in your own life.

CHAPTER 8

The Power of Essential Oils

How Plant-Based Medicine Can Help You Avoid Pharmaceuticals

When my mom was facing her second bout of cancer in 2005, we overhauled her diet by eliminating processed foods and sugar and building her daily meals around healthy fats, veggies, and tons of herbs. None of that may surprise you. But here's something that might: Essential oils were an indispensable aspect of her cancer-fighting approach as well. I had my mom start using frankincense oil every day, because it is strongly anti-inflammatory, protects healthy cells, stimulates the immune system, and eradicates germs and bacteria. But here's the kicker: It can even kill cancer cells, according to laboratory studies.[1] Myrrh oil can, too,[2] and my mom also used that daily. She diligently followed the diet and lifestyle regimen we created, and now she has been cancer free for fifteen years.

Essential oils weren't solely responsible for my mom's remarkable recovery. But I believe they played an integral role, and here's why: Just a few drops of these ancient substances are enough to have a healthy biological effect, and each oil has its own distinct benefits. Lavender oil, for instance, can take the edge off stress and anxiety.[3] Oregano is an effective way to kill fungus and battle candida and viral infections.[4]

The science supporting these remedies is recent, but humans have been using essential oils to heal a variety of ailments for thousands of years. These organic compounds, extracted from the flowers, leaves, bark, roots, resin, and peels of plants, were commonly used by the ancient Egyptians, including Cleopatra and the pharaohs, as medicines, beauty treatments, and embalming fluids. Entire Egyptian temples were dedicated to the production and blending of oils, and the recipes were written on the walls in hieroglyphics.

The ancient Chinese understood the power of essential oils as well. They began studying aromatics as early as 2700 BC and integrated oils into their elaborate medical system. A practitioner might use a yang essential oil, like ginger, which has warming properties, to aid in digestion and help clear dampness caused by candida or a cold, for instance.

In ancient Greece, Hippocrates prescribed aromatherapy to enhance the health benefits of massage and documented the action of two hundred different herbs. Others contributed to our essential oils knowledge base as well. Aristotle's successor, Theophrastus, for instance, investigated how specific scents affected emotions.

Essential oils are also an integral part of Ayurvedic medicine, and they are referenced more than 250 times in the Bible! In fact, the book of Exodus contains a recipe for the holy anointing oil—a blend of myrrh, cinnamon, calamus, cassia, and olive oil—that was routinely used for healing.

And these healing oils have been used in more recent history, as well. In 1910, the French chemist René-Maurice Gattefossé was working in a perfume plant when he burned his hand. He plunged it into the nearest vat of liquid, which turned out to be lavender oil. He felt instant relief—and his skin healed quickly, with minimal scarring. He then began his advanced studies on essential oils and wrote the groundbreaking aromatherapy textbook *Gattefossé's Aromatherapy*. In it, he shares the recipe for a disease-fighting blend called the Four Thieves—vinegar infused with a variety of herbs and spices, including sage, clove, rosemary, and wild marjoram. As legend has it, the antibacterial and antiviral formula was discovered by thieves in Europe during the seventeenth-century plague. They were robbing the dead and sick without becoming ill themselves. When they were caught, the authorities offered to pardon them in exchange for the formula. Modern versions of the Four Thieves recipe typically include clove, sage, thyme, rosemary, and garlic.

Why would an oil from a plant help you fight off illnesses? It's actually pretty simple. Plants are vulnerable to, and must fight off, many of the same pathogens that cause human disease, including viruses, bacteria, fungi, and parasites. So when you inhale, apply, or ingest their essential oils, your body utilizes the plant's protective compounds—and those substances work with your innate disease-fighting power to create a more powerful defense. Oregano and thyme are great examples. They contain compounds that naturally repel viruses, bacteria, and parasites—so when we use their essential oils, they bolster our ability to fight pathogens as well.

As a result, plant oils can be as helpful for modern health conditions as they were in older times. In fact, at least 8,500 studies have examined essential oils over the past 165 years. Many of my patients have used them in place of prescription medications, which makes a lot of sense. Not only are oils less expensive, they don't have toxic side effects like most medications do (although some oils can be dangerous if you don't use them correctly). What's more, they can have similar biological effects. Peppermint oil, for instance, has been proven to be effective at naturally treating irritable bowel syndrome (IBS). One study published in the journal *Digestive and Liver Disease* found a 50 percent reduction in IBS symptoms in 75 percent of patients who used it.[5] And in addition to the uses of frankincense I mentioned earlier, this "king of oils," as it's often called, is beneficial for those with chronic stress and anxiety—probably because it contains high doses of alpha-pinene, a substance that affects GABA, a brain chemical involved in mood regulation.

There's another way essential oils can bolster your overall health: You can use them in place of toxic household cleaning products and personal care products. Chelsea and I use lemon oil and tea tree oil, mixed with a few ounces of water and vinegar, as an effective and clean-smelling spray for our kitchen countertops. And when it comes to caring for your appearance, essential oils are preferable. Tea tree oil can effectively get rid of acne,[6] for example, and peppermint oil is a great way to freshen your breath.[7]

Coming up, I'll explain how essential oils can affect your body, as well as the benefits of a dozen of my favorite oils, and how to find the highest-quality options.

Essential oils provide many types of healing

Plants, like humans, have protective chemicals built into their systems to help them fight off bugs, pests, fungi, and other dangers. Those natural chemicals are what make vegetables and fruits such an indispensable part of our daily diets. Essential oils are similar, except they contain highly concentrated quantities of the most protective compounds in each plant. Created through a process of distillation, which captures the healing essence of each plant, the liquid in every small vial has tremendous therapeutic potential. A single 15-milliliter bottle of rose essential oil, for instance, contains *65 pounds* of distilled and condensed rose petals.

Because essential oils are so concentrated, they have a robust aroma. Remember when I explained the health benefits of terpenes, the scent chemicals found in hemp, back in chapter 7? Essential oils contain terpenes as well, and these compounds are responsible not only for the oils' relaxing and invigorating scents, but also for many of their medicinal properties. When you inhale an essential oil, terpene molecules plug into scent receptors in your nose, triggering effects that are relayed from your nervous system to your brain, where the tiny terpene molecules are able to cross the blood-brain barrier. The molecules also make their way to your lungs, where they're absorbed into your bloodstream. A single whiff, in some cases, is enough to trigger healthy emotional or physical changes. And when you apply oil topically, you not only inhale its effects, you also absorb the therapeutic molecules through your skin and into your bloodstream.

Natural healers knew this four thousand years ago, and practitioners of TCM and Ayurveda have been using aromatherapy as a cornerstone of treatment ever since. As evidence of essential oils' effectiveness piles up, Western healthcare professionals are taking notice. A number of hospitals around the country, from Nebraska to New Jersey, are using the substances to relax patients and staff. One study, published in *Evidence-Based Complementary and Alternative Medicine*, looked at the effect of inhaled lavender oil on patients in the intensive care unit. Researchers found that the treatment relieved patients' stress—which is typically high in ICU patients—and improved their sleep, an essential aspect of healing.[8] And that's just one example of hundreds of studies that are beginning to reveal why we all need essential oils in our medicine cabinets.

The 12 essential oils you can't live without

Essential oils are extremely versatile. You can diffuse them into the air, put a drop or two in the bathtub, rub a dab on your skin, or ingest a few drops, usually with water or a carrier oil, like coconut or olive oil. Oils that come from commonly consumed herbs, spices, roots, and berries—like ginger oil, turmeric oil, lemon oil, and peppermint oil—are safe to take orally; the common therapeutic dosage in medical studies is 1 or 2 drops, or approximately 60 milligrams.

But there are some caveats when using essential oils. Tree oils, including arborvitae, birch, cedarwood, cypress, eucalyptus, tea tree, white fir, and wintergreen, are dangerous to ingest. Other oils might cause a skin reaction if you apply them topically (I offer guidelines for safe usage below). If you experience any side effects, like dizziness or nausea, when using an oil, stop using it immediately. One more thing: It's extremely important to buy a high-quality product. Synthetic oils are worthless at best and unhealthy at worst. Make sure the package says the oil is certified USDA organic, 100 percent pure, therapeutic grade, and indigenously sourced.

Here are twelve of my favorite oils, along with the safest, most effective ways to use them. I'm thrilled to share them with you, so you can take advantage of some of the most beneficial remedies known to man.

■ *Lavender.* Recognized for centuries for its therapeutic and cosmetic value, lavender is the most widely used essential oil in the world. In a randomized, controlled trial, German researchers found that lavender oil capsules (they're available over the counter) actually work better than paroxetine, a commonly prescribed anti-anxiety drug, to treat generalized anxiety disorder.[9] Inhaling lavender oil has also been shown to relieve headaches[10] and improve sleep.[11] What's more, it's a natural antioxidant, so it helps prevent and reverse disease, and, according to a study in *Phytomedicine*, it actually bolsters the activity of some of the body's most potent antioxidants, including glutathione, catalase, and superoxide dismutase.[12] Putting a few drops in a diffuser every day may help you stay well and achieve better health overall. Lavender oil can also help calm acne and erase age spots. Just mix 3 to 4 drops with ½ teaspoon of a carrier oil, like coconut, jojoba, or grapeseed oil, and massage the mixture into your skin. Precautions: Lavender oil is safest and most effective when you inhale the scent or apply it topically. Don't use it in addition to a prescription or over-the-counter sleep aid, as it can exacerbate the sedative effects. Because it can relax muscles and affect hormones, avoid it in the third trimester of pregnancy—and use only infrequently in young children.

■ *Frankincense.* As you may remember, this essential oil plays an important role in the Bible. Along with gold and myrrh, it was one of the gifts the three wise men brought to the infant Jesus. In those days, it was used to strengthen the immune system, and studies today confirm its effectiveness in that regard.[13] So you can use it as part of your health regimen to fight colds and other viral and bacterial infections. With its lemony, woodsy scent, this ancient oil's numerous health benefits are due to a wide variety of terpenes, including boswellic acid, an anti-inflammatory that protects the health of your cells. I've already mentioned frankincense's anticancer properties. It has been shown to inhibit the aggressiveness or even kill breast cancer cells,[14] bladder cancer cells,[15] and skin cancer cells.[16] What's more, animal research suggests that frankincense oil improves memory and learning, and can improve cognition in those with Alzheimer's.[17] It also seems to be helpful for gut-related issues, like leaky gut, colitis, Crohn's disease, and irritable bowel syndrome.[18] To use frankincense for health, add 3 or 4 drops of oil to a diffuser or put a few drops of oil in a pot of boiling water. Frankincense can also improve skin, reducing pore size, preventing wrinkles, and even lifting and tightening skin. Mix 6 drops of oil in 1 ounce of unscented oil and apply it directly to the skin. It's most effective when you inhale the scent or apply it topically, but you can ingest small amounts as well.

■ *Oregano.* Hippocrates used oregano for treating respiratory and digestive diseases, and ancient Greeks used it to treat skin infections, sore throats, wounds, and viruses. In TCM, it has been used for thousands of years to treat diarrhea, parasites, and fungal infections—and many of those ancient uses are being validated today. Researchers are studying this oil as an alternative to antibiotics, which, as I explained in chapter 1, are dangerously overprescribed, a problem that is leading to widespread antibiotic resistance. Oregano oil—and particularly carvacrol, its most abundant chemical—has been shown to effectively inhibit a number of different viruses, including herpes, respiratory syncytial virus, and rotavirus.[19] To use it as a natural antibiotic or antiviral, put 4 drops in 1 teaspoon of olive oil and take it twice a day for ten days. Oral oregano oil was also able to get rid of intestinal parasites, according to a study in *Phytotherapy Research*,[20] and lower cholesterol, according to research published in *Evidence-Based Complementary and Alternative Medicine*.[21] Of all the essential oils, oregano is the best at treating athlete's foot.[22] To use it, add 3 drops to an antifungal powder made of 1 teaspoon of bentonite clay and ½ teaspoon of cayenne powder, then rub the powder onto the affected area. It is also great at getting rid of mold around your home, and can limit the survival of common food-borne pathogens, like listeria, salmonella, and *E. coli.*[23] To use it as a cleaning product, just add 5 to 7 drops to a spray bottle filled with water. Precautions: Don't take oregano oil orally for more than fourteen days in a row. Pregnant women shouldn't use it at all.

■ *Tea tree.* Derived from the plant *Melaleuca alternifolia,* tea tree oil has been used for thousands of years by the indigenous Bundjalung Aborigines of Australia, who use the leaves of the plant to treat common illnesses. The oil is essential to have on hand today during flu season, since it has potent antiviral properties. Inhaling the scent of the oil, for instance, can help you fight respiratory tract infections and coughs,[24] and diffusing it through the air may inactivate airborne flu virus particles.[25] Put 5 drops in a diffuser or boiling water, or inhale tea tree oil directly from the bottle. Tea tree oil has become popular around the world today because it is a powerful disinfectant and is effective for treating skin conditions. Indeed, it has the ability to inhibit the growth of bacteria and treat fungal infections, like athlete's foot and jock itch.[26] Mix 10 drops with 1 teaspoon of coconut oil and apply it to the affected area twice a day. It can also reduce acne when applied topically.[27] Mix 5 drops of tea tree oil with 2 teaspoons of raw honey, rub onto your face, and rinse off after one minute. And tea tree oil shampoo (there are a number on the market) has been shown to significantly reduce dandruff.[28] Precautions: Tea tree oil should never be ingested.

■ *Peppermint.* One of the oldest herbs used for medical purposes, peppermint's use dates to ancient Egypt, China, Japan, and Greece. It's also one of the most versatile oils and can help with everything from muscle aches to seasonal allergy symptoms. I explained earlier in the chapter that peppermint oil can relieve symptoms of irritable bowel syndrome. That's because it relaxes the muscles in the intestines,[29] and it can do the same with the muscles in the rest of your body. Because peppermint oil contains menthol, which increases blood flow and produces a cooling sensation, it also acts as an analgesic. To use it as a rub for sore muscles, mix 3 or 4 drops of peppermint oil with 1 teaspoon each of coconut oil and eucalyptus oil. Or add 5 to 10 drops to bathwater and soak in it. When you apply a drop or two to your forehead or temples, its refreshing scent can help ease migraines, too, according to a randomized, controlled trial published in the *International Journal of Clinical Practice*.[30] Similarly, inhaling peppermint oil can unclog stuffy sinuses and may reduce seasonal allergy symptoms. Put a few drops in a diffuser or boiling water, or apply topically to your temples, chest, and back of neck. Finally, you can use the scent to support weight loss, because peppermint suppresses cravings and improves digestive health.[31] Precautions: Peppermint oil can be inhaled, used topically, or taken orally, although you shouldn't ingest more than a drop or two. I also don't recommend using it on infants' skin, or on the skin of women who are pregnant or nursing.

■ *Lemon.* Ayurvedic medicine practitioners have been using lemon essential oil to treat a wide spectrum of health conditions for at least a thousand years. Made by cold-pressing the nutrient-dense peel, which contains a variety of terpenes and fat-soluble nutrients, the oil has a scent that can relieve nausea—studies have shown it's effective in pregnant women[32]—and constipation.[33] It can also decrease stress and anxiety, according to both animal[34] and human studies.[35] Moreover, ingesting lemon oil can promote detoxification. A 2016 animal study found that lemon oil reduced the aspirin-induced liver and kidney damage in rats.[36] To promote detoxification, add 1 or 2 drops to a glass of water daily for a week. Thanks to its strong antioxidant and anti-aging effects, lemon oil also protects the skin—and it can be helpful for everything from insect bites to athlete's foot.[37] Put 12 or so drops in ¼ cup of jojoba or coconut oil and apply to the affected area. Lemon oil is also useful as a home cleaning product, because it contains limonene and beta-pinene, two known antimicrobial agents. Add 40 drops of lemon oil and 20 drops of tea tree oil to a 16-ounce spray bottle filled with water and a dash of white vinegar. Precautions: Take no more than a drop or two a day orally. If you're applying it to your skin, test it on a small patch beforehand to make sure you don't develop a reaction. Because it can make your skin sensitive to sunlight, avoid direct sun for twelve hours after using.

■ *Rosemary.* The ancient Egyptians, Romans, and Greeks all considered rosemary sacred, and it was widely used to cleanse the air and prevent illnesses from spreading. Although the scent can't kill airborne pathogens, it is great for your brain. A study in the *International Journal of Neuroscience* found that inhaling the scent of rosemary oil can enhance memory and concentration[38]—and a paper in *Psychogeriatrics* showed that it may improve cognitive function in people with Alzheimer's.[39] Inhaling the scent can also reduce levels of the stress hormone cortisol,[40] which is helpful for anyone who is under a lot of stress or who is struggling with adrenal fatigue. Equally exciting, rosemary oil contains carnosol, which holds promise for its ability to kill cancer cells while leaving the healthy cells nearby unscathed—the gold standard for cancer treatments.[41] As of yet, there are no guidelines on how to use it for cancer prevention. With an oxygen radical absorbance capacity (ORAC) score of 11.07, rosemary has the same off-the-charts ability to fight free radicals as goji berries, so it's great for protecting your body from age-related disease as well. Finally, a study in the journal *SKINmed* found that rosemary oil increased hair growth in people with hair loss as well as the prescription drug minoxidil.[42] Precautions: When using topically, always dilute with a carrier oil, like jojoba, to avoid skin sensitivity. Don't use the substance on children, and don't take internally.

■ *Clary sage.* Medieval physicians called this herb "clear eye" (the Latin word *clarus* means "clear") for its ability to heal vision-related issues. In TCM, sage is used to strengthen the kidneys, adrenals, and women's reproductive organs. Long used as a folk remedy for relieving menstrual cramps (combine 5 drops of clary sage oil with 5 drops of jojoba oil and massage it into your abdomen), it also can be effective at relieving pain and anxiety for women during childbirth, according to a study by researchers in the United Kingdom.[43] Inhaling the oil's scent can also lower cortisol, the stress hormone, and improve mood in people diagnosed with depression, according to a study in the *Journal of Phytotherapy Research.*[44] Since stress is a major cause of insomnia, diffusing some clary sage oil into your bedroom (or putting 5 drops into your pre-bedtime bath) might help you sleep better. Moreover, a double-blind, randomized controlled trial found that clary sage aromatherapy can reduce blood pressure when you're under stress.[45] It also contains antifungal and antiseptic properties and boosts eye, hair, and skin health. Precautions: Avoid during pregnancy, because it can cause uterine contractions, and don't give it to infants or toddlers. Don't use it during or after drinking alcohol, as it can exacerbate alcohol's sedative effects. And don't ingest more than a drop or two.

■ *Holy basil.* In ancient India, tulsi, as it is also known, was considered a sacred plant and often called the elixir of life—and its essential oil has been used by Ayurvedic healers for years to help the body adapt (and not overreact) to stressful conditions. Indeed, holy basil works as an adaptogen and contains stress-fighting compounds, including ocimumosides A and B, that lower blood levels of the stress hormone cortisol.[46] Diffuse a few drops into the air during times of stress. Another paper, published in the *Journal of Ayurveda and Integrative Medicine*, explained that holy basil can counterbalance internal biological stress as well, by normalizing blood glucose, blood pressure, and lipid levels.[47] Indeed, in a randomized, placebo-controlled trial in people with non-insulin-dependent diabetes, holy basil decreased fasting as well as post-meal blood sugar levels.[48] Add 1 drop a day to a favorite recipe to reap the benefits. What's more, holy basil seems to bolster the immune system in a way that may offer protection from cancer.[49] Holy basil oil also contains eugenol, a potent antimicrobial, which is helpful for skin disorders—and it's anti-inflammatory, so it can lighten and brighten your skin. Put 2 or 3 drops in 1 teaspoon of coconut oil and use it on your skin. Precautions: Dab a drop on your skin before using it topically, because it may cause a rash in some people. Don't use it topically on children. People with clotting disorders should avoid it, because eugenol is an anticoagulant.

■ *Clove.* Clove has been used around the world for health purposes for more than 1,500 years, and we now know that it possesses an abundance of therapeutic properties thanks to its off-the-charts antioxidant score. It's actually ranked number one among herbs and spices. Per gram, cloves contain more antioxidants than blueberries—which means they have the ability to slow aging by reversing the damage caused by free radicals. Like holy basil, clove oil contains eugenol. This antimicrobial compound is responsible for the oil's strong fragrance and many of its medicinal qualities. Laboratory research shows it can suppress the infection potential of a common flu virus.[50] If you're exposed to someone with a cold or the flu, put a few drops in a diffuser and inhale the scent, or mix a few drops with 1 tablespoon of coconut oil and rub it on your neck and chest. What's more, clove oil can fight candida fungal infections as successfully as nystatin, a dangerous drug often prescribed for thrush (yeast infections in the mouth), according to a study in *Oral Microbiology and Immunology*.[51] To use, add 1 or 2 drops of clove oil to a few tablespoons of olive oil and swish it around your mouth 30 seconds. (It will help get rid of cavity-causing bacteria, too—and might relieve tooth pain.) You can also mix 1 drop with ½ teaspoon of coconut oil and rub it on a toddler's gums to relieve teething pain. (For children younger than age two, substitute peppermint oil for clove.) Precautions: Because it is an anticoagulant, don't use clove oil if you're taking blood thinners. It also may negatively interact with SSRIs, a commonly prescribed type of antidepressant; avoid it if you're taking one. Don't ingest clove oil.

■ *Eucalyptus.* Long a favorite in Australian Aboriginal folk medicine, eucalyptus oil is often used to relieve pain. It's effective thanks to its extremely high content of eucalyptol, which we now know to be a potent antioxidant and anti-inflammatory. A clinical trial published in *Evidence-Based Complementary and Alternative Medicine* found that the scent of eucalyptus oil can reduce pain after knee replacement surgery—and reduce blood pressure, too.[52] Diffuse a few drops to reap the benefits. Diffusing eucalyptus oil can also improve a variety of respiratory conditions, from asthma to the common cold, because it seems to open up the nasal passages, allowing air to flow more freely. Similarly, if you have a persistent cough, a substance in eucalyptus oil known as cineole (which has bronchodilating properties) can significantly decrease the frequency of coughing fits, according to a study published in the journal *Cough*.[53] Apply 2 or 3 drops to your chest and back of neck to relieve a cough. For a sore throat, apply several drops to your throat and chest. Here are two other pain-relieving uses: To get rid of headaches, rub 2 or 3 drops into your temples and the back of your neck. To relieve muscle pain, add 2 or 3 drops to 1 tablespoon of coconut oil and massage into your muscles. Precautions: Don't take eucalyptus oil orally. If applying it to children's skin, always dilute it with a carrier, like coconut oil.

■ *Cedarwood.* This tree oil has been used medicinally since ancient times. The Bible mentions cedar trees as a source of protection, wisdom, and abundance—and cedarwood oil does indeed have a surprising range of properties, from anti-inflammatory to antiseptic to sedative. Cedarwood oil is great for disinfecting wounds, thanks to its antiseptic activity. Just blend a few drops into 1 tablespoon of coconut oil and apply the mixture to cuts and scrapes to prevent infections. It also has calming effects, according to research published in *Planta Medica*,[54] and can relieve stress and tension. It may even promote sleep. Simply take a few sniffs of the bottle or diffuse a few drops. What's more, applying cedarwood oil in combination with the essential oils of thyme, rosemary, and lavender can improve hair growth.[55] Add 3 or 4 drops of cedarwood oil, along with 1 drop of thyme, rosemary, and lavender oil, to your shampoo, or mix the same amounts of essential oils with 1 tablespoon of coconut oil and massage it into your scalp. Let sit for 30 minutes, then shampoo. Precautions: Cedarwood oil shouldn't be taken orally. Don't use it if you're pregnant, and use sparingly on children.

11 other essential oils to treat common issues

While the oils described above are the ones I recommend the most highly, a number of others possess healing properties that I'd like you to know about. Here are eleven more ancient oils, along with their most important benefits.

■ *Helichrysum.* It's great for skin and can treat everything from hives to acne. Combine a few drops with a carrier oil and rub it onto the affected area. It's safe to ingest a drop or two.

■ *Sandalwood.* This is a go-to oil for enhancing mental clarity, mood, and calm. Just add 3 drops to a diffuser or rub 3 drops onto your ankles and wrists.

■ *Grapefruit.* Trying to lose weight? Grapefruit oil boosts metabolism, reduces appetite, and encourages your body to burn fat. Inhale the scent directly from the bottle. It's safe to ingest a drop or two.

■ *Turmeric.* The oil of this root has cancer-fighting properties and supports nerve regeneration in neurological diseases, like Parkinson's and Alzheimer's. Add 1 drop to a glass of water.

■ *Roman chamomile.* This calming oil eases anxiety and depression and improves sleep. Diffuse 5 drops or inhale the scent directly from the bottle.

■ *Ginger.* Ginger oil contains higher levels of the active ingredient gingerol than the edible root, which makes it even more effective for treating nausea, menstrual disorders, and digestion. Diffuse 2 or 3 drops or rub 1 or 2 drops into your abdomen. It's safe to ingest a drop or two.

■ *Myrrh.* This ancient Biblical oil can help fight bacteria and fungal infections of the skin. Add 3 drops to 1 teaspoon of jojoba oil to treat staph or athlete's foot.

■ *Ylang-ylang.* Use this as a natural energizer and mood stabilizer. Diffuse 3 drops or massage it into your temples.

■ *Bergamot.* Known to build confidence and enhance mood, bergamot is one of the best essential oils for depression. Diffuse 5 drops or rub 2 or 3 drops onto your stomach, feet, and the back of your neck.

■ *Lemongrass.* It's great for relieving muscle aches and cramps (add 3 drops to 1 teaspoon of coconut oil and rub it on the sore spots). It can also repel mosquitos—and fleas on pets. Add 5 drops to water and spray it on yourself or your pet. It's safe to ingest a drop or two.

■ *Vetiver.* Thanks to its relaxing and calming properties, it's been shown to be helpful for kids with attention deficit hyperactivity disorder. Diffuse 3 to 5 drops. It's safe to ingest a drop or two.

Consider this chapter your introduction to essential oils. Later in the book, I'll explain other important ways to use these potent medicines, and I'll go over some other oils that can be beneficial for your health. By understanding the basics of how and why these ancient therapeutic oils work, you can begin to experiment at home—and find the remedies that work best for you.

CHAPTER 9

Emotional and Spiritual Secrets for Breakthrough Healing

Ancient Ways to Align Mind, Body, and Spirit

Sixty to 80 percent of all doctor visits involve an illness or issue that can be traced at least partly to stress, according to a paper published in the *Journal of the American Medical Association*.[1] That statistic is not surprising. Stress is ubiquitous in modern life, and it can take a toll on every system in the body, from the cardiovascular, where it raises blood pressure and puts undue stress on your heart, to the gastrointestinal, where it weakens your gut wall, allowing toxins and food particles to enter the bloodstream.

Study after study has revealed the toxic nature of stress. And yet doctors rarely ask patients about it. The *JAMA* study found that just 3 percent of 33,045 office visits with primary care physicians included stress management counseling. Only the patients who were suffering from depression received counseling, leading the researchers to conclude that physicians may not recognize the role stress plays in other types of health conditions.

But in the ancient world, health practitioners knew that all emotional and physical issues have emotional and physical causes. In fact, the idea that the health of the mind is important to the health of the body is as old as medicine itself. It was a cornerstone of Hippocrates' philosophy, as well as TCM and Ayurvedic medicine. And that idea colors the approach of doctors who work in these traditions in dramatic ways. For instance, whereas a conventional modern doctor sees depression as a lack of serotonin in the brain (and treats it with a serotonin-boosting antidepressant), a TCM practitioner sees that the root cause of depression stems from unresolved emotional issues like hurt, guilt, shame, low self-worth, no sense of purpose, or few true friends—and would identify and treat those factors, with everything from herbs and diet to behavioral and lifestyle changes, to restore a patient to full health.

In ancient medicine, addressing the emotional causes of disease is the first priority, whereas in Western medicine it's the last—and signs of this lapse are everywhere. We're in the midst of a loneliness epidemic, with two in five people in the United States reporting that they sometimes or always feel lonely or socially isolated; Western doctors don't address this issue, even though loneliness can be as damaging to health as smoking fifteen cigarettes a day.[2] Likewise, the so-called deaths of despair—mortality from suicide, drugs, and alcohol—have recently surpassed anything seen in the United States since the dawn of the twentieth century, when alcohol-related deaths were high.[3] But Western medicine is ill-equipped to cope with the problem. And nearly three in five adults say they could use more emotional support than they received in the past year, according to the American Psychological Association's Stress in America 2019 survey—the highest proportion of adults who indicated that since the survey first asked the question in 2014. Why don't they receive it? Because Western medicine is so focused on using pharmaceuticals to treat physical and emotional symptoms that they ignore the simple truth that sometimes people just need emotional connection.

But it doesn't have to be that way. As you know by now, ancient medicine was designed to take the whole human being into account—body, mind, and spirit. As a result, early physicians created a variety of approaches to help patients cope with stress, bolster their spirits, and keep their bodies and minds in wholesome balance. By utilizing these approaches, you can do the same—and avoid the dangerous medicines modern doctors dole out as well.

A glimpse of the ancient approach in action

Not long ago, I consulted with a family friend, Julia, who had recently been diagnosed with breast cancer. Understandably, she was frightened and worried, and she wanted to do everything she could to fight the disease. So I gave her a laundry list of dietary changes I wanted her to try—including loading up on green juices, green foods, and herbal teas. I explained to her that from the ancient Chinese perspective, the root cause of cancer is blood and qi stagnation. When blood, nutrients, and energy are sluggish, your body doesn't clear toxins or neutralize abnormal cells as efficiently. The green foods and herbs I recommended can strengthen and mobilize qi.

But there's something else for qi (and cancer) that's equally important, something that Western oncologists almost never take into account: your emotions and sense of spirituality. Your body reacts to toxic thoughts and emotional trauma by churning out the stress hormone cortisol—and the result is the same as if you ate a diet of junk food: You develop chronic inflammation. Childhood trauma can be particularly damaging. The CDC-Kaiser Adverse Childhood Experiences Study found that emotional abuse, chronic neglect, and exposure to violence can lead to long-term changes in inflammation, immunity, and brain structure, putting children at risk for emotional problems as well as a host of chronic health conditions, including cancer, heart disease, and chronic obstructive pulmonary disease.[4]

But while long-term negative emotions contribute to stagnation and inflammation, uplifting feelings and the sense that you're connected to something larger than yourself can be the secret antidote that protects you from chronic health problems; helps you cope with sadness, anger, and stress; and gives you the resilience to handle life's inevitable challenges. Regardless of what you're dealing with, infusing your life with more positivity and healthy emotion is powerful medicine. In a study of more than seventy thousand women and four-teen hundred men, Harvard researchers found that over the course of ten years (for women) and twenty years (for men), those who scored highest on a standard test of optimism were the least likely to die.[5] And here's the best part: While emotions may seem like waves of feeling that are beyond your control, there are actually a number of simple strategies that can help you create healthy emotions and, as importantly, help you process and cope with negative emotions.

As I explained to Julia, lack of hope—understandably common in cancer patients—is a key cause of stagnation. When you hear the word *cancer*, it's natural to become fearful about your future. And the medical community often feeds this emotion by sharing worst-case survival statistics. As I chatted with Julia, I discovered that according to the five elements theory of Chinese medicine, her dominant element is wood, so she is prone to frustration and anger, both of which can contribute to stagnation. Those feelings were flaring up after her diagnosis because, like many people with cancer, Julia felt like all the hard work she'd done in trying to achieve her life goals was being thwarted by something that was outside her control.

To counteract the stagnating effect of these emotions, I had several phone calls with Julia, and we worked on shifting her focus from fear and frustration to her hopes and dreams for the future. In addition, I asked her to start each day with positive affirmations: "I am strong and resilient and my body is getting healthier every day," for instance, or "I am filled with love, joy, and gratitude for my family, my friends, and my future." I also asked her to spend time reading the Bible or a favorite book about spiritual growth. Finally, I suggested she start a meditation practice focused on patience and gratitude, spend time with uplifting people, pray for healing, and try, as best she can, to accept that while she can't control everything in life, she can have faith that she's done everything she can and that her fate is in God's hands. The goal: to help her feel more joy, hopefulness, gratitude, and love—even during her difficult ordeal—because those emotions can reignite the qi and serve as a potent catalyst for healing.

Nine months after her diagnosis, I reached out to Julia to see how she was faring. She had opted to get a mastectomy, she told me, but had declined chemo. She said that thanks to her healthy diet, she had lost twenty pounds, had energy to spare, and was feeling better than she had in years. What's more, she said, all the emotional strategies she'd added to her daily life had helped her turn her attitude around. She was feeling optimistic and excited about her future. And, while she continued to get regular checkups to ensure that her health was stable and the cancer hadn't reappeared, she said she could actually feel her body healing.

By supporting the best of Western medicine—cutting-edge surgery—with powerful ancient remedies, Julia was able to restore not only her health but also her faith in her body's ability to heal.

The risks of toxic emotions—and the ones that are the most likely to affect you

Julia's experience wouldn't have been surprising to ancient physicians. Early TCM practitioners believed that fear causes disease in your reproductive organs, anger allows toxicity to build up in your liver, depression weakens your immune system, worry destroys your digestive health, and anxiety harms your heart and brain. The goal in TCM is to live calmly, between emotional extremes.

Similarly, early practitioners of Ayurveda believed that the main cause of emotional imbalance is the inability to process emotions effectively. The word *ama* refers to toxic sludge that clogs and poisons your system. If food moves too slowly through your body, it causes ama; if negative emotions sit in your heart and brain, they do the same. Depression, anger, and anxiety are emotional ama—and ancient Ayurvedic practitioners understood that it was important to face those emotions head on to reduce their intensity.

We'd all rather avoid difficult feelings, but when we ignore, suppress, or numb our suffering, it doesn't go away; it *grows*—and spills over in ways that affect our ability to function in the world. A number of studies show that suppressing your emotions can affect your body and mind. In one, researchers from the Harvard School of Public Health found that people who scored highest on a standard scale of emotional suppression had a 70 percent greater chance of dying from cancer in the ensuing twelve years—and a 35 percent greater risk of dying prematurely from any cause—than those who were least likely to inhibit their emotions.[6] Those who suppressed anger were particularly vulnerable.

The study provides support for what TCM has long theorized about cancer: that it is caused in part by emotions that get stuck in a particular organ. According to TCM, cancer in the left breast often stems from giving too much of yourself to others, which our culture encourages women to do, even though it is depleting; cancer in the right breast can stem from yin deficiency, which can, in some women, be caused by an internal struggle or discomfort with an aspect of their feminine side. Ovarian cancer can come from shame regarding sexuality, especially in those who are (or have been) sexually abused. The emotional cause of lung and colon cancer is clinging to the past and living in a state of grief, shame, or guilt. In prostate cancer, kidney yang is stagnant, a condition caused by fear. One common fear—fear of failure—makes you feel stuck, unexcited, and unfulfilled, and that emotional sense of being stuck plays out in your body, slowing the movement of blood and qi to the prostate; eventually, it leads to mutations in cells. Cancer is almost always linked to the liver, which is responsible for the movement of blood, as well as the lungs, which promote the flow of qi. So if you want to prevent and fight cancer, you need to consume herbs and foods that move qi and blood. Some examples are turmeric, cilantro, fennel, cayenne, onions, garlic, cabbage, and broccoli. At the same time, you need to make an effort to bolster healthy, qi- and blood-moving emotions, like forgiveness, faith, hope, love, joy, and optimism.

Lack of forgiveness, or holding a grudge, is one of the most damaging—and carcinogenic—emotions you can experience. This toxic combination of resentment and rumination over past hurts or insults affects the two systems that are responsible for fighting cancer. Resentment, like anger, affects the detoxification system (the liver and gallbladder), and living in the past affects the immune system (the lungs and colon).

Emotions are incorporated into TCM's five elements theory as well. Identifying your dominant element(s)—if you haven't done so yet, take the quiz in chapter 3—can help you understand which negative emotions you are most likely to be overwhelmed by, along with the emotions that can counteract their ill effects. Check out this chart to get some insight into your particular emotional strengths and weaknesses.

Element	Vulnerable to...	Counteract with...
Wood	anger, guilt, frustration, rage	hope, faith, optimism, creativity
Earth	worry, low self-worth, discouragement	happiness, harmony, security, support
Fire	anxiety, depression, loneliness, jealousy	joy, love, gratitude, passion
Water	fear, exhaustion, inadequacy	peace, self-confidence, wisdom
Metal	grief, hurt, regret, judging, shame	cheerfulness, humility, forgiveness

Just as physical pain is a sign there's something wrong with your body and you need to uncover the root cause so you can heal it, emotional pain is your cue to slow down, identify the underlying problem, and do what you need to do to cope with it. Yes, it can be difficult to face your issues. That's why so many people numb their fear, anxiety, and sadness with drugs, alcohol, technology, shopping, or work. But none of those things are effective in the long run. In fact, they're flimsy emotional Band-Aids, which allow the underlying emotional problems to fester—and usually create new challenges of their own.

The key to rooting out emotional problems is to deal with them head on. There's no one single approach that works for everyone. But I've found that the following five-step process can be incredibly effective for helping people understand what's happening to them emotionally—and overcome it. My friend Dr. Caroline Leaf, a neuropsychologist who has written a number of books, including *Switch on Your Brain*, created this approach, and it dovetails with ancient emotional philosophies. When I'm feeling stuck in my own life, this is my go-to strategy to get back on track—and I highly recommend you try it, too:

1. Discover the source of the trauma, toxic thought, or memory. Keeping a journal and writing about your thoughts and emotions can help, as can meditation and prayer. Tracing the source of your pain is the first step toward acknowledging it and easing its grip on your life.

2. Connect with a pastor, mentor, trained emotional coach, psychologist, or mental health professional who can serve as a wise guide and sounding board as you face your past hurts or toxic emotions and work through them.

3. Accept what happened by acknowledging it aloud to yourself or your mentor or therapist. You could say, "I was bullied" or "I was abused" or "I was told I wasn't smart." Speaking the truth out loud allows you to both face your pain and defuse its power. In fact, researchers at UCLA discovered that naming an emotion—sadness, anger, jealousy, resentment—actually calms the amygdala, the brain's fear center, which is often activated when you're experiencing negative emotions.[7]

4. Choose to use your challenges for good. For instance, if you were bullied you can volunteer for an organization that fights bullying or speak out against bullying on social media. If you were told you weren't smart, you could tutor children with learning issues or write an article about your experience that might help others. By using your trauma for good, you not only transform your own suffering but also become a world-changer who can encourage, inspire, and aid those who struggle with the same issue.

5. Create daily habits that build positive emotions, like faith, joy, and gratitude. Find the way that works best for you. Some techniques that I often recommend—and use in my own life—include positive affirmations, prayer, meditation, reading personal growth or spiritual growth books, spending time with supportive friends and family, and practicing gratitude.

How age-old emotional techniques can help you get—and stay—well

Adopting habits to help you deal with emotions doesn't mean you should never feel bad or ignore sadness, pain, or fear. Quite the opposite. It's natural to feel out of sorts or overwhelmed at times; we all experience an array of negative emotions every day. The key is to recognize the ones that are most likely to trip you up and face them, because the longer they linger, the more likely they are to become toxic. There are a number of time-tested mind-body practices that can help you stay on top of your feelings. And here's the best news of all: You don't need a prescription in order to add these life-changing practices to your daily routine. They don't cost a dime. They're risk free. And you have the power to adopt them right now.

The following ancient techniques are specifically designed to help you consciously recognize when you've become stuck in negativity, and they give you the tools you need to restore your emotional equilibrium so your feelings don't derail your health.

■ *Meditation.* This practice is truly ancient. Its roots in Judaism and India extend back six thousand years. It has lasted through the ages and is astoundingly popular in the United States today for one reason: It actually changes the structure of your brain, training it to become not only more aware of your moment-by-moment feelings, but also to be more resilient and calm. At its core, meditation involves letting your thoughts rest on a single point of focus—your breath, for instance, or a word like *love*. When your focus drifts, acknowledge it, then return your mind, without judgment, to your breath. Practicing this basic type of meditation can make you more adept at recognizing emotions as they come up. It also helps you understand a vital concept: Your emotions aren't *you*—they're passing feelings that come and go like clouds in the sky. That simple but profound notion helps loosen the grip of toxic emotions. A slightly different version of the practice, known as loving-kindness meditation, which was described in the Bible and has roots in Buddhism and Judaism, goes even further by actively shifting the mind from fear, anxiety, irritation, or anger to love, empathy, and compassion. By doing so, loving-kindness meditation not only protects you from toxic emotions, it also helps you be a better spouse, parent, partner, friend, and colleague. In a landmark study, researchers from the University of North Carolina at Chapel Hill had a group of working adults practice loving-kindness meditation five days a week for seven weeks. At the end, the study found that the meditation group experienced increased love, joy, contentment, and gratitude, and also felt a greater sense of purpose in life, increased social support, and decreased illness symptoms.[8] Other research has shown that meditating on compassion and kindness is linked to an increase in positive social behaviors, like generosity.[9] Sound appealing? Here's how to do it: Sit comfortably in a quiet place, close your eyes, and bring your awareness to your breath for a few inhales and exhales. Once you feel settled, think of someone who loves—or loved—you unconditionally. Feel the sensation of their love in your heart and breathe it in. Visualize that love flowing throughout your whole body, circulating just like blood and qi. Allow yourself to marinate in that feeling for at least ten breaths. Then, imagine sending that feeling to someone else. Hold on to an image of that person, and repeat in your mind, "May you be safe, may you be happy, may you be healthy, may you be at peace." When I do this practice, I meditate on how I can be more loving, often with a help of a verse from the Bible. I ask God to fill my heart with his love, and I think about how I can be a more loving spouse, parent, business partner, and friend. Even five minutes a day fills me with a sense of calm and helps me feel more connected to the people I love. Not only can loving-kindness meditation increase your equanimity, over time it will also decrease the intensity of chronic, harmful emotions and amplify the healing feelings of compassion, kindness, and love.

■ *Spiritual triathlon.* I do this trio of ancient practices every day. It centers me, grounds me, gives me hope, and helps me consciously think about—and appreciate—the good things in my life. The spiritual triathlon was a cornerstone of my mom's anticancer plan, and I routinely recommend it to patients, friends, and family. My spiritual triathlon begins with ten minutes of gratitude: writing down or just thinking about things I'm grateful for. Spending time in gratefulness helps me savor the good things in my life and focus less on negative emotions. What's more, studies show it can enhance your physical and psychological health, boost your happiness and life satisfaction, and protect you from materialism and burnout.[10] Next, I do ten minutes of Bible reading. I like to read scripture because the Bible's ancient wisdom guides me and helps me live in accordance with my values and beliefs. But you can choose your own form of spiritual reading—any text that makes you think about living a life of purpose and depth will do the trick. Having purpose in life is more than just a new age concept, by the way. It integrates who you are as a human being with what you do in your everyday life—and it gives you a reason to get out of bed in the morning. What's more, a feeling of purpose is fundamental to happiness, fulfillment, passion, productivity, and overall health. For a recent study published in the *Journal of the American Medical Association Network Open*, researchers from the University of Michigan measured sense of purpose in seven thousand people over the age of fifty. Over the ensuing four years, those with the greatest sense of purpose were less likely to develop heart, circulatory, and blood conditions, and were significantly less likely to die of any cause.[11] The final leg of my spiritual triathlon is ten minutes of prayer, a practice that helps me find peace no matter what is happening in my life. Research shows it can reduce stress,[12] and people who pray are less likely to experience worry, fear, self-consciousness, and social anxiety, according to research published in the journal *Sociology of Religion*.[13] Meditation works, too, as does a walk in the woods. Choose the practice that most consistently grounds you, helps you feel connected to something greater than yourself, and counterbalances the daily onslaught of stress.

■ *Affirmations.* You might recall that one of the things I asked Julia, who was diagnosed with cancer, to do was recite daily affirmations. The practice has been lampooned over the years, but it continues to be widely used because it is an effective way to shore up your private image of yourself, which has a number of positive effects. Research in the *Journal of Experimental and Social Psychology*, for instance, found that self-affirmation helps you structure information and focus on the big picture.[14] And other research has shown that self-affirmations restore your sense of competence when it has been rocked in some way (whether you've lost your job, been diagnosed with cancer or another scary disease, or are in the midst of a divorce). What's more, sedentary people who practice self-affirmations are more likely to begin exercising.[15] To use affirmations to reverse negative thought patterns, first write down the negative messages you're sending yourself—"I am going to die of this disease" or "I'm not going to be able to afford my mortgage." Then write a powerful statement that counteracts it, like "I'm going to live a long, vibrant life" or "I'm going to find a lucrative job that's better suited to me than my last one." Repeat the affirmation aloud for three minutes in the morning and at night.

■ *Random acts of kindness.* As Lao Tzu, an ancient Chinese philosopher, said, "Kindness in words creates confidence. Kindness in thinking creates profoundness. Kindness in giving creates love." What we now know is that kindness boosts happiness and optimism, bolsters your self-esteem, supports your immune system, improves the health of your heart, and promotes healthy aging. For instance, a study published in the *Journal of Social Psychology* found that performing small kindnesses for seven days increased study participants' happiness—and the more kind acts they performed, the greater the boost.[16] Kindness doesn't have to be expensive, time-consuming, or involved. It can include holding the door for someone, complimenting a stranger, picking up litter in your neighborhood, paying for someone's coffee, mowing your elderly neighbor's lawn, or writing a letter to a mentor or friend expressing your gratitude for how they've positively influenced your life. Research shows that being kind feels good because it affects a range of mood-related hormones, bolstering oxytocin, the love hormone, and serotonin, a happiness-related chemical, while decreasing cortisol, the stress hormone. Even better: Kindness is contagious. Merely witnessing an act of kindness can make you happy—and more likely to do something kind yourself.

Protecting yourself from illness, and fighting deadly diseases, requires more than just physical medicine. It requires *emotional* medicine. The ancients knew this. And now that you understand why your emotional health is inseparable from your physical health, I hope you can appreciate the benefits of their age-old emotional remedies, too. Integrating these strategies into your own life will give you something no pill ever can: an increased sense of happiness, peace, and hope that not only enhances your day-to-day well-being, but also safeguards and supports your health.

CHAPTER 10

Ancient Therapies and Lifestyle Medicine for Modern Health Woes

Deepening Your Mind-Body Connection

Several years ago, a friend of mine confessed to me that he was having trouble with erectile dysfunction. Colton was only forty and was taking Viagra—and was embarrassed to even bring it up. I reassured him the problem was common, and we began an ongoing conversation about other things he could do to help treat it. His problems, I told him, stemmed from low testosterone, a symptom of low qi and low yang. He was a triathlete, so he got tons of cardiovascular exercise, and he ate mostly raw veggies and a little meat. I suggested he start eating foods that boost testosterone, like ginseng and fenugreek, as well as nuts (brazil nuts, almonds, pumpkin seeds), which support yang; mulberries and goji berries, which are good for stimulating qi; and fish, red meat, liver, bone broth, healthy fats, and cooked vegetables, all of which can build qi.

But I also recommended a number of other treatments that I was certain would help turn his problem around. The first was acupuncture. It's one of the best cures for releasing blocked qi and restoring healthy energy levels—and research shows it can be helpful for erectile dysfunction. One placebo-controlled trial published in the *International Journal of Impotence Research* found that nearly two-thirds of patients receiving acupuncture improved significantly, compared to 9 percent in the placebo group.[1]

I also suggested he start lifting heavy weights two to three times a week, doing squats, deadlifts, rows, pull-ups, bench press, shoulder press, and planks. While aerobic exercise is wonderful for the cardio-vascular system, the best way to build yang (testosterone) is a combi-nation of strength training and short bursts of cardio — a technique called high-intensity interval training (HIIT). In addition, I recom-mended that he sit in front of an infrared light first thing in the morn-ing and just after sunset to help his body get on a healthy circadian rhythm. Syncing his body with healthy, natural rhythms would also help restore qi and yang. When I saw him again several months later, he was happy to report that he was about 70 percent better, and well on his way to feeling fully himself again — all without Viagra or any other prescription medications.

Nearly 74 percent of medical appointments and 80 percent of emergency room visits end with the doctor jotting down a prescrip-tion.[2] Medication is by far the most commonly used tool in Western medicine — with surgery coming in second — even though there are a number of ancient therapies, treatments, and lifestyle habits that can decrease pain, heal wounds, improve strength and balance, bolster mood, reduce stress and inflammation, and offer myriad other types of healing. These alternative therapies are far less expensive than most prescription meds — and have far fewer side effects.

Exercise is a perfect example. It is deeply embedded in ancient medical practice. In 600 BC, an Ayurvedic physician named Susruta was the first in recorded history to prescribe daily exercise to patients. He said that "diseases fly from the presence of a person habituated to regular physical exercise." Hippocrates prescribed exercise to ancient Greeks as well, as did Galen for Romans in the sixteenth century.

But according to the CDC, only one-third of adults say their doc-tor has raised the topic of exercise[3] — which is absurd given its widely known and thoroughly documented benefits. Studies have shown that exercise reduces the risk of depression, anxiety, heart disease, stroke, type 2 diabetes, obesity, and many cancers. If it were a pill, it would be a billion-dollar pharmaceutical, and doctors would prescribe it to everyone.

And exercise is just one of a number of ancient approaches that can bolster overall wellness in times of health, give your body the strength it needs to fight disease, and help you get well more quickly if you do get sick.

Five qi-strengthening therapies that support sustained health and well-being

While Western treatments still dominate the medical landscape, a handful of ancient practices are gaining popularity as more and more people—within and outside the medical community—realize how effective they are. It's still rare that a mainstream doctor will mention any of these options. But each of the following treatments strengthens qi and offers its own unique benefits. Like most ancient remedies, they target the root cause of problems, rather than fixing the most obvious symptom. As a result, they confer broad benefits that extend well beyond the apparent ailment.

■ *Acupuncture.* Developed by ancient Chinese practitioners about two thousand years ago, acupuncture spread to Japan and Korea over the next few centuries, and by the late 1600s, a handful of doctors in the West were starting to use it. Today in the United States there are at least thirty-five thousand licensed acupuncturists,[4] a number that attests to its growing acceptance among the lay public, if not the medical establishment. In one study of people who used acupuncture, 45 percent initially tried the treatment because a friend or family member recommended it, while 27 percent had received a recommendation from a healthcare provider.[5] As you probably know, acupuncturists insert tiny needles (so small you often don't feel them at all) into the outer layer of your skin to stimulate certain well-defined points that lie along the fourteen major energy channels, known as meridians, in your body. Different conditions require different needle placement—but they all stimulate qi and can move blood and nutrients to an area to aid in healing. Most studies of acupuncture have focused on its potential for pain relief. For instance, Cochrane reviewed twenty-two trials (including nearly five thousand patients) using acupuncture to prevent migraines and concluded that it is as effective as commonly prescribed prophylactic drugs.[6] It has also proved to be effective in those with chronic low back pain[7] and neck pain.[8] And in a 2018 review, an international team of researchers led by two scientists at Memorial Sloan Kettering Cancer Center concluded that acupuncture is effective for treating chronic musculoskeletal, headache, and arthritis pain; that treatment effects persist over time; and that "referral for a course of acupuncture treatment is a reasonable option for a patient with chronic pain."[9] Acupuncture can also be helpful for a variety of other conditions, including insomnia,[10] cancer (it can help manage symptoms like nausea and pain in patients undergoing treatment),[11] and postpartum depression.[12] It also works well as a basic wellness strategy, because it improves digestion, bolsters immunity, balances hormones, and can protect you from the cold and flu and also relieve their symptoms. Chelsea and I go to our acupuncturist once or twice a month, whether we're sick or not. Some insurance plans cover the treatment, so be sure to check before booking an appointment. To find a good acupuncturist, ask your doctor or friends for a referral. The American Academy of Medical Acupuncture has a list on its website as well (medicalacupuncture.org/Find-an-Acupuncturist).

■ *Cupping.* Used in China as early as 3000 BC, cupping uses special suction cups that are strategically placed on the skin to reduce pain and inflammation and bolster relaxation, well-being, and blood flow. Cupping works by expanding the capillaries, increasing blood circulation, and strengthening the flow of qi. Although cupping hasn't been well studied, a literature review published in *PLOS One* concluded that the therapy can be effective for respiratory issues, like bronchitis, viral infections, and pneumonia, as well as shingles, Bell's palsy (a form of facial paralysis), acne, herniated discs, and age-related wear and tear on the spine.[13] Anecdotally, patients say it helps reduce pain and ease stress and tension, too—and increasing numbers of athletes are using it to bring blood flow to muscles to encourage recovery and repair. I attended the 2012 Olympics because in prior years I had been the physician for some of the professional swimmers, and a number of the swimmers I worked with—as well as Michael Phelps—were using cupping to heal their muscles and stay in peak competitive shape.

■ *Gua sha.* This ancient Chinese technique involves scraping the skin with a massage tool to stimulate blood flow. It's usually performed on the legs, back, neck, butt, and arms, but there's also a gentle version that can be helpful for facial skin. More research is needed, but it appears to be effective for a range of conditions. One study of forty-eight patients with chronic neck pain found it was more helpful in reducing pain than a heating pad,[14] while another literature review found it was helpful for easing the symptoms of perimenopause.[15] What's more, a randomized, controlled trial published in *Complementary Therapies in Clinical Practice* reported that gua sha relieved symptoms in patients with diabetic peripheral neuropathy.[16] Another randomized controlled trial determined that it relieved pain and improved overall health in patients with low back pain.[17]

■ *Chiropractic.* For thousands of years, medical practitioners have recognized the important role the spine and nervous system play in overall health. In fact, evidence of spinal manipulation dates back more than two thousand years to ancient Greece, when Hippocrates said, "Look well to the spine for the cause of disease."[18] In 1656, a book called *The Complete Bone Setter* described manipulative techniques as well.[19] But the practice of chiropractic as we know it today began in the late 1800s. As I mentioned in chapter 5, Thomas Edison hypothesized, "The doctor of the future will give no medicine, but will interest his patient in the care of the human frame, in diet, and the cause and prevention of disease." And this is what doctors of chiropractic aim to do: treat the spine, along with diet and lifestyle, to help the body heal naturally. As you probably know, chiropractors use hands-on adjustments of the spine to restore proper alignment, which can effectively treat a number of problems, including migraines,[20] neck pain,[21] and sciatica,[22] constipation,[23] and asthma.[24] In addition, it's great for low back pain, acid reflux, high blood pressure, and epilepsy—and it can help you avoid back surgery, according to a paper in *Journal of the American Medical Association*.[25] Many professional sports teams have doctors of chiropractic on staff, because their treatments can enhance athletic performance, improve recovery, and prevent injuries. The reason: Aligning the spine can reset your nervous system to its healthy, natural state, which improves breathing, digestion, and organ function, and reduces inflammation. In effect, chiropractors remove unhealthy interference from the nervous system so patients' bodies can heal and function in the way they were intended to. Many doctors of chiropractic are also highly trained in nutrition as well as certain types of physical therapy, because chiropractic colleges, unlike medical schools, include courses on these subjects in their curricula. In fact, there's a unique form of chiropractic known as applied kinesiology that's particularly effective. It combines chiropractic, nutrition, and acupressure, a practice that's similar to acupuncture but uses manual pressure instead of needles. My friend, Dr. Christopher Motley, has had enormous success treating hypothyroidism, autoimmune disease, and Lyme disease and other chronic infections with this approach. To find a capable chiropractor, go to the International Chiropractors Association's website, which has a list of licensed practitioners (chiropractic.org/find-a-doctor).

■ *Red light therapy.* Light therapy has ancient roots in various medical traditions, including those of Egypt, Greece, China, and India. In this contemporary version, low-power red light waves are emitted through the skin. (Red light is part of the visible spectrum and doesn't penetrate the body as deeply as infrared, which is part of the invisible spectrum.) Red light, which doesn't have age- and cancer-promoting UVA or UVB rays, can be absorbed to a depth of 8 to 10 millimeters, allowing it to penetrate into the dermis, the skin layer where most of your collagen—a vital component of youthful skin—resides. As a result, it can promote wound healing, tissue repair, and skin rejuvenation. It can also decrease inflammation.[26] And because it seems to affect mitochondria, the energy-generating bodies in cells, it's being studied for rehabilitation after stroke, traumatic brain injury, degenerative brain disease, and spinal cord injury.[27]

The 10 ancient habits that can maintain—and restore—your health

Exercise is at the top of the list of ancient lifestyle habits that confer health benefits. Find something you love, whether it's walking, cycling, swimming, or kickboxing, and do it regularly. There are a number of other deeply restorative habits that are (or are becoming) widely available. I encourage you to explore these options to find ones that suit you and your lifestyle and provide the type of healing you need.

■ *Yoga.* The word *yoga* was first mentioned in the oldest sacred text of India, the Rig Veda. The fact that it is enormously popular today attests to its effectiveness. I'm a fan of this contemplative movement practice because it's exercise with an intentional side. Moving through the poses helps you get in touch with your body—which parts are tight, where you're holding tension—and stay centered in the present. As a result, it improves your balance, strength, and flexibility—both physically and emotionally. Here's the impressive list of yoga's benefits, according to the National Institute of Health's National Center for Complementary and Integrative Health: stress relief, improved sleep, pain relief, reduced anxiety and depression, weight loss, and improved quality of life in people who are struggling with chronic disease.[28] If you're new to the practice, find a good teacher for your first few classes, so you can be sure you're doing the poses correctly. After that, you can easily follow a yoga video at home.

■ *Tai chi.* One of ancient China's early martial arts, this mind-body practice is often called moving meditation, because it's a series of slow, gentle motions that are patterned after the movements of nature.

The practice elevates qi, allowing you to feel rested yet energized. It is a wonderful option if you're new to fitness, dealing with or recovering from an illness, or if you have physical challenges that prevent you from moving with ease. Traditionally, you perform the deliberate movements standing up, but you can easily do a modified seated version. Either way, it has innumerable benefits. Research shows it can improve balance and stability in older people and those with Parkinson's, reduce pain in those with arthritis and fibromyalgia, and bolster mood in people with heart failure and cancer.[29] Find a class online or, even better, check your local park or senior center for group classes.

■ *Functional strength.* You might not guess that building body strength has anything to do with your brain, but it actually affects both your mood and your brain structure in powerful ways—and it's a great way to build qi. A study in *Molecular Psychiatry* found that six months of strength training improved cognition and increased the size of associated brain regions.[30] Other research has shown it can relieve anxiety[31] and depression.[32] I like functional strength training because it doesn't require a gym membership or any equipment. You just use your body weight to build strength and fitness, by doing moves like burpees, planks, and wall sits. (Online programs can show you how to do these moves, which you can tailor to suit your fitness level.) As with any exercise, start slowly and build strength gradually. The simple act of setting small goals—and meeting them—can be uplifting, too.

■ *Walking in nature ("forest bathing").* Here's a quick eye-opening exercise: Set down this book, step outside, look up at the sky, and take a few deep breaths. You feel a little different, right? More energetic, more focused, calmer, happier? There's something about being in the natural world, as opposed to hunched over your computer, that releases feel-good chemicals in the brain and rebalances your body's qi. And when you immerse yourself in nature, by walking in a local park or remote forest, you reap even more benefits. The Japanese have a particularly wonderful name for this: forest bathing. A study in the journal *Environmental Health and Preventive Medicine* found that people who strolled through a forest had lower blood pressure and levels of cortisol afterward than those who walked around a city.[33] If you live in a city, a walk in the park or near a body of water can serve the same purpose. Immersing yourself as best you can in the natural world can reduce stress, improve your mood, bolster creativity, and enhance the activity of your immune system, too. What's more, it can enhance your spiritual life, by inspiring feelings of awe, wonder, gratitude, and reverence, emotions that make you feel better and can motivate you to be more generous, cooperative, and kind.[34]

▪ *Relaxation and downtime.* There's a new health problem that's afflicting more and more people in our fast-paced culture: burnout—the most modern example of qi deficiency. In a Gallup poll of nearly 7,500 full-time employees, 23 percent said they felt burned out at work very often or always, while another 44 percent felt that way sometimes—and that feeling has real health consequences.[35] Burned-out employees are 63 percent more likely to take a sick day and 23 percent more likely to visit the emergency room.[36] And Brazilian researchers found that burnout is a significant predictor of heart disease, headaches, gastrointestinal issues, and respiratory problems, as well as mortality in those younger than forty-five.[37] You might have experienced this yourself. It's something our ancestors didn't have to contend with, but taking a page from their slower, less distracted lifestyle can give us the balance we need. The secret: Build relaxation into your day. Go outside at lunch, sit on a bench, and do *nothing*. Just watch the world go by. At night, instead of bingeing the latest Netflix series, get in bed and read a novel or relax in front of the fire or light some candles and soak in the tub. The Dutch call this idea *niksen*. This kind of relaxation can effectively counterbalance stress, and allowing your mind to wander also fosters creative problem solving—a gift that's stifled in our always-on-the-go lives.[38]

▪ *Digital fasting.* The average adult in the United States spends about eleven hours every day interacting with technology—whether it's reading or watching something online, scrolling through social media, or listening to a podcast.[39] Does that sound familiar? If you're constantly tethered to technology, you never fully relax, and that's hard on your body and mind. You undoubtedly already know this. In the American Psychological Association's annual Stress in America survey, 18 percent of adults said technology use was a significant source of stress[40]—and stress drains qi. Not surprisingly, technology use has also been linked to depression, anxiety, and insomnia. So putting your phone and laptop aside for an hour, a day, a weekend, or a week can give your brain and body time to relax and rejuvenate, which allows your qi to recover as well. It also makes sense to purge your social media feeds of unsettling or irritating influences—and add uplifting ones. I did this, and it made a surprisingly noticeable difference in my day-to-day well-being. Those little hits of anger and outrage add up. Protect yourself by replacing them with things that bring you joy.

■ *Sleeping (and scheduling your life) according to your circadian body clock.* Circadian rhythms are built-in physical, mental, and behavioral changes that occur naturally according to a daily cycle, like sleeping at night and being awake during the day. In Western medicine, circadian rhythms are viewed primarily through the lens of the sleep-wake cycle. But traditional Chinese medicine takes the concept much further, linking nearly every bodily function and organ to the time of day when it's most energized. The twenty-four-hour circadian clock can be a helpful guide for planning your day and for understanding why you might feel a little off at one time or another. For instance, your heart energy is at its highest from 11 a.m. to 1 p.m., so that's a good time to get together with loved ones and close friends, or to talk with them on the phone. Likewise, your large intestine becomes active between 5 a.m. and 7 a.m., making those hours an ideal time to wake up and ease into your day. TCM endorses a slow transition from sleep to waking. Meditating or praying first thing in the morning can allow your mind and body to ease into wakefulness and set a positive tone for the whole day. Take a look at the 24-Hour Circadian Clock chart to find a more in-depth tool for shaping your days. In ancient times, people went to bed when it got dark and rose when it was light. Our bodies' internal clocks are still set to those same circadian dials,

CHINESE MEDICINE 24-HOUR CIRCADIAN CLOCK

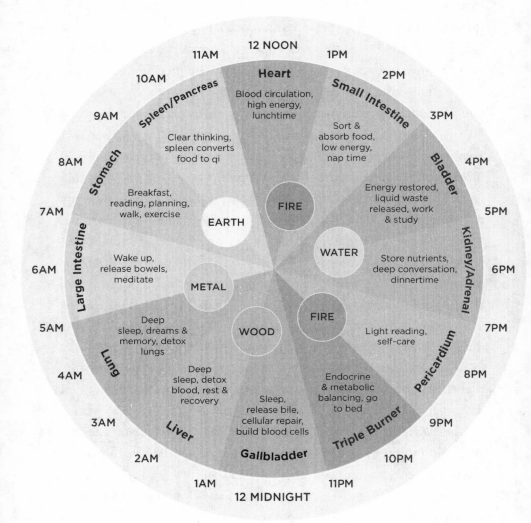

even though we routinely ignore them. But there are reasons to be more mindful about getting seven to eight hours of sleep most nights. According to ancient Chinese medicine, you should be relaxing by 8 p.m. and sleeping by 11 p.m. One key reason: When you're asleep, both your gallbladder, which controls your emotions and judgment, and your liver, which is responsible for emotional well-being, are undergoing repairs. When you sleep too little, both those organs suffer. Indeed, research shows that sleep deprivation impairs your ability to think clearly, and it makes you feel cranky, irritable, and depressed, which means you're more likely to react negatively when something doesn't go well.[41] If your work or travel schedule doesn't permit you to sleep within these hours, try to maintain the most consistent sleep schedule you can. So long as it has a regular schedule, the body is remarkably adaptable. One way to get more sleep, regardless of your sleep timing: Put your phone and devices away a couple of hours before bed and do something relaxing. The blue light emitted from screens can interfere with your natural sleep-wake cycle. That one change can help you live more in sync with your body's natural circadian rhythms.

■ *Grounding and earthing.* This therapeutic practice involves activities like walking barefoot outside, lying on the grass or the beach, or wading in a lake or ocean to do what our ancestors did naturally all the time: connect physically to the earth. The benefits, which include enhanced red blood cell fluidity[42] (great for cardiovascular health), reduced muscle pain after exercise,[43] and reduced stress, depression, and fatigue,[44] derive from the fact that the earth emits electric charges that have positive effects on your body. Although research is still in its infancy, it appears that the electric charge affects the living matrix between your cells, resulting in decreased inflammation.[45] It couldn't be simpler to do—and it may actually allow your body to recalibrate its internal settings and enhance your health.

■ *Crystals.* Similar to grounding, crystals are lovely stones taken from the earth that carry electrical energy. Although there's no contemporary research on their effectiveness, they have been used throughout history to improve health. And while I don't believe they are miraculous in any way or that they are an actual cure for any health issue, I do believe they have subtle health benefits. There are a number of types of healing crystals—from clear quartz, which is known as the master healer, to obsidian, which protects you from emotional and physical negativity—but the idea is to select the one that's right for you. You can read about the different qualities of each type and purchase one online that seems to suit your needs. Or you can choose a crystal by going into a store and holding different stones in your hand, one at a time. Many people say they can sense which one is right for them. To benefit from your crystal's energy, you can meditate with the stone, put it in your bath, carry it in your pocket, or place various stones around your house.

■ *Rain, ocean, and other nature sounds.* Research is revealing that physically connecting with the earth is healthy, and listening to its sounds can be, too. Natural sounds have long been linked with relaxation, and now studies are starting to validate that long-held theory. Research has shown that the sounds of streams, birdsong, and fountains improve both adults' and children's cognitive performance,[46] for instance. And in a study published in *Scientific Reports*, researchers used fMRI brain scans and heart rate monitors to determine how various sounds affected people. What they found: When listening to artificial sounds, like traffic and highway noise, people's cognitive attention was focused inward, as it is when we're worrying or ruminating, and their reaction times were slower than when they listened to natural sounds, which elicited more external-focused attention. On the flip side, the study found that natural sounds were more likely to trigger a relaxing, parasympathetic nervous system response, and an associated drop in heart rate, blood pressure, and stress levels.[47] People seemed to reap the greatest benefits from natural sounds that were familiar, so it makes sense to find a playlist, app, or noise machine that has sounds you're used to, whether it's rain or waves or burbling creeks. Or, if you don't live in a city or near a busy street, just throw open your windows and enjoy the natural, relaxing symphony outside your home.

I understand that life is busy, and it may feel overwhelming at first to adopt a new lifestyle habit — or even find a good acupuncture or chiropractic practitioner. But each of the strategies I've outlined above enhances qi by giving you calm, sustainable energy. And when your qi is strong, you're better able to handle all your other responsibilities.

In other words, these approaches make you feel better, and in doing so they actually make life feel *easier.* Commit to even one of them for a few weeks, and you'll see what I mean. When you take the time to calm your mind, reset your body, and feed your soul, you bring your whole being into greater harmony and enhance your ability to enjoy, appreciate, and fully engage in life.

PART III

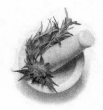

Ancient Prescriptions

CHAPTER 11

Understanding the Five Organ Systems of TCM

How to Use the World's First Truly Holistic Approach to Health and Diet

When I first opened my functional medicine clinic in Nashville many years ago, I was on a mission to change healthcare. After seeing how ancient remedies saved my mom's life, I was inspired to do everything I could to help my patients prevent illness by using food as medicine and heal the root cause of their diseases with an array of ancient remedies. From early on, I was gratified to see that the majority of the people I treated had incredible results. But not everyone responded as robustly as I hoped—and I wasn't sure why. Interestingly, a health problem of my own helped lead me to the answer.

Three years after opening my clinical practice, I was working sixty or more hours a week and on the go all the time. I'd discovered my life's purpose, and I was impatient to help as many people as I could. When I wasn't at the clinic, I read book after book about nutrition, medicine, and personal growth—all in the interest of getting better at the art of healing. I'd work all day, come home for dinner, then open my laptop at 7 p.m. and work till 10 p.m. or later. One day, out of the blue, I developed digestive issues—alternating loose stools and constipation—and they didn't go away. My symptoms didn't make sense. I had an extremely nutritious diet, full of fresh vegetables, bone broth, salmon, and other ancient health foods, with no unhealthy processed foods. I tried to tweak my eating in various ways, but nothing had a lasting effect on my gut problems.

During my search for a cure, I met Gil Ben-Ami, a local acupuncturist who also practices herbal medicine and had studied in Israel under one of the world's leading TCM teachers. Gil told me that an imbalance in my liver was the root cause of my gut issues. My impatience, overwork, and frustration were putting undo stress on this vital organ. In TCM, he explained, those emotions, along with anger, are toxic to the liver. And when the liver becomes overstressed, it starts to affect the digestive system, including the pancreas, spleen, and stomach. Gil advised me to do the one thing I couldn't bring myself to do on my own: Work fewer hours and unplug for an hour or two every day. "You have to turn your brain off," he told me. "Read a novel. Schedule daily downtime." He also suggested I spend more time in prayer while walking in nature, and practice giving my worries over to God rather than trying to control everything in my life. He had me come for acupuncture sessions twice a month, and he recommended herbs, like astragalus and milk thistle, to support my liver.

His advice to unplug wasn't easy to follow. I felt guilty for not spending every waking minute on my practice and lazy just lying around the house reading non-work-related books. But after a few weeks, I noticed something interesting: The more relaxed I became, the more creative and productive I was at work. Chelsea noticed the change, too. She told me that I was more carefree and connected at home. In other words, by working less and bringing more balance into my life, I became a better doctor and a better spouse. What's more, after following Gil's plan for three months, my digestive symptoms cleared up, and my usual high energy and good health returned.

As Gil advised me on my health issues and became a good friend, he provided the missing wisdom I needed to discover the root cause of my patients' symptoms—and my own! I knew about TCM's five elements, but he explained this system in greater detail, focusing specifically on the way the five organs affect one another within this nourishing or depleting cycle, and how toxic emotions can affect your organs. I was fascinated—and eager to learn everything I could about the five elements protocol. I started reading everything I could get my hands on, from Chinese medicine textbooks to clinical studies from around the world proving this ancient approach's effectiveness. As I slowly began to integrate the five elements approach into my practice, my patients who had not responded to my initial treatments started getting better as well.

Now I want to share these concepts, in simplified form, with you. This isn't a crash course in Chinese medicine. The practice is far too complex. I'm still learning more about it every day, as are the world's most renowned Eastern medicine practitioners. But I want to demystify this ancient system, which has been misunderstood in the West for far too long. What's more, by having a grasp of how and why this system works, you can begin to use this ancient form of healing to guide your everyday health, diet, and lifestyle choices—and feel comfortable seeing a TCM practitioner when health issues arise.

How the five organ systems create a cycle of nourishment or harm

In chapter 3, I explained the five elements: fire, earth, wood, metal, and water. If you took the quiz in that chapter, you've already identified your dominant element or elements. You may also recall that each element is connected with particular organs. It's these organs—or, more specifically, organ systems—that I want to explore in more depth. Here's a graphic that depicts the connections between the elements and the organ systems.

As you can see from the graphic's arrows, each system influences the next. Your digestive system influences your immune system, which consists of the lungs, colon, and skin; your immune system influences your hormonal, or endocrine, system; your hormonal system directly affects your detoxification system, including your liver

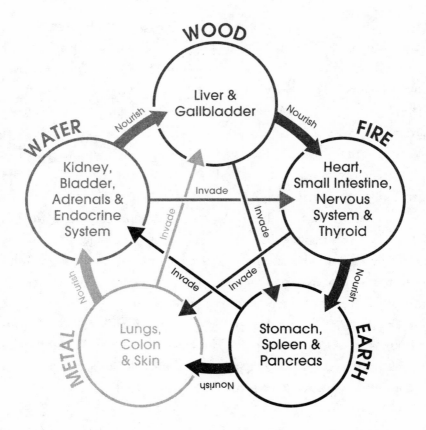

and gallbladder; and your detoxification system influences your neuro-cardiovascular system, which in turn feeds back into your digestive system. These organ systems affect one another in two ways. The first is the nourishing, or generating, connection. In Chinese medicine this is known as the mother-child organ relationship, in which one healthy organ system helps feed and nourish the next one, just as a mother nourishes a child.

Here's another way to think of it, using the metaphor of the five elements:

Wood generates fire. Think of burning logs to fuel a stove.

Fire creates earth. As a fire's ashes blend with the soil, they nourish it and make it more fertile.

Earth generates metal. As earth ages, rich minerals form deep below its surface.

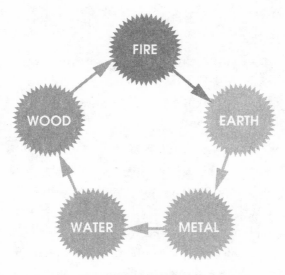

Generating (Sheng) Cycle

Metal generates water. Think of this as a natural spring emerging from deep within the mountains.

Water generates wood. Water is necessary for plants and trees to grow.

Similarly, each organ system nourishes the next. For instance, your digestive system nourishes and supports your immune system, which means that when your gut is healthy, your immune system can function optimally. Indeed, we know this is true from scientific research, which has confirmed that 70 percent of your immune system resides in your gut.

But the nourishing cycle is just one aspect of the relationship. The other is a cycle of weakness and damage, which can lead to disease. For instance, if an imbalance or weakness arises in your digestive system (earth element) due to poor diet or excessive worry, it will deplete your immune system. In other words, signs of digestive weakness, like gas and bloating, can eventually lead to immune-related issues, like inflammatory bowel disease or autoimmune disease, or even lung symptoms, like sinusitis or chronic lung congestion. As a result, in order to heal the root cause of an immune-related condition (your metal element), you need to strengthen your digestive system. By examining your pulse and tongue, TCM practitioners can identify the source of the problem.

Imbalance can also occur when one organ system becomes too dominant or overactive and overwhelms another system—although in this case it doesn't usually affect its nearest neighbor. This is called the invading cycle, and it follows the thin, straight arrows going across the middle of the diagram on page 190. For instance, when your water element (adrenals) becomes overactive due to chronic stress, your fire element (which includes your thyroid) may become weak, causing thinning hair, anxiety, and hypothyroidism. I saw this pattern in many of my patients. I learned that when someone has hypothyroidism, the problem isn't usually the thyroid itself. The root cause is more often overactive adrenals pumping out too much of the stress hormone cortisol and overwhelming the thyroid. Or, in the case of Hashimoto's thyroiditis, two underlying problems are often to blame: The adrenals are stressed, and the immune system (metal element) is weak (remember, metal nourishes water), which causes autoimmune disease, which impacts the thyroid.

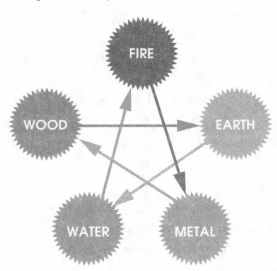

It's easy to understand the invading cycle if you think of it from the five elements perspective. It's kind of like a physiological game of rock, paper, scissors:

Water invades fire, dousing its flames.

Fire invades metal, melting it with its heat.

Metal invades wood, like an axe felling a tree.

Wood invades earth, like roots holding a tree in place and absorbing the soil's nutrients.

Earth invades water, like a dam in a river, slowing or stopping its flow.

In most cases, people have two or three of these invading patterns going on at the same time, along with one or two of the pernicious influences I explained in chapter 2, like cold or dampness or stagnation. For instance, if you have digestive issues, it's often caused by a combination of wood (an overactive or malfunctioning liver or gallbladder) invading fire (your spleen and digestive system), plus several pernicious influences, like a spleen-pancreas qi deficiency, dampness, and sometimes too much cold internally as well. I know this is a bit complicated—and there's no need for you to understand all the connections. It takes years of study. But I do want you to have a sense of how this ancient system works, to help you see that it's actually a far more comprehensive and holistic approach than what we have in the West. The five elements' broad mind-body-spirit approach is more effective than Western medicine for supporting health, because the system is based on a complex, interconnected web—one that reflects the true nature of the body itself.

As Plato said, "The part can never be well unless the whole is well." The "whole" includes not just the body, but the mind, emotions, and spirit. That's why TCM and other ancient approaches are known as *holistic* medicine. Understanding the links between every organ system in your body is a way of seeing the bigger picture, including emotions, that allows you to treat illness at its source.

And there's another unexpected benefit I haven't pointed out yet. In my practice I've observed that merely taking a TCM approach to patients' illnesses can offer emotional healing. Here's what I mean. In Western medicine, you're diagnosed with a single condition, be it ulcerative colitis or hypothyroidism, and typically told there is no cure. Over time, that condition can become part of your identity. If you have diabetes, you might even start saying, "I am a diabetic," as if you're a different species.

But let's say you have hypothyroidism and you see a holistic physician who understands TCM. You'll be diagnosed with a qi and yang deficiency, the root causes of hypothyroidism—both of which can be corrected. You won't be labeled as someone with a chronic disease, but rather told that you have a correctable imbalance. You'll understand that you have the ability to change your internal environment, and to heal. Because of this, you'll stay hopeful. In other words, this ancient system *empowers* you. And that can be surprisingly meaningful for your health.

Research shows that people who think positively about their lives, including their health, are actually healthier overall—with lower blood pressure, blood sugar, weight, and incidence of heart disease. In fact, a large study in the *American Journal of Epidemiology* found that optimism was correlated with a decreased risk of death, a link that persisted even in people with cancer, heart disease, stroke, respiratory disease, and infections.[1] And you've surely heard of the placebo effect, in which patients given a sugar pill in place of a real drug actually feel better. They improve because the mind itself has the power to heal the body.

TCM harnesses this power by helping you believe in your body's innate ability to heal. In that way, it's similar to Biblical medicine, which teaches that faith and hope can help you heal. Just as beneficial, your faith in your body's self-healing ability can work hand in hand with the ancient herbs, holistic treatments, and lifestyle approaches I've shared in prior chapters—and together, they can create an upward spiral of health and healing.

Bringing harmony to the five organ systems

In Western medicine, we view an organ according to its immediate and isolated function. The spleen, for instance, is an organ on the outside of the pancreas that is involved in the destruction of old blood cells and the production of certain types of white blood cells. But ancient medicine views the spleen, pancreas, and stomach together as a holistic system responsible for the entire digestive process. So as you read the following sections, keep in mind that when your TCM practitioner refers to an organ, whether it's the heart or lung, this refers not only to the anatomical structure, but also to a network of inter-related organs. Opening your mind to Chinese and other forms of ancient medicine doesn't necessarily mean fully rejecting the Western paradigm. But it does mean broadening your perspective to include new ideas and concepts.

With that in mind, here's a rundown of the five organ systems and how they can affect your health, plus specific foods and meal plans to nourish each organ system and its corresponding element.

Earth: Digestive System

In TCM, the main organs of the digestive system are the stomach, spleen, and pancreas. They absorb the nutrients in food and nourish the body by transforming those nutrients into blood and qi; they transport qi to your lungs, and blood to your liver, providing the fuel that keeps every system functioning.

Symptoms of spleen-pancreas imbalance: Gas, bloating, loose stools, yeast overgrowth, sugar cravings, bad breath, fatigue, and loss of appetite. You might also bruise easily and have pale lips, heavy menstrual blood flow, or miscarriage.

Emotions that impair digestive function: Chronic stress, worry, anxiety, and obsessing or overthinking harm your digestive function.

Most common dysfunctional digestive system patterns:

■ *Spleen qi deficiency.* Also known as "weak digestion," this imbalance leads to symptoms like gas, bloating, and loose stools. The root causes of this pattern are excess worry or stress; overeating, especially of sugar and refined grains, which taxes the pancreas; and a diet that doesn't contain sufficient amounts of the nutrients that strengthen the pancreas, like pumpkin and cinnamon. Other common problems, like hypothyroidism, anemia, chronic fatigue, sleep disorders, and diabetes can result from spleen qi deficiency as well. Spleen deficiency is the cause of most cases of anxiety and panic, as one worry builds on another. And if the deficiency is chronic, it can eventually lead to lung, colon, and hormonal problems.

■ *Spleen-pancreas dampness.* The spleen manages fluid balance, and dampness—the perfect condition for candida overgrowth—is a sign of a weak spleen. Lifestyle factors, like overeating sugar, dairy, and wheat; mold exposure; and emotional or physical exhaustion contribute to the problem.

■ *Stomach heat.* Stress, frustration, and fiery foods, like hot spices, sauces, and coffee can build heat in the stomach, leading to acid reflux and heartburn.

■ *Blood deficiency.* Blood is derived mostly from food qi and is produced by the spleen, so if there's a weakness in this system, the blood can become weak as well, resulting in anemia.

■ *Liver heat.* When the liver gets too hot, usually from eating fried foods and exposure to toxins, it expends too much energy on detoxifying and less on moving blood and qi to digestive organs. This causes loose stools, poor nutrient absorption, and sometimes nausea.

Easy, everyday strategies to support digestive health: Find ways to manage your worry, whether it's meditation, exercise, or talking with friends or a therapist. Eat mostly cooked foods. When consuming grains, cook them in a slow cooker overnight, for instance, and routinely incorporate soup, which is easy on the system, into your diet. Try not to eat after 7 p.m. so you have plenty of time to digest before lying down to sleep.

Foods that nourish the earth element and digestive system:

- *Vegetables:* Carrots, cabbage, rutabaga, spinach, sweet potatoes, squash (acorn, butternut, spaghetti), and pumpkin
- *Fruits:* Apples, cherries, peaches, pineapple, mango, and papaya
- *Grains and starches:* Corn, barley, millet, and oats
- *Meat and Fish:* Bone broth, beef, veal, salmon, and tuna
- *Nuts and seeds:* Macadamia nuts, pine nuts, and walnuts
- *Legumes:* Chickpeas, fava beans, and peas
- *Herbs and spices:* Cinnamon, fennel, ginger, and nutmeg
- *Other:* Dates, stevia, monk fruit, and maple syrup

7-Day Eating Plan to Heal Digestive System (Earth) Imbalance

Monday
Breakfast: Pumpkin Smoothie (page 290)
Lunch: Chicken thighs with roasted sweet potato
Dinner: Short Rib Tacos (page 338)

Tuesday
Breakfast: Oatmeal with walnuts, collagen protein, and manuka honey
Lunch: Chicken, vegetable, and rice soup
Dinner: Grass-fed burger with steamed vegetables and tahini

Wednesday
Breakfast: Sweet Potato Hash Bowl (page 297)
Lunch: Beef Stew (page 305)
Dinner: Salmon Cakes (page 333) with roasted vegetables

Thursday
Breakfast: Vanilla Cherry Smoothie
Lunch: Steamed rice noodles with salmon and vegetables
Dinner: Carrot Ginger Soup (page 307) with chicken thighs

Friday

    Breakfast: Apple Pie Sauce (page 301)

    Lunch: Coconut Chicken Tenders (page 329) with roasted vegetables

    Dinner: Spaghetti Squash with Grass-Fed Beef Meatballs (page 327)

Saturday

    Breakfast: Blueberry Pumpkin Pancakes (page 299)

    Lunch: Chicken thighs with steamed vegetables and Israeli Hummus (page 325)

    Dinner: Steak with grilled asparagus and broccoli

Sunday

    Breakfast: Congee (page 294) with pistachios and dates

    Lunch: Butternut Squash Bisque (page 306) with Grass-Fed Beef Meatballs (page 327)

    Dinner: Shepherd's Pie (page 335)

Metal: Immune System

In TCM, the lungs and colon are responsible for immunity, and the two work together as a team: The lungs take in qi from the air, then circulate it throughout the body; the colon eliminates waste. The lungs also provide protection from invading toxins, bacteria, and viruses. The colon plays a significant role in immune function as well, since it's where the majority of your gut microbes live, and they impact immunity. The colon also works with your liver to cleanse the body.

Symptoms of lung and colon imbalance: Shortness of breath and shallow breathing, excessive sweating, fatigue, cough, runny nose, sneezing, congested sinuses, frequent colds and flu, allergies, and asthma. Autoimmune disease, inflammatory bowel disease (IBD), dry skin, constipation, and depression can be lung- and colon-related as well.

Emotions that can impair lung-intestine function: Grief, sadness, holding a grudge, and hanging onto hurts from the past.

Most common dysfunctional immune system patterns:

■ *Lung qi deficiency.* Characterized by a chronic cough, shortness of breath, fatigue, weak voice, and a tendency to catch colds, lung qi deficiency can be caused by long-term asthma or other lung disorders, as well as spleen qi deficiency.

■ *Lung yin deficiency or lung dryness.* This imbalance crops up as a result of chronic lung infection or inflammation. It's usually related to a deficiency of kidney yin, because the kidneys support the yin of the entire body, and can manifest as a dry cough, sore throat, intermittent fever, chronic thirst, red cheeks, and night sweats.

■ *Lung dampness.* Typically caused by weak digestion, which creates mucus throughout the system, dampness in the lungs can also result from mucus-promoting foods, like dairy, peanuts, soy products, and sugar and other sweeteners.

Easy, everyday strategies to protect lung function: Work on letting go of emotional issues from the past that are weighing you down by turning your attention to the future and making plans that instill a sense of hope and excitement. Stay warm when the weather gets cold. Swaddle your neck and chest with warm layers to preserve lung energy. Do yoga or qigong, both of which can expand and protect your lungs.

Foods that nourish the metal element and immune system:

■ *Vegetables:* Asparagus, bok choy, broccoli, cauliflower, cabbage, carrots, onions, radishes, parsnips, pumpkin, and watercress
■ *Fruits:* Pears, mulberries, and baked fruit, like apples
■ *Grains:* Rice, oats, and spelt
■ *Meat and fish:* Chicken broth, chicken, beef, tuna, and mackerel

- *Nuts and seeds:* Almonds, coconuts, and walnuts
- *Legumes:* Chickpeas and white beans
- *Herbs and spices:* Fennel, garlic, ginger, horseradish, mustard seed, and thyme
- *Other:* Shiitake and wild mushrooms, honey, miso, and probiotic-rich dairy, like goat milk kefir

7-Day Eating Plan to Heal Immune System (Metal) Imbalance

Monday
Breakfast: Baked pears with walnuts, cinnamon, and collagen protein
Lunch: Chicken, vegetable, and rice soup
Dinner: Dr. Axe Immunity Bowl (page 304)

Tuesday
Breakfast: Sweet Potato Hash Bowl (page 297)
Lunch: Steamed rice noodles with salmon and vegetables
Dinner: Grass-fed burger with mashed faux-tatoes (cauliflower)

Wednesday
Breakfast: Oatmeal with walnuts, collagen protein, and manuka honey
Lunch: Butternut Squash Bisque (page 306) with Grass-Fed Beef Meatballs (page 327)
Dinner: Chicken or salmon with roasted vegetables

Thursday
Breakfast: Vanilla Blueberry Smoothie (page 289)
Lunch: Chicken thighs with steamed vegetables and Israeli Hummus (page 325)
Dinner: Cauliflower Soup (page 308)

Friday
Breakfast: Congee (page 294) with macadamia nuts and honey

Lunch: White Bean Soup (page 312)

Dinner: Spaghetti Squash with Grass-Fed Beef Meatballs (page 327)

Saturday

Breakfast: Mushroom and Kale Frittata (page 298)

Lunch: Watercress salad

Dinner: Coconut Lemongrass Soup

Sunday

Breakfast: Coconut Yogurt Parfait (page 302)

Lunch: Turkey burger, romaine lettuce, tomato, and avocado mayo on spelt bread

Dinner: Carrot Ginger Soup (page 307) with chicken thighs

Water: Hormonal System

The water element's organs are the kidneys—the key organ for sustaining life—the adrenals, bladder, reproductive organs, bones, and endocrine system, which churns out hormones that respond to stress, promote fertility, and help maintain your body's balance. In TCM, the kidney system is viewed as having profound influence over health. It's the foundation of the body, governing the sex organs and reproduction, and providing qi and warmth to whatever part of the body needs it. Your adrenal glands, which sit atop the kidneys, are responsible for your stress response, among other things. Kidneys are also associated with the health of bone tissue, ears, and hair.

Symptoms of kidney-adrenal imbalance: Bone problems (including osteoporosis and problems with the knees, lower back, and teeth); low libido; reproductive issues, including infertility and low testosterone; adrenal fatigue; hypothyroidism; ringing in the ears; hearing loss; poor growth and development; frequent urination; urinary incontinence; dry mouth; and premature aging, including early graying.

Emotions that can impair kidney-adrenal function: Fear, exhaustion, inadequacy, insecurity, and isolation.

Most common dysfunctional hormonal system patterns:

▪ *Kidney yin deficiency.* Caused by an inadequate supply of yin fluids, this imbalance can occur because organs like the heart, liver, and lungs are drawing too much yin from the kidneys. Symptoms include dizziness, ringing in the ears, dry throat and mouth, low back pain, weak legs, and spontaneous sweating.

▪ *Kidney yang deficiency.* This occurs when the kidney's ability to warm and energize the rest of the body is impaired, and is often caused by digestive issues, which inhibits yang absorption. It can cause cold arms, legs, hands and feet, pale complexion, lethargy, and low sex drive.

Easy, everyday strategies to support kidney-adrenal health: Get eight hours of sleep at night and regular movement throughout the day. Vinyasa yoga (a flowing form of yoga, in which you move from one posture to the next while focusing on your breath), tai chi, and swimming are great options to nourish these organs. Also, stomping your feet slowly for a few minutes every day stimulates kidney meridians that run through the soles and heels of your feet. Creating weekly downtime is also critical. To optimize your adrenal health, you must recharge your adrenal batteries. Meditation, prayer, and reading, along with meaningful, one-on-one conversations with close friends support and protect kidney-adrenal health.

Foods that nourish the water element and
the hormonal system:

Vegetables: Asparagus, kale, green beans, beets, peas, squash, and sea vegetables, like nori and kombu

Fruits: Blueberries, blackberries, goji berries, cranberries, acai berries, grapes, and figs

Grains: Black rice, wild rice, buckwheat, and quinoa

Meat and fish: Wild-caught fish, caviar, bone broth, and eggs

Nuts and seeds: Chestnuts, chia seeds, walnuts, and black sesame seeds

Legumes: Kidney beans, black beans, adzuki beans, and organic soybeans

Herbs and spices: Cinnamon, fennel, fenugreek, licorice, holy basil, sage, and thyme

Other: Shiitake mushrooms, miso, bee pollen, tamari, soy sauce, and natto

7-Day Eating Plan to Heal Hormonal System (Water) Imbalance

Monday

Breakfast: Vanilla Blueberry Smoothie (page 289)

Lunch: Kale Salad with Cranberries and Pine Nuts (page 318)

Dinner: Quinoa, Black Bean, and Mushroom Burger (page 342)

Tuesday

Breakfast: Mushroom and Kale Frittata (page 298)

Lunch: Chicken thighs and Rice Noodles with Miso Pesto (page 343)

Dinner: Chicken or salmon with roasted vegetables

Wednesday

Breakfast: Oatmeal with walnuts, chia seeds, collagen protein, and manuka honey

Lunch: Salmon Teriyaki (page 328) with quinoa

Dinner: Stuffed Bell Peppers (page 345)

Thursday

Breakfast: Goji Collagen Smoothie (page 291)

Lunch: Arugula Salad with Beets and Goat Cheese (page 314)

Dinner: Grilled chicken with cauliflower rice

Friday

Breakfast: Congee (page 294) with macadamia nuts and honey

Lunch: Chicken, vegetable, and rice soup

Dinner: Salmon Cakes (page 333) with steamed vegetables and tahini

Saturday
> **Breakfast:** Coconut Yogurt Parfait (page 302)
> **Lunch:** Ancient Grains Bowl (page 332)
> **Dinner:** Spaghetti Squash with Grass-Fed Beef Meatballs (page 327)

Sunday
> **Breakfast:** Acai bowl
> **Lunch:** Ahi Tuna Salad (page 318)
> **Dinner:** Coconut Chicken tenders with roasted asparagus, broccoli, and cauliflower

Wood: Detoxification System

The liver is the organ most affected by chronic stress and toxic emotions. As a result, it is often one of the most congested organs. Your liver is involved in the smooth flow of blood and nutrients throughout the body and mind. It also regulates bile secretion, stores blood, and has an influence on the health of the tendons, nails, and eyes.

Symptoms of liver imbalance: If you're often irritable, your liver is telling you it is out of balance. You might also suffer from headaches, PMS, cancer, gallstones, high cholesterol, dizziness, joint pain, neck pain, tendonitis, and eye conditions, including redness and dryness.

Emotions that can impair liver function: Anger, frustration, impatience, irritability, bitterness, and resentment.

Most common dysfunctional patterns:

- *Liver qi stagnation.* Commonly caused by eating too much rich, greasy food, liver qi stagnation occurs when the liver becomes sluggish and is unable to freely circulate qi throughout the body. When liver qi stagnates, it causes swelling in other areas, including the gallbladder and abdomen, where it can cause bloating. It also can make your tendons less supple, and can cause eye problems, including cataracts, glaucoma, and red or dry eyes.

■ *Liver fire (heat).* Liver heat is a direct cause of liver qi stagnation. Fueled by the consumption of unhealthy fats (like margarine or vegetable shortening) or excessive fat, it can cause everything from inflamed eyes to anger to migraines, dizziness, and high blood pressure.

■ *Blood stasis.* Caused by a combination of liver qi stagnation and low yin fluids (which can be caused by a jam-packed, overly busy lifestyle), blood stasis causes symptoms that can include irregular blood flow during periods (too much or too little), anemia, muscle spasms, pale skin and fingernail beds, and dark spots (also known as floaters) in your vision.

Easy, everyday strategies to support liver health: Avoid fried foods and unhealthy fats and avoid alcohol (no more than one glass of wine or one cocktail once or twice a week), since it is difficult for the liver to metabolize. At the same time, engage in moderate exercise, like swimming, hiking, walking, easy cycling, rock climbing, yoga, and tai chi to protect the elasticity of your tendons and liver. Counteract anger and frustration with meditation, prayer, and deep breathing—and make time to do things that bring you joy.

Foods that nourish the liver:

■ *Vegetables:* Artichokes, asparagus, beets, broccoli, brussels sprouts, carrots, celery, green beans, green leafy vegetables, spinach, sprouts, squash, turnips, zucchini, and small amounts of sauerkraut

■ *Fruits:* Plums, grapefruit, lemon, lime, raspberries, blueberries, and goji berries

■ *Grains:* Sprouted oats, sprouted rice, and sprouted rye

■ *Meat and fish:* Bone broth, chicken, liver, and wild-caught fish

■ *Nuts and seeds:* Flaxseed, hemp seeds, and pumpkin seeds

■ *Legumes:* Mung beans, lima beans, peas, and green lentils

■ *Herbs and spices:* Cardamom, cilantro, cumin, ginger, fennel, peppermint, and turmeric

■ *Other:* Olives, wheatgrass juice, matcha green tea, shiitake mushrooms, and honey

7-Day Eating Plan to Detox and Heal Liver (Wood) Imbalance

Monday

    Breakfast: Vanilla Blueberry Smoothie (page 289)

    Lunch: Kale Salad with Cranberries and Pine Nuts (page 318)

    Dinner: Salmon Teriyaki (page 328) and vegetable stir-fry

Tuesday

    Breakfast: Oatmeal with hemp seeds, collagen protein, and manuka honey

    Lunch: Detox Soup (page 309)

    Dinner: Dr. Axe Immunity Bowl (page 304)

Wednesday

    Breakfast: Detox Shake (page 291)

    Lunch: Grilled salmon with steamed asparagus, broccoli, and radishes with Israeli Hummus (page 325)

    Dinner: Carrot Ginger Soup (page 307) with chicken thighs

Thursday

    Breakfast: Apple Pie Sauce (page 301)

    Lunch: Arugula Salad with Beets and Goat Cheese (page 314)

    Dinner: Grilled fish with baked vegetables

Friday

    Breakfast: Goji Collagen Smoothie (page 291)

    Lunch: Ancient Grains Bowl (page 332)

    Dinner: Salmon Cakes (page 333) with steamed vegetables and tahini

Saturday

    Breakfast: Coconut Yogurt Parfait (page 302)

    Lunch: Chicken, vegetable, and rice soup

    Dinner: Spaghetti Squash with Grass-Fed Beef Meatballs (page 327)

Sunday

    Breakfast: Pumpkin Smoothie (page 290)

Lunch: Ahi Tuna Salad (page 318)

Dinner: Coconut Chicken Tenders (page 329) with roasted broccoli and cauliflower with tahini

Fire: Neurological and Cardiovascular Systems

In the West, we think of heart health as cardiovascular fitness. That's certainly an important part of the equation, but true heart health requires happiness, love, and a sense of contentment with your life's journey. TCM healing recognizes that the heart is the emotional and mental epicenter of your well-being. Indeed, in ancient medicine theory, your body has three brains: the first is in your central nervous system, the second is in your gut, and the third is in your heart. And research today confirms that those are the three areas of your body with the most nerve tissue. The Chinese word for heart, *xin*, is often translated as "heart-mind." So in addition to governing blood circulation, the heart regulates things like sleep, memory, consciousness, and spirit, and is closely linked to the nervous system and the brain.

Symptoms of heart-neurological imbalance: Difficulty concentrating, insomnia, heart palpitations, high blood pressure, poor long-term memory, and emotional problems, like depression.

Emotions that can impair heart-neurological function: Lack of enthusiasm, low vitality, despair, and not having a life passion, mission, or sense of purpose.

Most common dysfunctional neurological and cardiovascular patterns:

■ *Heart yin deficiency.* Often, heart yin deficiency results from an unhealthy liver that is consuming more than its share of the body's yin. But it also may be caused by a weakness in the kidneys. It manifests as an "unstable spirit," with insomnia, excessive dreaming, memory loss, and racing or irregular heartbeat.

◼ *Heart fire.* This can occur when the liver fails to nourish the heart with blood, nutrients, and qi. Your nails and eyes can become dry, and you may develop insomnia, anxiety, and heart palpitations.

Easy, everyday strategies to support heart-neurological health: Practice gratitude by writing down, or just thinking about, a few things you're grateful for before you drift off to sleep. And do things that stimulate your heart and lift your spirits—smile at neighbors and people you meet on the street; sing your favorite songs at the top of your lungs; make connections with people in your community; plan adventures and social activities with friends; and make a list of people that you love to be around—and spend more time with them!

Foods that nourish the fire element and neurological and cardiovascular systems:

◼ *Vegetables:* Arugula, asparagus, beets, broccoli, brussels sprouts, chard, chives, eggplant, endive, green leafy vegetables, okra, red bell peppers, red cabbage, tomato, parsley, and spinach
◼ *Fruits:* Avocados, olives, cherries, goji berries, pomegranate, raspberries, and strawberries
◼ *Grains and starches:* Barley, corn, oats, and quinoa
◼ *Meat and fish:* Bone broth, beef, lamb, liver, fatty fish, and poultry
◼ *Nuts and seeds:* Coconut, pistachios, sunflower seeds, and walnuts
◼ *Legumes:* Red lentils, chickpeas, and kidney beans
◼ *Herbs and Spices:* Cinnamon, black pepper, garlic, rosemary, and turmeric
◼ *Other:* Coffee, dark chocolate, and shiitake mushrooms

7-Day Eating Plan to Heal Cardio-Neuro (Fire) Imbalance

Monday
Breakfast: Chocolate Cherry Shake (page 290)

Lunch: Arugula Salad with Beets and Goat Cheese (page 314)

Dinner: Grass-fed burger with steamed vegetables and tahini

Tuesday

Breakfast: Oatmeal with walnuts, collagen protein, and dates

Lunch: Beef Stew (page 305)

Dinner: Chicken or salmon with roasted vegetables

Wednesday

Breakfast: Sweet Potato Hash Bowl (page 297)

Lunch: Turkey burger, avocado, and tomato in a lettuce wrap

Dinner: Steak with grilled asparagus and broccoli

Thursday

Breakfast: Goji Collagen Smoothie (page 291)

Lunch: Salmon Teriyaki (page 328) and vegetable stir-fry

Dinner: Short Rib Tacos (page 338)

Friday

Breakfast: Two fried eggs with avocado and chicken sausage

Lunch: Arugula Salad with Beets and Goat Cheese (page 314)

Dinner: Paleo Meatloaf (page 337)

Saturday

Breakfast: Congee (page 294) with pistachios and dates

Lunch: Butternut Squash Bisque (page 306) with Grass-Fed Beef Meatballs (page 327)

Dinner: Eggplant Lasagna (page 339)

Sunday

Breakfast: Coconut Yogurt Parfait (page 302) and Turmeric Golden Milk (page 293)

Lunch: Coconut Chicken Tenders (page 329) with roasted vegetables and Israeli Hummus (page 325)

Dinner: Spaghetti Squash with Grass-Fed Beef Meatballs (page 327)

If you are a vegan or vegetarian, here is a link to a plant-based meal plan that is nourishing to all organ systems. In addition, I recommend using the following supplements to address nutritional deficiencies that are common with vegetarian diets: vegan protein powder, vitamin B-complex, and probiotics. Vitamin D, zinc, iron, and omega-3 fatty acids are also essential. http://draxe.com/ancient-remedies-bonuses/

Ancient medicine is the future of medicine

I envision a world in which holistic, nourishing treatments become the norm, regardless of what condition you have—a world in which synthetic drugs are prescribed rarely, practitioners work together to help patients achieve optimal results, and doctors rely on holistic treatments to support and augment the body's own miraculous ability to heal. In that world, your doctor would prescribe a personalized diet, herbal supplements, and lifestyle adjustments designed to heal the root cause of your illness or condition. Rather than drugs and surgery, your doctor would recommend therapeutic modalities like acupuncture, chiropractic, and *gua sha*. And your doctor would not only ask you how you feel emotionally—whether you're stressed or sad or overburdened at work—but also suggest emotional strategies to help you heal, or refer you to a therapist who understands how to treat the emotional roots of health issues without medication.

This is the future I see. It's a future where supposedly incurable diseases are healed, where patients are empowered with hope, and where doctors treat the whole person, in all their emotional, physical, and spiritual complexity. Now that you've come this far with me on your ancient remedies journey, I hope you can envision that healthy, wholesome future, too. If we have the ability to imagine this alternate reality together, we have the capacity to create it—and bring a new level of healing to the world.

CHAPTER 12

Prescriptions for 70+ Conditions

A Comprehensive Guide to Healing
with Ancient Remedies

Now that you have a solid introduction to ancient remedies, it's time to take action with personalized health protocols designed for you. In this chapter, you'll find seventy-five common health conditions, from acid reflux to weight gain, along with the ancient perspective on the underlying root cause of each condition and the most effective treatments, including diet, herbs, lifestyle habits, and essential oils. These age-old antidotes can help you eliminate your health issues by restoring your body's natural balance—and avoid pharmaceuticals and their damaging side effects.

As you begin using these approaches, it's wise to enlist the support of a doctor who understands herbalism, TCM, or functional medicine, so you can consult with them if you have lingering symptoms. In addition, if you are on medications, please consult with your healthcare provider about how they might interact with herbs and supplements. If you have a diagnosis or health problem that's not listed here, go to draxe.com and search my website, or type "Dr. Axe" into your search engine, along with the name of your condition.

I pray you are blessed with extraordinary health!

ACID REFLUX. Also known as gastroesophageal reflux disease (GERD), acid reflux happens when stomach acid leaks back into the esophagus, causing a burning sensation in the chest. Poor diet, pregnancy, and hiatal hernias are common causes.

Ancient perspective: The root cause is weak stomach qi and liver stagnation. Worry, overthinking, emotional stress, and frustration will make these symptoms worse.

Foods That Harm	Foods That Heal
Chocolate, alcohol, spicy food, fried food, tomatoes, citrus, soda, energy drinks, artificial sweeteners, mint, dressings, oils, refined grains	Ginger, fennel, aloe vera, honey, cooked vegetables, pumpkin, squash, oatmeal, bone broth, organic chicken, wild-caught fish, rice, oats, apples, pears

Top 5 ancient prescriptions:
1. Licorice root. Soothes the stomach. Take 500 to 1,000 mg daily.
2. Ginger. Balances stomach acid. Take 500 mg or drink 1 cup of tea twice daily.
3. Probiotics. Clears out bad bacteria. Take 25 to 50 billion IU daily.
4. Apple cider vinegar or baking soda. Both neutralize stomach acid. Drink 1 tablespoon of apple cider vinegar in a glass of water, and at another meal try ¼ teaspoon baking soda dissolved in a glass of water. See which one gives more relief and continue.
5. Fennel. Reduces stomach inflammation. Take 500 mg 2 or 3 times daily.

Other remedies: Try acupuncture,[1] eat small portions, chew thoroughly, avoid food 3 hours before bed, control stress with deep breathing, meditation, yoga, or exercise.

Essential oils: Add 1 drop of ginger or fennel oil to food or drink before meals.

ACNE. Skin breakouts happen when pores get clogged. It's caused by hormones, poor diet, stress, and some medications.

Ancient perspective: In TCM, the underlying cause is damp heat in the spleen and liver.

Foods That Harm	Foods That Heal
Conventional dairy, sugar, gluten and wheat, chocolate, fried food, fast food, hydrogenated oils, processed food, packaged snacks	Leafy greens, asparagus, broccoli, cauliflower, celery, green beans, pumpkin, squash, berries, apples, rice, oats, organic chicken, omega-3-rich foods (salmon, tuna), zinc-rich foods (pumpkin seeds, beans)

Top 5 ancient prescriptions:
1. Probiotics. Improves gut health and clears out candida, which can reduce acne. Take 25 to 50 billion IU daily.
2. Zinc. Has been shown in clinical studies to significantly reduce acne. Take 15 to 30 mg of a whole food–based zinc supplement daily.
3. Guggul. Fights cystic acne in particular. Take 25 mg twice daily.
4. Vitex. Treats hormonally induced acne. Take 400 mg daily before breakfast.
5. Fish oil. Reduces inflammation, a primary cause of acne. Take 1,000 to 2,000 mg daily.

Other remedies: Drink holy basil tea and consider supplements of vitamin A, vitamin B complex, burdock, and milk thistle. Reducing stress and worry are keys to reducing acne. Practice meditation, spiritual growth reading, walking in nature, or yoga daily.

Essential oils: Mix 4 to 8 drops of tea tree oil (or lavender or clary sage oil) with 1 teaspoon coconut oil and 1 teaspoon manuka honey and use a cotton ball to dab onto pimples.

ADRENAL FATIGUE. The adrenals are integral to the body's stress response, and in our high-stress culture, they're being overtaxed. Signs include body aches, moodiness, depression, weight gain, food cravings, difficulty waking up, and hair loss.

Ancient perspective: Kidney qi deficiency is the underlying cause, according to TCM.

Foods That Harm	Foods That Heal
Caffeine, sugar, artificial sweeteners, refined grains, starchy carbs, processed food, hydrogenated oils	Leafy greens, asparagus, broccoli, cauliflower, carrots, peas, pumpkin, berries, goji, figs, pomegranates, rice, oats, quinoa, coconut oil, chestnuts, chia seeds, hemp seeds, wild-caught fish, bone broth, grass-fed beef, chicken, seaweed, miso, green beans, kidney beans, chickpeas

Top 5 ancient prescriptions:
1. Ashwagandha. Supports a healthy stress response. Start with 500 mg daily and increase gradually up to 1,250 mg.
2. Rehmannia. Strengthens adrenal qi. Take up to 350 mg daily.
3. Schisandra. Boosts energy and clarity and keeps cortisol in check. Take 1 to 3 g daily.
4. Holy basil. Counters metabolic stress by normalizing blood glucose and blood pressure. Drink 1 or 2 cups of holy basil tea daily.
5. Reishi, chaga, and cordyceps mushrooms. Lowers cortisol. Take 1,000 mg of each daily.

Other remedies: Try meditation, spiritual reading, prayer, digital fasting, walking in nature, yoga, and gratitude. Build downtime into your day and get 8 hours of sleep a night.

Essential oils: Diffuse 2 or 3 drops of lavender or chamomile oil to promote relaxation.

ALLERGIES. Allergies develop when the immune system overreacts to an environmental trigger, whether it's pollen, dust, food, or bee stings. Food sensitivities to gluten, lactose, tyramine, or additives aren't allergies and don't involve the immune system.

Ancient perspective: In TCM, lung qi deficiency causes sneezing, and liver qi deficiency causes itchy, red eyes. Stress and lack of sleep contribute.

Foods That Harm	Foods That Heal
Gluten, conventional dairy, hydrogenated oils, eggs, processed food, alcohol, caffeine, sugar	Fresh vegetables, asparagus, cauliflower, celery, citrus fruits, berries, pears, wild-caught fish, chicken, bone broth, rice, oatmeal, flaxseed and chia seeds, ginger, raw local honey, seaweed, miso, fermented foods

Top 5 ancient prescriptions:
1. Stinging nettle. Has antihistamine properties. Take 300 to 500 mg twice daily.
2. Butterbur. Combats excess mucus and hay fever. Take 500 mg daily.
3. Quercetin and vitamin C. Lowers histamine. Take 1,000 mg of each 3 times daily.
4. Probiotics. Improves immunity and gut health. Take 50 billion IU daily.
5. Reishi mushrooms. Contains triterpenes, which reduce allergies. Take as directed.

Other remedies: Try acupuncture and/or chiropractic, consume 1 to 2 teaspoons local honey and bee pollen year-round to build a tolerance to regional pollen, drink 8 glasses of water a day, and sleep 8 hours a night. Use a neti pot to thin mucus and flush nasal passages. Also, eating locally and spending more time outdoors in nature during non-allergy season will help.

Essential oils: Diffuse 3 drops of peppermint, eucalyptus, lemon, or tea tree oil.

ALZHEIMER'S DISEASE. This form of dementia impairs memory, reasoning, judgment, and word-finding. Risk factors include age, family history, and genetics. Some research suggests that a diet rich in fat and low in carbohydrates, like a ketogenic diet, can help.

Ancient perspective: In TCM, the root cause is kidney qi and kidney yin depletion.

Foods That Harm	Foods That Heal
Food additives, alcohol, sugar, refined grains, food in aluminum packages	A diet high in healthy fats (coconut oil), omega-3-rich foods (wild-caught fish, walnuts, chia seeds), eggs, grass-fed beef, avocados, olive oil, tahini, leafy greens, cruciferous vegetables, berries

Top 5 ancient prescriptions:

1. Ginkgo biloba. A meta-analysis showed it's beneficial for cognition.[2] Take 120 mg daily. (Bacopa has similar benefits and can help, too.)
2. CBD oil. Its antioxidant capacity can protect memory. Take 40 to 160 mg daily.
3. Vitamin D3. Supports nerve tissue regeneration. Take 5,000 to 10,000 IU daily.
4. Turmeric. May slow the disease's progression. Take 500 to 2,000 mg daily.
5. High-DHA fish oil. Reduces brain inflammation. Take 1,000 to 3,000 mg daily.

Other remedies: Try acupuncture, spiritual reading, yoga, socializing, and walking in sunlight. Get 8 hours of sleep a night.

Essential oils: Diffuse a few drops of frankincense, cedarwood, and/or rosemary oil, all of which enhance memory.

ANEMIA. Anemia occurs when the blood has too few red blood cells, or if the cells don't have enough hemoglobin. Signs include fatigue, weakness, shortness of breath, brain fog, cold hands and feet, and headaches.

Ancient perspective: In TCM, anemia is seen as blood deficiency. Blood is derived from food qi and produced by the spleen, so nourishing the spleen is the focus of treatment.

Foods That Harm	Foods That Heal
Sugar, processed food, dairy, bran (it removes iron), foods that block iron absorption (chocolate, soda, coffee, black tea)	Beef or chicken liver, grass-fed beef or bison or lamb, egg yolks, leafy greens, beets, blackstrap molasses, vitamin C–rich foods, broccoli, red bell peppers, cherries, figs, raspberries, prunes, kidney beans, spleen-nourishing foods (carrots, pumpkin, acorn squash, butternut squash)

Top 5 ancient prescriptions:
1. Dong quai. The best herb for strengthening blood. Take 1 g 3 times daily.
2. Iron. Boosts iron in the blood. Take 10 to 30 mg daily of a food-based supplement, along with 1,000 mg of vitamin C.
3. Astragalus. Great for blood building and spleen support. Take 500 to 2,000 mg daily.
4. Probiotics. Helps the gut stay healthy so it can absorb more iron. Take 50 to 100 IU daily.
5. Desiccated liver. High in iron and B vitamins. Take 3 grams daily.

Other remedies: Try acupuncture, exercise, walk in nature, get plenty of rest, and find things that bring you joy to counteract worry and support spleen health.

Essential oils: Add 1 or 2 drops each of cinnamon and ginger oil to food or a smoothie daily.

ANXIETY. Characterized by excessive worry or fear, anxiety is commonly caused by emotional trauma, physical trauma, life stressors, and genetics.

Ancient perspective: If you're having insomnia, it's due to heart deficiency; if you're fearful, the cause is kidney deficiency; excess worry is linked to spleen deficiency.

Foods That Harm	Foods That Heal
Sugar, refined grains, artificial sweeteners, caffeine, alcohol, and processed carbs	Leafy greens, carrots, pumpkin, squash, beets, healthy fats, nuts and seeds, coconut oil, wild-caught fish and other omega-3-rich foods, walnuts, foods high in B vitamins (eggs, fermented dairy)

Top 5 ancient prescriptions:
1. CBD. Reduces anxiety. Take 20 to 80 mg daily.
2. Valerian. Improves sleep. Take 1 teaspoon of a tincture daily.
3. Ashwagandha. Helps keep cortisol in check. Take 300 to 500 mg daily.
4. Magnesium. Calms the nervous system. Take 250 to 600 mg daily.
5. Chamomile. Calms the nervous system. Drink 1 or 2 cups of tea daily, or take a supplement as directed.

Other remedies: Meditate, pray, try acupuncture, do yoga, exercise, get 8 hours of sleep a night, walk in nature, listen to nature sounds, perform random acts of kindness, practice gratitude, try digital fasting, and make time for activities and people who bring you joy. Additional herbs that are helpful: astragalus, kava kava, lemon balm, and dong quai.

Essential oils: Diffuse a few drops of lavender, chamomile, or ylang-ylang oil to promote relaxation.

ARTHRITIS. Arthritis occurs when the cartilage cushioning the joints wears down, causing pain and inflammation. It strikes the lower back, hips, knees, feet, neck, and fingers.

Ancient perspective: In TCM, arthritis is caused by liver qi deficiency as well as liver fire and blood stagnation.

Foods That Harm	Foods That Heal
Sugar, artificial sweeteners, gluten, processed food, packaged snacks, refined carbs, dairy, red meat, fried food, nightshade vegetables (tomatoes, potatoes, eggplant, and bell peppers)	Omega-3-rich wild-caught fish (salmon, sardines, mackerel, tuna), chicken bone broth, leafy greens, broccoli, kiwi, pineapple, blueberries, figs, walnuts, flaxseed, chia seeds, olive oil, coconut oil, green tea, turmeric, ginger, rosemary

Top 5 ancient prescriptions:

1. Turmeric. Eases pain and contains curcumin, which has anti-inflammatory benefits. Best taken in combination with black pepper or piperine. Take 1,000 to 3,000 mg daily.
2. Bone broth protein. Contains collagen, hyaluronic acid, glucosamine and chondroitin, which repair connective tissue. Take 20 g daily.
3. Boswellia (frankincense). Cuts inflammation. Take 500 to 1,500 mg daily.
4. Fish oil. Reduces inflammation. Take 1,000 to 3,000 mg daily.
5. Bromelain. Anti-inflammatory found in pineapple. Take 500 mg daily.

Other remedies: Try acupuncture, meditate, do low-impact exercise (yoga, swimming, cycling, and walking in nature), take time for spiritual reading and affirmations.

Essential oils: Mix 3 drops of frankincense and myrrh oil with ¼ teaspoon coconut oil; apply to affected area. Add 1 or 2 drops of ginger oil or turmeric oil to soup or smoothies.

ASTHMA. A respiratory condition in which environmental irritants trigger narrowing and swelling of the airway, asthma causes wheezing, coughing, and shortness of breath.

Ancient perspective: Asthma is usually caused by dampness in the lungs, kidney qi deficiency, and excess mucus caused by spleen imbalance. Dry asthma (the key sign is a dry, nonproductive cough) is caused by liver qi deficiency, which causes lung dryness.

Foods That Harm	Foods That Heal
Sugar, packaged food, processed carbs, conventional dairy, additives and preservatives, frozen food, fast food, refined grains, casein, gluten, refined vegetable oils	Orange and red fruits and vegetables (sweet potatoes, pumpkin, squash, carrots, berries, tomatoes), celery, broccoli, cauliflower, wild-caught fish and other omega-3-rich foods, chicken, folate-rich foods (leafy greens, beans, nuts), citrus, pears, honey

Top 5 ancient prescriptions:

1. Licorice root. Strengthens lung qi. Take 1,000 mg daily as a capsule or tea.
2. Reishi. Contains triterpenes, which reduce asthma. Take 2 to 9 g daily.
3. Astragalus. Builds the immune system and lung health. Take 1,000 mg daily.
4. Slippery elm and marshmallow root. Moistens the lungs. Take as directed.
5. Peppermint. Effective for dampness in the lung. Take as directed.

Other remedies: Try acupuncture or chiropractic, spiritual reading to reduce stress, deep breathing (into your belly), qi gong, and aerobic exercise—running, cycling, or walking.

Essential oils: Diffuse 3 drops of peppermint or eucalyptus oil, both of which open the airways and relieve congestion. You can also apply topically to the chest and neck.

ATTENTION DEFICIT HYPERACTIVITY DISORDER (ADHD). This childhood neurodevelopmental disorder features a pattern of inattentiveness and/or hyperactivity and impulsivity. It may be caused by exposure to toxins, chemical additives in diet, and genetics. But question the diagnosis. Some kids with these symptoms may just be bored, or kinesthetic learners.

Ancient perspective: The root cause, in TCM, is damp heat in the spleen and liver.

Foods That Harm	Foods That Heal
Sugar, artificial sweeteners, gluten, nitrites, conventional dairy, food dyes, caffeine, MSG, hydrogenated oils, and hydrolyzed vegetable protein	Bone broth, grass-fed beef, poultry, eggs, spinach, kale, broccoli, cauliflower, carrots, squash, berries, apples, rice, oats, sweet potato, probiotic-rich foods, coconut oil, avocados, salmon and other omega-3-rich foods

Top 5 ancient prescriptions:

1. Probiotics. ADHD can be linked to gut issues caused by sugars and antibiotics, so probiotics may help. Take 25 to 100 billion IU daily.
2. CBD oil. May reduce hyperactivity, impulsivity, and inattention.[3] Try 10 mg daily; experiment to find an effective dose, up to 100 mg daily.
3. Fish oil. Omega-3 fats improve brain function. Take 1,000 mg daily.
4. Multivitamin. Zinc, iron, magnesium, and B vitamins may improve symptoms. Take as directed.
5. Bone broth or collagen protein. Supports gut. Take 10 to 30 mg daily.

Other remedies: Exercise, pray, get 8 hours of sleep a night, and spend time in nature.

Essential oils: Take 3 inhales of vetiver, rosemary, or cedarwood oil 3 times daily.

AUTISM. This developmental disorder affects children's development of language, behavior, and social skills. The cause is still unknown but may include genetics and exposure to toxins and antibiotics in utero or in infancy.

Ancient perspective: In TCM, the root cause is a lack of fire depleting the spleen, liver qi deficiency, and heart qi deficiency. Frustration is a key sign of liver involvement, and poor digestion a sign of spleen qi deficiency.

Foods That Harm	Foods That Heal
Gluten, conventional dairy, sugar, hydrogenated oils, food additives and dyes, and soy	Unprocessed foods, bone broth, wild-caught fish, poultry, beef, cooked vegetables, carrots, pumpkin, squash, rice, applesauce, blueberries, healthy fats from coconut

Top 5 ancient prescriptions:
1. Probiotics. Restores healthy gut bacteria. Take 50 billion IU daily.
2. CBD oil. Research shows it can relieve symptoms.[4] Take 4.6 mg per kilogram of body weight daily.
3. Astragalus. Helps heal gut-brain connection. Take 500 mg twice daily.
4. Bone broth or collagen protein. Supports gut health. Take 10 g daily.
5. Fish oil. Reduce brain and body inflammation. Take 1,000 mg daily.

Other remedies: Try acupuncture or chiropractic, exercise, spend time in nature, walk barefoot on the grass, listen to nature sounds, and try occupational therapy.

Essential oils: Vetiver oil can balance brain waves, lavender oil can benefit the nervous system, and frankincense oil supports neurological development. Diffuse 5 drops of each.

BRONCHITIS. Bronchial tube inflammation causes coughing and develops after a respiratory infection. Chronic bronchitis is due to environmental irritants.

Ancient perspective: In TCM, bronchitis is caused by lung qi deficiency with dampness.

Foods That Harm	Foods That Heal
Sugar, artificial sweeteners, gluten, nitrites, conventional dairy, food dyes, processed food, chocolate, fried food, eggs, oils	Organic vegetables and fruit, whole grains, beans, bone broth, wild-caught fatty fish, probiotic-rich fermented foods, fresh herbs and spices, plenty of warm fluids with manuka honey, miso, ginger, rice congee, pears

Top 5 ancient prescriptions:
1. Echinacea. Shown to improve bronchitis in studies. Take 250 to 400 mg twice daily.
2. Astragalus. Strengthens the lungs. Take 500 mg twice daily.
3. Panax ginseng. Improves lung function. Take 500 mg twice daily.
4. Probiotics. Heals the gut and protects the lungs. Take 25 to 50 billion IU daily.
5. Andrographis. Dries dampness. Take 500 to 1,000 mg 3 times daily.

Other remedies: Take licorice root, mullein, or N-acetylcysteine (NAC); try acupuncture; use a humidifier in your bedroom while you sleep to loosen mucus; use prayer, spiritual growth reading, digital fasting, and daily downtime to reduce stress.

Essential oils: Add 10 drops of eucalyptus oil to a pan of boiled water. Lean over the pan, drape a towel over your head, and inhale for 5 to 10 minutes. Take a few whiffs of peppermint straight from the bottle. Or take 1 or 2 drops of oregano oil once daily for no more than 2 weeks.

BRUISING. Bruising occurs when blood from damaged blood vessels collects near the skin's surface. Blood thinners, aging, nutrient deficiencies, and leukemia increase risk.

Ancient perspective: Liver blood stagnation causes bruises to heal slowly, and chronic susceptibility to bruising is caused by spleen qi deficiency.

Foods That Harm	Foods That Heal
Sugar, processed food, gluten and wheat, fast food, alcohol	Vitamin K–rich foods (kale, collard greens, spinach), vitamin C–rich foods (citrus, colorful fruits and veggies), zinc-rich foods (grass-fed beef, pumpkin seeds), 4 to 5 ounces of protein per meal, pineapple

Top 5 ancient prescriptions:

1. Cold and heat. On days 1 and 2, apply a cold compress for 10 minutes 5 to 6 times. On day 3, alternate warm and cold compresses for 15 minutes 3 to 5 times daily.
2. Elevate. Prevents blood pooling. In first 24 hours, elevate for 20 minutes 3 to 5 times.
3. Arnica gel. Apply a fingertip-size portion to the area twice daily.
4. Turmeric. A potent anti-inflammatory. Take 1,000 to 3,000 mg daily.
5. Astragalus. Strengthens the spleen. Take 1,000 mg once or twice daily.

Other remedies: Use compression to prevent vessels from leaking; apply aloe vera gel and witch hazel to reduce pain and inflammation; stretch or walk to keep blood moving.

Essential oils: Apply 2 drops of frankincense oil to the area 3 times daily. Add 2 drops of cypress oil to ¼ teaspoon of coconut oil and apply to the area 3 times daily. Lavender, rosemary, helichrysum, and yarrow oil may help as well.

BURNS. First-degree burns damage the outer skin layer. Second-degree burns affect deeper layers and often blister. Third-degree burns, which involve all skin layers, and fourth-degree burns, which affect muscle and bone, are medical emergencies, as are all electrical burns. Use these home remedies to treat first- and second-degree burns that are less than 3 inches in diameter and not on the face or hands.

Ancient perspective: It dovetails with conventional—burns are caused by heat.

Foods That Harm	Foods That Heal
Sugar, artificial sweeteners, refined grains, hydrogenated oils, processed food, too much sodium	Vitamin C–rich foods (citrus, colorful fruits and veggies, leafy greens, carrots, berries, pumpkin), zinc-rich foods (grass-fed beef, pumpkin seeds), bone broth, omega-3-rich wild-caught fish, walnuts, chia seeds, flaxseed, liver

Top 5 ancient prescriptions:

1. Cool water. Run cool (not cold) water over the burn for 20 minutes, then wash with soap and water. Apply cool compresses for 5 minutes 5 to 10 times daily.
2. Lavender essential oil. Promotes healing. Apply 2 to 5 drops 3 times daily. Also, apply 3 drops of peppermint oil as needed to reduce pain.
3. Aloe vera gel. Stimulates wound healing. Apply a thin layer to the burn once daily until it is healed. Use a product without additives.
4. Manuka honey. A natural antibacterial. Apply a thin layer topically once daily until skin begins to heal.
5. Zinc. Critical for healing the skin. Take 30 mg 2 times daily.

Other remedies: Try acupuncture, limit sun exposure, and don't pop blisters.

CANCER. Mutated cells divide uncontrollably, invading nearby tissue. Causes include environmental toxins, poor diet, genetics, stress, inflammation, and radiation.

Ancient perspective: The root cause is poor diet and unhealthy emotions; they deplete liver qi, which leads to blood and qi stagnation.

Foods That Harm	Foods That Heal
Processed food, sugar, artificial sweeteners, gluten, nonorganic produce, alcohol, food with hormones or antibiotics, fried food, charred meat	Organic leafy greens, cruciferous vegetables, asparagus, carrots, celery, beets, pumpkin, berries, goji, citrus, wild-caught fish, bone broth, liver, fermented foods, seeds, olives, coconut, shiitake and other wild mushrooms, miso, onion, garlic, green tea, herbs, spices

Top 5 ancient prescriptions:
1. Turmeric. Protects against many cancers, including gastrointestinal, lung, brain, breast, and bone. Take 1,000 to 3,000 mg daily.
2. Reishi and maitake mushroom. Studies show it has tumor-inhibiting effects.[5] Take as directed.
3. Chlorella and spirulina. Support cellular health and cleansing. Take 1 tablespoon daily.
4. Astragalus. Aids the immune system. Take 1,000 to 3,000 mg daily.
5. Galangal. Has significant cancer-fighting effects. Take 3 to 6 g daily.

Other remedies: Vitamin D3, vitamin C, ginseng, milk thistle, and proteolytic enzymes have anticancer properties. Reduce stress with prayer, meditation, and exercise. To tame unhealthy emotions, practice gratitude, forgiveness, and loving others. Visualize a hopeful future. Consider natural treatments such as acupuncture, massage, chelation therapy, hyperbaric chamber, Gerson therapy, and Budwig protocol.

Essential oils: Diffuse 5 to 10 drops of frankincense and myrrh oil.

CANDIDA. If the body's pH balance is off, this yeast can grow out of control. Symptoms include headaches, sugar cravings, fatigue, and gastrointestinal problems.

Ancient perspective: In TCM, candida overgrowth is caused by dampness, spleen qi deficiency, and a weak digestive system. Excessive worry will make it worse.

Foods That Harm	Foods That Heal
Cold or raw foods, refined carbs, sugar, wheat, dairy, egg whites, oils, nut butters, banana, fruit juices, alcohol, soy, tofu, fried food, and pork	Bone broth, cooked vegetables, asparagus, radishes, celery, carrots, squash, pumpkin, stewed apples and pears, fermented foods, beef, chicken, salmon, beans, rice, oats, barley, onions, cinnamon, ginger, bitter foods and herbs

Top 5 ancient prescriptions:
1. Pau d'arco. Strong anti-yeast and antifungal properties. Drink 1 to 3 cups of tea daily, with warming bitter herbs like cinnamon and ginger.
2. Alisma. Clears candida and dampness from the body. Take as directed.
3. Astragalus. Stimulates the immune system. Take 1,000 mg daily.
4. Probiotics. Can reduce candida overgrowth.[6] Take 50 billion IU daily.
5. Garlic. Helps fight fungal infections and boosts the immune system.[7] Take 2 capsules or consume 2 fresh garlic cloves daily.

Other remedies: Control stress with spiritual triathlon (see page 167), meditation, yoga, exercise, digital fasting, and walking in nature. Herbs like grapefruit seed, poria, and sage may also help.

Essential oils: For oral thrush, add 3 drops of either clove or oregano oil to 1 tablespoon of coconut oil, swish for 2 minutes, then spit out.

CARDIOPULMONARY LUNG DISEASE (COPD). COPD is a respiratory disease in which the lungs become inflamed, restricting airflow, most often caused by smoking. Symptoms include shortness of breath, chronic cough, wheezing, chest tightness, and mucus accumulation.

Ancient perspective: In TCM, the cause is lung yin deficiency, known as "wilting lung."

Foods That Harm	Foods That Heal
Conventional dairy, processed food, sugar, additives, preservatives and food dyes, simple carbs, fried food, salt, apples, stone fruits	Organic vegetables, fruits (especially citrus, which contains quercetin), mulberries, mango, rice, oats, sweet potatoes, beets; omega-3-rich foods (wild-caught salmon, flaxseed, chia seeds), poultry, eggs, healthy fats (avocados, coconut products, olive oil), tahini, honey

Top 5 ancient prescriptions:
1. Panax ginseng. Improves lung function. Take 500 mg twice daily.
2. Astragalus. Has anti-inflammatory properties and supports lung function. Take 1,000 mg daily.
3. Ginger tea. Its antioxidant content is good for lungs. Cut up a 2-inch knob of ginger; steep in 4 cups of hot water. Drink throughout the day.
4. Probiotics. Healing the gut aids the lungs. Take 50 billion IU daily.
5. CBD oil. Reduces inflammation in lung cells.[8] Take 160 mg daily.

Other remedies: Try acupuncture; do qi gong "pursed-lip" breathing exercises (inhale through nose for 2 to 3 seconds, then exhale through pursed lips for 4 to 6 seconds); reduce stress with yoga and spiritual reading; avoid smoke, perfume, and insect spray.

Essential oils: Diffuse 5 drops of eucalyptus oil, which improves lung function in COPD.

CHOLESTEROL (HIGH). This naturally occurring substance is used to repair damaged arteries. It travels in fat cells through the blood and can build up on artery walls, decreasing blood flow—and increasing the risk of heart attack or stroke.

Ancient perspective: According to TCM, spleen qi deficiency causes excess dampness, leading to internal obstruction, while anger can lead to liver stagnation, causing heat.

Foods That Harm	Foods That Heal
Hydrogenated oils, sugar, refined grains, gluten, full-fat dairy, pork, bacon, and other processed meats, alcohol, caffeine, fast food	Leafy greens, vegetables, berries, nuts and seeds (especially flaxseed and walnuts), beans, sweet potatoes, wild-caught fish (especially salmon), avocados, olive oil, coconut, green tea, small amounts of gluten-free grains, oats, rice

Top 5 ancient prescriptions:
1. Hawthorn. Can lower bad (LDL) cholesterol and increase good (HDL) cholesterol. Take 500 to 1,500 mg daily.
2. Garlic extract. Can lower cholesterol. Take 500 mg daily.
3. Red yeast rice. Contains a substance that's identical to the active ingredient in a prescription cholesterol-lowering drug. Take 1,200 mg twice daily.
4. Turmeric. Reduces LDL cholesterol. Take 1,000 to 3,000 mg daily.
5. Fish oil. Reduces artery inflammation. Take 1,000 to 3,000 mg daily.

Other prescriptions: Niacin, CoQ10, reishi, and green tea can help keep cholesterol in check. Reduce stress with yoga, walking in nature, prayer, and meditation, and drink 100 ounces of water a day. Strength training and interval cardio increase HDL and lower LDL.

Essential oils: Mix 3 drops of lavender oil and rosemary oil and rub on neck and chest.

COMMON COLD. The common cold is a contagious respiratory illness caused by any of more than two hundred viruses. Symptoms include runny nose, stuffy nose, sneezing, sore throat, cough, and low fever.

Ancient perspective: In TCM, the virus takes hold due to wind, dampness, or excess cold.

Foods That Harm	Foods That Heal
Sugar (including fruit juice), conventional dairy, egg whites, packaged and processed foods, refined grains	Cooked vegetables, carrots, celery, squash, pumpkin, vitamin C–rich fruits (citrus, kiwi, goji, amla, camu camu), fermented foods, miso, rice congee, bone broth, chicken, salmon, beef, lamb, garlic, onions, thyme, sage, oregano, ginger

Top 5 ancient prescriptions:

1. Echinacea. Prevents and treats colds. Take 5 ml twice daily for 10 days.
2. Elderberry. Can shorten illness duration. Take as directed.
3. Astragalus. Strengthens the immune system. Take 1,000 mg 1 to 4 times daily.
4. Turkey tail and reishi mushrooms. Boosts the immune system. Take as directed.
5. Zinc. Strengthens the immune system. Take 30 mg 3 to 4 times daily.

Other remedies: Take vitamin C, vitamin D3, andrographis, and ginseng to support immune health. Make homemade chicken bone broth soup, with warming herbs like garlic and ginger, and drink hot water with honey, cinnamon, and a squeeze of lemon. Do light exercise (gentle yoga or walking in nature) and aim for 9 to 10 hours of sleep a night.

Essential oils: Take 1 or 2 drops of oregano oil and/or myrrh oil for no more than 10 days; diffuse 3 drops of thyme, lemon, eucalyptus, or clove oil.

CONSTIPATION. Characterized as fewer than three bowel movements a week, constipation has symptoms that include gas, bloating, and back pain. Too little water and dietary fiber, stress, inactivity, hypothyroidism, and magnesium deficiency are common causes.

Ancient perspective: The root causes are liver stagnation, and heat and dryness in the large intestine. Overwork and emotions related to frustration contribute as well.

Foods That Harm	Foods That Heal
Refined flour, sugar, pasteurized dairy, fried food, eggs, red meat, pork, alcohol, caffeine	High-fiber food, cooked vegetables, leafy greens, okra, carrots, fruits, apples, bananas, blueberries, prunes, figs, coconut, pumpkin, sweet potatoes, beans, seeds, omega-3-rich fish

Top 5 ancient prescriptions:

1. Probiotics. Help maintain a healthy intestinal tract, which supports the normal movement of food waste. Take 25 to 50 billion IU daily.
2. Slippery elm and marshmallow root. Reduce heat and moisten the colon. Take as directed.
3. Chia seeds and flaxseed. Lubricate the colon. Take 2 to 3 tablespoons daily with water.
4. Magnesium. Boosts intestinal motility. Take 250 mg 2 or 3 times daily.
5. Triphala. Strengthens the colon. Take as directed.

Other remedies: Exercise, such as brisk walking, yoga, and jumping on a mini trampoline. Meditate and pray daily to reduce frustration and impatience, and read spiritual growth books. Drink 8 ounces of carrot juice with 2 tablespoons flaxseed oil upon awakening. Drink 100 ounces of warm liquids throughout the day.

Essential oils: Take 1 or 2 drops of ginger or fennel oil with water twice daily.

DEPRESSION. Characterized by low mood and energy; symptoms include sadness, anger, sleep issues (too little or too much), loss of appetite and libido, and suicidal thoughts.

Ancient perspective: The root cause is lung qi deficiency, liver qi weakness, and heart qi deficiency, which is made worse by dwelling on the past and a lack of hope and joy.

Foods That Harm	Foods That Heal
Wheat, hydrogenated fats, packaged food, processed oils, caffeine, alcohol, sugar	Coconut, omega-3-rich foods, wild-caught fish, walnuts, avocados, olive oil, bone broth, grass-fed beef, organic chicken, vegetables, leafy greens, broccoli, asparagus, beets, onions, wild mushrooms, seeds, berries

Top 5 ancient prescriptions:

1. CBD. Affects the brain receptors that produce an antidepressant effect.[9] Take 40 to 160 mg daily.
2. St. John's wort. Can improve mild to moderate depression. Take 300 mg 3 times daily with meals.
3. Fish oil. Omega-3s support brain health and mood. Take 1,000 to 3,000 mg daily.
4. Ginkgo biloba. Supports brain health and qi circulation. Take 100 to 250 mg daily.
5. Ashwagandha. Balances stress. Take 300 to 500 mg daily.

Other remedies: Take time for prayer, exercise, gratitude, spiritual growth reading, affirmations, making future plans, volunteering, and connecting with supportive friends. Uplifting community events, like church, sporting events, or music performances, are also helpful.

Essential oils: Diffuse a few drops of chamomile, lavender, ylang-ylang, or bergamot oil to boost mood and induce feelings of relaxation.

DIABETES (TYPE 2). Characterized by high blood sugar, type 2 diabetes occurs when the body doesn't produce enough insulin. Symptoms include frequent urination, excessive thirst, fatigue, and tingling or numbness in hands and feet.

Ancient perspective: In TCM, it's caused by a spleen qi deficiency or kidney yin deficiency caused by stress, worry, and overeating carbohydrates.

Foods That Harm	Foods That Heal
All sugar, dried fruit, packaged snacks, conventional dairy, alcohol, white potatoes, white bread, pasta, rice	Leafy greens, cruciferous vegetables, pumpkin, carrots, squash, berries, wild-caught fatty fish (salmon, sardines), poultry, grass-fed beef, eggs, coconut oil, olive oil, avocados, seeds, nuts, dark chocolate, stevia, liver, bone broth, tahini, asparagus, monk fruit

Top 5 ancient prescriptions:
1. Cinnamon. Research shows it can reduce blood sugar levels.[10] Stir 1 to 2 teaspoons daily into your morning coffee or smoothie.
2. Gymnema. Known as the "destroyer of sugar." Start by taking 100 mg once daily and gradually increase up to 4 times daily.
3. Chromium. Balances blood sugar. Take 100 to 400 mcg daily.
4. Fenugreek. Improve glucose metabolism. Take as directed.
5. Holy basil. Lowers inflammation and blood sugar. Take 500 to 2,000 mg daily.

Other remedies: Exercise, do yoga, walk in nature, and reduce stress and worry through meditation, spiritual triathlon (see page 167), and making time for things that bring you joy. For additional herbal support, try bitter melon, ginseng, astragalus, and rehmannia.

Essential oils: Diffuse 3 drops of coriander, cinnamon, ginger, or lavender oil.

DIARRHEA. Caused by food allergies, infections, and stress, as well as a number of digestive disorders, including irritable bowel, and medications like antibiotics.

Ancient perspective: In TCM, diarrhea is most commonly caused by spleen dampness and coldness, which can be brought on by candida (see Candida for how to treat) or by worry, stress, or overwork. Also, hot diarrhea (which feels like you've eaten spicy food) can be caused by stomach fire.

Foods That Harm	Foods That Heal
Conventional dairy, raw food, fats, oils, sugar, caffeine, and common allergens (soy, gluten, dairy, shellfish, nuts)	Bone broth, coconut water, rice congee, cream of rice, long-cooked oatmeal, bananas, applesauce, pears, butternut squash, cooked carrots, ginger, flaxseed oil

Top 5 ancient prescriptions:

1. Probiotics. Research shows they can reduce the length of a bout of diarrhea.[11] Take 50 billion IU daily.
2. Astragalus. Supports colon to reduce symptoms. Take 1,000 mg once or twice daily.
3. Ginger. Eases gut inflammation. Take 500 mg 1 to 3 times daily in tea or capsules.
4. Bone broth or bone broth powder. Strengthens the gut lining. Take 10 to 20 mg once or twice daily.
5. Cinnamon. Warms the colon and balances blood sugar. Take 500 mg twice daily.

Other remedies: Chronic stress, worry, and exhaustion contribute to the problem, so exercise, meditate, spend time in nature, pare back your schedule, and get 8 hours of sleep a night. For hot diarrhea, consume aloe vera juice and steamed vegetables.

Essential oils: Take 1 or 2 drops of peppermint oil in water, or mix 2 or 3 drops of clove or ginger oil with 1 teaspoon of coconut oil and rub on the abdomen.

DIVERTICULITIS. With age, some people form small pouches, or diverticula, in their digestive tract. They can get inflamed or infected, causing pain, fever, and nausea.

Ancient perspective: In TCM, diverticulitis is caused by spleen qi deficiency and damp heat.

Foods That Harm	Foods That Heal
Popcorn, corn, nuts, seeds, gluten, conventional dairy, sugar, refined flour, spicy food, peanut butter, garlic, ice-cold drinks, ice cream, hydrogenated oils, coffee, alcohol, caffeine	Cooked vegetables, leafy greens, asparagus, cauliflower, carrots, pumpkin, butternut squash, peas, bone broth, miso, organic meat, fish, chicken, coconut kefir, baked pears, applesauce, coconut, rice congee, cardamom

Top 5 ancient prescriptions:

1. Chamomile. Expels heat and calms the gut lining. Drink 1 or 2 cups of tea daily, or take a supplement as directed.
2. Cardamom. Strengthens intestines and digestion. Take as directed.
3. Aloe vera juice. Eliminates heat. Take ¼ cup twice daily before meals.
4. Licorice root. Soothes the intestinal tract. Take 500 to 1,000 mg daily.
5. Probiotics. Improves gut health and fights infection. Take 50 to 100 billion IU daily.

Other remedies: Exercise moderately every day to promote bowel movement; drink at least eight 8-ounce glasses of water or clear fluids daily to keep stool soft; for pain, try acupuncture, yoga, meditation, spiritual triathlon, and nature walks; eat foods that can reduce inflammation and fight infection, including garlic, green tea, ginger, and turmeric; take digestive enzymes as directed to relieve abdominal pain.

Essential oils: For pain, mix 3 drops of lavender oil with ½ teaspoon coconut oil and rub on abdomen once or twice daily, or diffuse 5 drops as needed.

EAR INFECTION. These bacterial or viral illnesses cause pain, fever, and fatigue.

Ancient perspective: In TCM, the root cause is excess wind and heat. Chronic infections point to kidney qi deficiency.

Foods That Harm	Foods That Heal
Processed food, sugar, artificial sweeteners, gluten, common food allergens (soy, peanuts, eggs, conventional dairy)	Chicken bone broth, omega-3-rich foods (salmon, chia seeds, flaxseed), cooked vegetables (carrots, broccoli, cauliflower, asparagus, celery, squash), pears, kiwi, oranges, rice congee, coconut, miso, onions, garlic, ginger, breast milk (for babies)

Top 5 ancient prescriptions:

1. Garlic mullein oil. Eases pain. Put 3 to 7 drops of slightly warm oil in the affected ear. Rest with the affected ear facing up for 5 to 10 minutes. Repeat 2 or 3 times daily.
2. Elderberry. If given when symptoms first appear, it can shorten the duration of viruses. Take ¼ teaspoon twice daily.
3. Probiotics. Boosts immune function and can prevent recurrent infections. Take 25 to 50 billion IU daily.
4. Echinacea. Can help fight viruses and bacteria. Take ¼ teaspoon twice daily.
5. Astragalus. Has antiviral and antibacterial properties. Take 1,000 mg once or twice daily.

Other remedies: Chiropractic care can help improve ear infections. To reduce pain, put a warm hot water bottle wrapped in a towel on the affected ear.

Essential oils. Combine 2 or 3 drops of tea tree, basil, or oregano oil with 1 teaspoon coconut oil and massage into the skin around the ear area, but not in the ear.

ECZEMA. Also called atopic dermatitis, this rash presents itself as red patches that are flaky and itchy. They can occur all over the body and are caused by food allergies, chemical sensitivities, leaky gut, genetics, stress, and immune deficiencies.

Ancient perspective: In TCM, eczema is caused by heat in the lungs, dampness in the spleen, and/or heat in the blood and liver yin deficiency.

Foods That Harm	Foods That Heal
Additives and preservatives, gluten, lactose and other allergens, peanuts, margarine and conventional dairy, soy, tomatoes, nuts, seeds, refined grains, corn, eggs	Bone broth, fish, poultry, fermented foods, miso, cooked vegetables, carrots, leafy greens, cauliflower, cabbage, celery, broccoli, squash, pumpkin, mulberries, pears, apples, blueberries, coconut oil, oatmeal, rice congee, grass-fed beef, sweet potatoes

Top 5 ancient prescriptions:
1. Sun therapy or vitamin D3. Calms inflammation and reduces itching. Get 10 to 15 mins of sun (without sunscreen) daily. For D3, take 2,000 to 10,000 IU daily.
2. Dead Sea salt bath. Increases hydration and reduces inflammation. Take a warm (not hot) bath once or twice daily. Follow package instructions for adding salt.
3. Probiotics. Heals gut, reduces flares. Take 50 billion IU daily.
4. Peony. Nourishes blood and decreases heat. Take as directed.
5. Burdock. Reduces skin inflammation. Take as directed.

Other remedies: Apply this skin-soothing salve before bed: ¼ cup aloe vera gel, ¼ cup manuka honey, 40 drops lavender or chamomile oil. Wash off in the morning. Calendula can heal skin too. Other helpful supplements include lonicera, fish oil, peppermint, and zinc. Acupuncture can control itchiness. Reduce stress with fun activities outdoors.

Essential oils: Mix 1 teaspoon coconut oil, 5 drops tea tree oil, and 5 drops lavender oil; apply to rash.

ENDOMETRIOSIS. This condition, in which the endometrium (the tissue lining the uterus) grows on the ovaries, fallopian tubes, or pelvic lining, causes pelvic pain and infertility.

Ancient perspective: In TCM, it's caused by qi stagnation and blood stasis.

Foods That Harm	Foods That Heal
Processed food, sugar, artificial sweeteners, dairy, refined grains, hydrogenated oils, raw food, ice-cold food, fried food, gluten, alcohol, meat or dairy with hormones or antibiotics, produce with pesticides	Organic leafy greens, asparagus, beets, broccoli, cauliflower, carrots, pumpkin, squash, berries, goji, figs, kiwi, pineapple, chia seeds, flaxseed, bone broth, wild-caught salmon, grass-fed beef, avocados, olive oil, coconut oil, green tea, turmeric, ginger, rosemary

Top 5 ancient prescriptions:

1. Dong quai. It's anti-inflammatory and promotes blood movement. Take as directed.
2. Vitex. Reduces pain and bleeding. Take 400 mg daily.
3. Rehmannia. Boosts qi and blood movement. Take up to 350 mg daily. (Avoid if you're pregnant or breastfeeding.)
4. Turmeric and skullcap. Both reduce inflammation. Take as directed.
5. Bupleurum. Encourages movement of qi. Take as directed.

Other remedies: Try acupuncture, take fish oil supplements, exercise, meditate, pray, read spiritual growth books, practice gratitude, and, if your condition is causing emotional issues, talk to a therapist or join a support group.

Essential oils: Mix 3 drops each of clary sage, rose, and lavender oil with 1 teaspoon coconut oil and rub on abdomen twice daily.

ERECTILE DYSFUNCTION. The inability to get or sustain an erection can be caused by low testosterone, poor diet, depression, fatigue, and heavy metal poisoning.

Ancient perspective: In TCM, erectile dysfunction is caused by kidney yang deficiency and liver qi stagnation.

Foods That Harm	Foods That Heal
Refined vegetable oils, processed food, sugar, artificial sweeteners, caffeine, alcohol, fatty food, fried food	High-fiber food, omega-3-rich foods (wild-caught salmon, tuna, walnuts), vitamin E–rich foods (sunflower seeds, almonds, brazil nuts, avocados, spinach), zinc-rich foods (liver, pumpkin seeds, beans, eggs, grass-fed beef), bone broth, coconut oil, gluten-free grains, rice, oatmeal, sweet potatoes, cherries, figs, cinnamon, ginger

Top 5 ancient prescriptions:
1. Fenugreek. Boosts testosterone. Take 500 to 2,000 mg daily.
2. Panax ginseng. Known as herbal Viagra, it can promote healthy erectile function. Take 600 to 1,000 mg daily for 4 to 12 weeks.
3. Saw palmetto extract. Supports testosterone levels. Take the recommended dose.
4. Epimedium ("horny goat weed"). Facilitates blood flow. Take as directed.
5. Rhodiola. Improves sexual function. Take 150 to 200 mg daily for 3 months.

Other remedies: Do strength training and high-intensity interval training; try acupuncture; reduce stress through prayer, meditation, and yoga; get 8 hours of sleep a night; practice gratitude. Zinc, tribulus, cordyceps, and maca can also help.

Essential oils: Add 3 drops of sandalwood oil, a natural aphrodisiac, to 1 teaspoon of coconut oil and rub it on your abdomen, back of neck, and bottoms of feet. Diffuse 5 drops of rose oil, which tames stress and anxiety, or rub 2 drops on your neck before sex.

FIBROMYALGIA. This chronic illness is marked by body-wide muscle pain, fatigue, impaired memory, depression, anxiety, headaches, sleep apnea, and irritable bowel syndrome.

Ancient perspective: In TCM, spleen qi deficiency contributes, and the root cause is past trauma, lack of sympathy, and unhealed emotional pain.

Foods That Harm	Foods That Heal
Cold or raw foods, refined carbs, sugar, wheat, dairy, egg whites, oils, nut butters, bananas, fruit juices, alcohol, soy, tofu, fried food, pork	Magnesium-rich foods, cooked spinach, kale, asparagus, broccoli, cauliflower, carrots, pumpkin, squash, blueberries, apples, pears, rice congee, omega-3-rich foods (salmon, walnuts, flaxseed, coconut oil, avocados), grass-fed beef, poultry, bone broth

Top 5 ancient prescriptions:
1. Magnesium. Relaxes muscles. Take 250 to 600 mg daily.
2. Astragalus. Strengthens organ systems. Take 1,000 mg daily.
3. Ashwagandha. Keeps cortisol balanced and aids sleep. Take 500 to 1,000 mg daily.
4. Turmeric. Relieves inflammation and pain. Take 1,000 mg daily.
5. CBD. Reduces pain and inflammation. Take 20 to 100 mg daily.

Other remedies: Try acupuncture, chiropractic, cupping, and/or massage; pray; meditate; read for spiritual growth; exercise; do yoga; get daily sunshine; walk in nature; practice gratitude and affirmations; seek therapy to work through trauma and difficult emotions.

Essential oils: Diffuse 3 drops of lavender, frankincense, ylang-ylang, or peppermint oil, or add 3 drops of any of those oils to 1 teaspoon coconut oil and rub into painful muscles.

FLU. This contagious respiratory illness is caused by a variety of viruses, and can cause mild to severe illness with fever, chills, cough, and body aches.

Ancient perspective: In TCM, the flu is caused by excess wind. Qi deficiency contributes.

Foods That Harm	Foods That Heal
Cold or raw foods, refined carbs, sugar, wheat, dairy, egg whites, oils, fried food, spicy food, bananas, dried fruit, cold water, caffeine, alcohol	Light and easy-to-digest foods (bone broth soups, cooked vegetables), celery, carrots, rice, parsley, garlic, onions, miso, shiitake mushrooms, herbal teas, licorice tea, ginger tea

Top 5 ancient prescriptions:

1. Elderberry. Stimulates the immune system. Take as directed.
2. Echinacea. Eases upper respiratory symptoms. Take 1,000 mg 2 or 3 times daily.
3. Probiotics. Bacillus bacteria has anti-flu activity. Take 50 billion IU daily.
4. Astragalus. Strengthens the gut and immune system. Take 1,000 mg 2 or 3 times daily.
5. Bone broth. Supports immune health. Drink 3 to 4 cups daily.

Other remedies: Take zinc, vitamin C, vitamin D, and turkey tail mushrooms; get acupuncture and chiropractic care; sleep as much as possible; reduce stress; breathe fresh air; use a humidifier at night; gargle with salt water; drink ginger tea (cut up a 2-inch knob of ginger, steep in 4 cups of hot water, and add 1 tablespoon honey and lemon); cook with wind-expelling herbs (sage, oregano, thyme, galangal, and garlic); drink plenty of water throughout the day.

Essential oils: Take 1 or 2 drops of oregano oil daily for no more than 14 days; rub 3 drops of peppermint or frankincense oil onto your neck and soles of your feet; mix 1 drop of clove oil with ¼ teaspoon coconut oil and take once daily for no more than 14 days.

FOOD SENSITIVITIES. A food sensitivity is an adverse reaction to certain foods that can cause diarrhea, bloating, constipation, gas, eczema, and acne. The most common offenders are lactose and casein (in cow's milk), gluten (in wheat, barley, and rye), soy, corn, eggs, peanuts, tyramine (in cheese, sour cream, beer, red wine, sausage, avocado, and chocolate), and preservatives and additives. To diagnose, eliminate all items in the "foods that harm" list below for 3 weeks. Then, introduce one food group at a time. Eat it every day for 1 week. If your symptoms return, eliminate the food again. If your symptoms go away, you'll know that's the culprit.

Ancient perspective: In TCM, the cause is spleen qi deficiency and dampness.

Foods That Harm	Foods That Heal
Gluten, dairy, soy, corn, peanuts, citrus fruits, hydrogenated oils, added sugars, alcohol, caffeine, nightshades (potatoes, tomatoes, bell peppers, eggplant)	Fill your plate with 40% organic fresh vegetables, 30% clean protein (bone broth, grass-fed beef, wild-caught fish, pastured chicken), 20% healthy fat (coconut oil, olive oil, ghee, almond butter), and 10% whole food carbs and fruit (rice congee, oatmeal, applesauce, pears, blueberries).

Top 5 ancient prescriptions:
1. Bone broth. Collagen and amino acids heal gut lining. Drink 2 or 3 cups daily.
2. Astragalus. Strengthens the digestive system. Take 500 to 2,000 mg daily.
3. Probiotics. Replenishes beneficial bacteria. Take 50 to 100 billion IU daily.
4. Digestive enzymes. Aids digestion. Take as directed.
5. Digestive bitters. Aids digestion and reduces dampness. Take as directed.

Other remedies: Try acupuncture and supplements of L-glutamine, gentian, thyme, and MSM. Reduce stress with meditation, yoga, and nature walks.

GALLBLADDER DISEASE. Characterized by gallstones (a hardened deposit in the gallbladder) and mild inflammation, this condition causes pain in the upper right abdomen near the rib cage.

Ancient perspective: In TCM, this problem is linked to damp heat in the liver and gallbladder. Anger, frustration, overwork, and overthinking make it worse.

Foods That Harm	Foods That Heal
Spicy food, garlic, pepper, high-fat food, hydrogenated oils, fast food, fried food, dairy, butter, chocolate, peanuts, shrimp, pork, red meat, vinegar, citrus fruits, coffee, alcohol	Organic artichokes, asparagus, broccoli, beets, celery, carrots, radish, zucchini, pumpkin, cilantro, apples, berries, plums, pears, beans, rice, oatmeal, quinoa, lean protein, bone broth, chicken, wild-caught fish, matcha green tea, liver

Top 5 ancient prescriptions:
1. Digestive bitters. Clears liver heat and toxins. Take as directed.
2. Ox bile salts. Helps digest fat and dissolve gallstones. Take 1 or 2 capsules daily with meals.
3. Lipase enzymes. Bolsters fat digestion. Take as directed.
4. Milk thistle. Promotes liver and gallbladder health. Take 150 mg 2 or 3 times daily.
5. Artichoke and turmeric. Both improve bile flow. Take as directed.

Other remedies: For spasms, take wild yam root as directed every hour. To ease gallbladder pain, apply a warm compress to the area for 10 to 15 mins, repeating throughout the day as needed. Also helpful for pain: Stir 2 tablespoons apple cider vinegar into warm water and sip. Exercise regularly to reduce cholesterol and prevent gallstones. Reduce stress with meditation, acupuncture, yoga, spiritual triathlon (see page 167), walks in nature, and daily downtime.

GOUT. A complex form of arthritis, gout is characterized by sudden, severe pain in joints, usually in the big toe, feet, ankles, knees, hands, and wrists. Caused by a buildup and crystallization of uric acid in the joints.

Ancient perspective: Root causes are liver heat and dampness and kidney qi deficiency.

Foods That Harm	Foods That Heal
High-purine foods (red meat, wild game, tuna, sardines, scallops, trout), nightshades (tomato, eggplant), organ meat, packaged snacks, sodium, alcohol, refined carbs, high-fructose foods (soda, fruit juice)	Organic artichokes, celery, cucumber, radish, broccoli, cauliflower, carrots, zucchini, pumpkin, parsley, apples, cherries, blueberries, kiwi, watermelon, seeds, rice, coconut, olive, flaxseed oil, coffee, matcha green tea, eggs, chicken, wild-caught salmon, bone broth

Top 5 ancient prescriptions:

1. Celery seed extract. Decreases uric acid buildup. Take as directed.
2. Black cherry juice. Reduces the number of attacks.[12] Drink 1 or 2 cups daily.
3. Nettle tea. Clears uric acid. Drink 1 or 2 cups daily.
4. Fish oil. Reduces inflammation. Take 1,000 to 2,000 mg daily.
5. Burdock. Cleanses the liver and uric acid. 1,000 to 2,000 mg daily.

Other remedies: Try acupuncture, exercise, do yoga, walk in nature, and work on stress reduction. Soak your foot in epsom salt bath for 30 minutes 3 times daily. Magnesium, vitamin C, dandelion, milk thistle, chlorella, and bromelain can also help.

Essential oils: Add 3 drops of wintergreen, birch, or peppermint oil to ¼ teaspoon of coconut oil and apply to the painful joints.

HAIR LOSS. This can be caused by hormonal changes, genetics, stress, thyroid conditions, and some medications. Male pattern is usually a receding hairline. Female pattern is balding at the top of the head.

Ancient perspective: In TCM, hair loss is caused by kidney qi and yin deficiency.

Foods That Harm	Foods That Heal
Hydrogenated fats, sugar, refined grains, processed food, soy, fried food, alcohol	Wild-caught salmon, sardines, mackerel, eggs, chicken, bone broth, chia seeds, flaxseed, pumpkin seeds, almonds, walnuts, berries, mulberries, goji, figs, mango, spinach, broccoli, beets, sweet potatoes, coconut, avocados, rice, oats, beans, mushrooms, green tea, spirulina

Top 5 ancient prescriptions:

1. Fo-ti. Historically known for stopping hair loss. Take 1,000 to 2,000 mg daily.
2. Saw palmetto. Good for male pattern loss. Take according to package directions.
3. Bone broth. High in collagen and hair-building amino acids. Drink 2 cups daily.
4. Panax ginseng. Stimulates hair follicles. Take 500 mg twice daily.
5. Ashwagandha. Balances cortisol and promotes hair growth. Take 500 mg daily.

Other remedies: Acupuncture can help, as can supplementing with biotin, rehmannia, and omega-3s. Also, to clear blocked follicles, apply 2 tablespoons aloe vera juice to the scalp twice daily; allow to sit for 1 hour before shampooing.

Essential oils: Add 3 drops of rosemary oil to ¼ teaspoon coconut oil and massage into scalp to promote growth; add 3 drops each of peppermint, rosemary, and sage oil to 1 tablespoon olive oil and massage into scalp to stimulate new hair growth.

HASHIMOTO'S THYROIDITIS. In this autoimmune disorder, the immune system attacks the thyroid. Signs are fatigue, depression, digestive issues, infertility, and low libido.

Ancient perspective: Weak lung qi (metal) causes weakness in the kidney and endocrine system (water). Stress and adrenal fatigue are contributing factors.

Foods That Harm	Foods That Heal
Sugar, gluten, refined flour, packaged and processed foods, conventional dairy, raw food, hydrogenated oils, alcohol, excess caffeine	Wild-caught salmon, bone broth, chicken, grass-fed meat, coconut oil, fermented foods, cooked asparagus, broccoli, cauliflower, celery, pumpkin, squash, sweet potatoes, berries, pears, goji, rice, oats, beans, miso, seaweed, chia seeds, flaxseed

Top 5 ancient prescriptions:
1. Ashwagandha. Balances stress and thyroid hormones. Start with 500 mg daily and increase gradually to 1,250 mg.
2. Astragalus. Strengthens the organ systems and fights stress. Take 1,000 mg once or twice daily.
3. Pinella. Stabilizes the nervous system and calms the immune system. Take as directed.
4. Probiotics. Supports gut health and reduces inflammation. Take 50 billion IU daily.
5. CBD oil. Reduces inflammation. Take 40 to 160 mg daily.

Other remedies: Try acupuncture and stress reduction through exercise, prayer, meditation, spiritual growth reading, yoga, walking in nature, digital fasting, and spending time with a community of supportive friends. The mushroom chaga also helps the thyroid.

Essential oils: Diffuse 3 drops of frankincense, holy basil, or lemongrass oil. Combine 1 drop each of frankincense and myrrh oil with 1 teaspoon coconut oil; apply below the Adam's apple.

HEMORRHOIDS. Everyone has veins inside and outside their anus, but when they become enlarged, they cause itching, pain, mucus discharge, and bleeding.

Ancient perspective: Intestinal qi deficiency and qi stagnation.

Foods That Harm	Foods That Heal
Fried food, spicy food, oil, fatty food, gluten and other allergens, caffeine, alcohol	High-fiber food, small meals, fermented foods, cooked artichokes, cauliflower, carrots, asparagus, celery, red cabbage, green beans, peas, pumpkin, squash, apples, blueberries, cherries, goji, grapes, raspberries, wild-caught salmon

Top 5 ancient prescriptions:
1. Butcher's broom. Reduces swelling and helps veins contract. Take 200 mg 2 or 3 times daily.
2. Horse chestnut. Promotes blood flow and reduces swelling. Take 100 to 150 mg of aescin (the active ingredient) daily. Most extracts are 20% aescin.
3. Bilberry. Reduces hemorrhoid-related pain and swelling. Use an extract according to package directions.
4. CBD suppositories. Reduces pain and inflammation. Take as directed.
5. Witch hazel. Relieves inflammation and itching. Apply a small amount topically.

Other remedies: Try acupuncture and movement, whether it's yoga, walking, running, swimming, or other exercise. Since constipation is a cause, counteract it with daily prayer, meditation, and spiritual growth reading to reduce frustration and to build hope and faith. Drink plenty of fluids throughout the day.

Essential oils: Mix 3 drops of cypress or helichrysum oil with 1 teaspoon coconut oil and apply with a cotton ball to affected area.

HERPES. This viral infection causes small blisters to develop on the skin and mucus membranes. HSV-1 causes cold sores around the mouth. HSV-2 affects the genitals.

Ancient perspective: In TCM, excess liver heat is at the root, often caused by suppressed emotions. Emotional distress is a common trigger for outbreaks.

Foods That Harm	Foods That Heal
Packaged food, sugar, acidic food, alcohol, foods that contains L-arginine (nuts, seeds, meat, legumes, seaweed)	Zinc-rich foods (eggs, liver, pumpkin seeds); wild-caught fish (sardines, cod); asparagus, broccoli, cauliflower, spinach, carrots, pumpkin, squash, red bell peppers, blueberries, apples, kiwi, citrus, miso

Top 5 ancient prescriptions:

1. Licorice root. Contains glycyrrhizic acid, a compound that can kill cells infected with the virus. Take 500 to 1,000 mg daily.
2. Propolis. Studies show it helps heal herpes. Take according to package directions.
3. L-lysine, zinc, and vitamin C. These nutrients boost immunity and studies show they reduce herpes. Take according to package directions.
4. Garlic. Potent antiviral. Take 2 tablets or eat 2 fresh garlic cloves daily.
5. Elderberry syrup. Prevents and shortens outbreaks. Take as directed.

Other remedies: Apply a warm compress to reduce pain and swelling. Reduce stress with meditation, spiritual growth reading, exercise, walks in nature, and daily downtime.

Essential oils: Apply 1 or 2 drops of Melissa oil (lemon balm) to a cold sore 3 times daily. Add 1 drop of tea tree oil to ¼ teaspoon coconut oil and apply to sore 3 times daily.

HIGH BLOOD PRESSURE. Blood pressure is the measure of the force of blood pushing against the walls of the arteries. When it's too high (aka hypertension), it puts you at risk of heart attack and stroke.

Ancient perspective: In TCM, high blood pressure is caused by liver yang rising, which is related to stress, or kidney yin deficiency, which is linked to poor diet or a sedentary lifestyle.

Foods That Harm	Foods That Heal
High-sodium food, sugar, refined grains, caffeine, processed meats, canned food, alcohol	Salmon and other wild-caught fish, cage-free eggs, grass-fed meat, leafy greens, asparagus, broccoli, beets, spinach, beans, walnuts, seeds, coconut oil, avocados, blueberries, goji, raspberries, pomegranates, oats, dark chocolate

Top 5 ancient prescriptions:
1. Hawthorn. Can reduce blood pressure. Take 1,200 mg of an extract daily.
2. Garlic. A natural vasodilator, it can reduce blood pressure. Take 500 mg daily.
3. Fish oil. Reduces blood pressure. Take 1,000 to 3,000 mg daily.
4. CBD. Research shows it reduces blood pressure.[13] Take 100 to 160 mg daily.
5. Ginger tea. Lowers blood pressure by blocking calcium channels. Steep 1 tablespoon of grated fresh ginger in 2 cups of boiling water. Sip throughout the day.

Other remedies: Try acupuncture, prayer, meditation, yoga, walking in nature, exercise, and other lifestyle habits to lower stress, like spiritual growth reading, gratitude, digital detox, and building downtime into your day. Magnesium and potassium may also help.

Essential oils: Diffuse 3 drops of lavender, ylang-ylang, rosemary, or frankincense oil. You can also apply frankincense oil to your chest, back of neck, or bottoms of feet.

HYPERTHYROIDISM. Also known as Graves' disease, this autoimmune disorder causes an overproduction of thyroid hormones. Signs include insomnia, sensitivity to heat, hand tremors, irregular periods, digestive problems, weight loss, and mood changes.

Ancient perspective: In TCM, hyperthyroidism is caused by spleen qi and yin deficiency, particularly related to the wood element. The goal is to restore yin/yang balance.

Foods That Harm	Foods That Heal
Packaged food, sugar, gluten, refined grains, flour, conventional dairy, spicy food, citrus fruits, vinegar, caffeine, alcohol	Bone broth, wild-caught fish, chicken, duck, eggs, spinach, kale, green beans, carrots, celery, zucchini, seaweed, apples, blueberries, blackberries, goji, peaches, mango, beets, pumpkin, squash, sweet potatoes, rice, oats, millet, beans, coconut oil, olive oil, flaxseed, mushrooms

Top 5 ancient prescriptions:
1. Bugleweed. Can suppress the thyroid. Take 2 ml of a tincture 3 times daily.
2. Lemon balm. Lowers thyroid hormone. Take 2 ml of a tincture 3 times daily.
3. Rehmannia. Supports thyroid qi and yin. Take up to 350 mg daily. (Avoid if you're pregnant or breastfeeding.)
4. CBD oil. Calms thyroid and builds yin. Take 160 mg daily.
5. Astragalus. Supports thyroid. Take 1,000 mg daily.

Other remedies: Try acupuncture, meditation, and aerobic exercise. To further reduce stress (which can ignite autoimmune reactions), try digital fasting, walking in nature, walking barefoot on the grass, and spiritual growth reading.

Essential oils: Apply 2 or 3 drops each of Melissa (lemon balm), frankincense, and myrrh oil below your Adam's apple (where your thyroid is) twice daily.

HYPOTHYROIDISM. An underactive thyroid can cause moodiness, weight gain, fatigue, feeling cold, constipation, stiffness, and rough skin.

Ancient perspective: In TCM, the cause is qi deficiency and spleen or kidney yang deficiency, so the goal is to restore yin/yang balance. Hypothyroidism is exacerbated by stress.

Foods That Harm	Foods That Heal
Goitrogrens (raw cruciferous vegetables, red wine, beer, soy, peanuts), sugar, gluten, refined grains, processed food, conventional dairy	Bone broth, fish, chicken, beef, lamb, leafy greens, cooked green beans, asparagus, seaweed, pumpkin, squash, sweet potatoes, berries, goji, stewed fruit, beans, chickpeas, fermented foods, chia seeds, walnuts, brazil nuts, coconut oil, beans, rice, oats, dates, cinnamon, ginger

Top 5 ancient prescriptions:
1. Ashwagandha. Balances cortisol and thyroid hormones. Start with 500 mg daily and increase gradually, up to 1,250 mg.
2. Astragalus. Supports thyroid function. Take 1,000 mg daily.
3. Probiotics. Treats leaky gut and reduces nutrient deficiencies that contribute to thyroid problems. Take 25 to 50 billion IU daily.
4. Kelp. Contains iodine for thyroid support. Consult with holistic doctor on iodine supplementation. Spirulina and chlorella are also beneficial; take as directed.
5. Schisandra. Supports adrenals and lowers stress. Take according to package directions.

Other remedies: Try acupuncture, prayer, meditation, walking in nature, and building downtime into your day. Strength training can help build yang. Selenium and vitamin B complex can also improve symptoms.

Essential oils: Rub 2 to 4 drops of frankincense and lemongrass oil on the thyroid.

IMMUNE SYSTEM WEAKNESS. Meant to rid the body of bacteria, viruses, and mutated cells, your immune system is most effective when it's strong. If it's weak, you fall prey to many seasonal bugs. Stress, age, poor diet, and lack of sleep can lower immunity.

Ancient perspective: In TCM, immunity can be bolstered by strengthening lung and spleen qi.

Foods That Harm	Foods That Heal
Gluten and other food allergens, sugar, processed carbs, additives and preservatives, produce with pesticides, meat and dairy with antibiotics and hormones, alcohol	Cooked asparagus, broccoli, cauliflower, cabbage, carrots, celery, kale, spinach, squash, and pumpkin; vitamin C–rich fruits (citrus, kiwi, goji, amla, blueberries, strawberries); fermented foods (miso, ama); rice congee, bone broth, chicken, salmon, beef, shiitake mushrooms, garlic, onions, thyme, oregano, ginger

Top 5 ancient prescriptions:
1. Probiotics. SBO probiotics like bacillus species strengthen the gut and the immune system. Take 25 to 50 billion IU daily.
2. Elderberry. A natural immune booster. Take as directed.
3. Reishi. Enhances antibody response. Take as directed.
4. Astragalus. Strengthens the gut and immune system. Take 1,000 mg twice daily.
5. Bone broth. Supports gut health. Drink 1 or 2 cups daily.

Other remedies: Try acupuncture; exercise; get 8 hours of sleep a night; reduce stress with prayer, meditation, spiritual growth reading, exercise, walking in nature, and daily downtime; bolster joy by being with people and doing activities you love. Take turkey tail mushroom, schisandra, zinc, and vitamin D.

Essential oils: Take 1 drop orally of frankincense, lemon, and ginger oil daily to support immune health.

INFERTILITY. Defined as an inability to conceive after trying for at least one year, infertility can be caused by hormonal issues, stress, poor nutrition, excessive exercise, and obesity.

Ancient perspective: Kidney yin deficiency and, for those who can conceive but can't maintain a pregnancy, spleen qi deficiency.

Foods That Harm	Foods That Heal
Hydrogenated oils, processed meats, sugar, soda, low-fat dairy products, refined grains, fast food, fish with mercury, pesticide-laden produce, alcohol, caffeine	Wild-caught fish, bone broth, liver, grass-fed beef, chicken, eggs, walnuts, pumpkin seeds, brazil nuts, sesame tahini, coconut, olives, avocados, asparagus, broccoli, spinach, carrots, peas, pumpkin, squash, sweet potatoes, beans, rice, oatmeal, blueberries, figs, goji, grapes, dark chocolate, fennel, fenugreek, cinnamon, ginger

Top 5 ancient prescriptions:
1. Vitex. Can normalize menstrual cycles. Take 160 to 240 mg daily.
2. Dong quai. Bolsters blood flow to reproductive organs. Take 1,000 mg daily.
3. Rehmannia. Bolsters adrenals and reproductive organs. Take up to 350 mg daily.
4. Panax ginseng. Increases sperm count in men. Take 500 to 1,000 mg daily.
5. Astragalus. Helpful for men and women. Take 1,000 mg daily.

Other remedies: Try acupuncture; reduce stress and build faith with yoga, prayer, meditation, digital fasting, and spiritual reading; get 8 to 10 hours of sleep a night; do weight training; spend time around encouraging friends. Other supplements for women: maca, shatavari, ashwagandha, and evening primrose; for men: tribulus and fenugreek.

Essential oils: Diffuse 5 drops of sandalwood or ylang-ylang oil in the bedroom, or apply 2 drops of each to the temples, wrist, and chest. They're aphrodisiacs for both men and women.

INFLAMMATION. Caused by chronic immune reactions, inflammation is associated with many health conditions, from Alzheimer's to heart disease to cancer.

Ancient perspective: In TCM, inflammation is caused by excess yang or a yin deficiency, both of which are associated with excess heat.

Foods That Harm	Foods That Heal
Packaged food, fried food, sugar, artificial sweeteners, grains, gluten, flour, processed meat, dairy and meat with hormones or antibiotics, soybean oil	Leafy greens, asparagus, broccoli, cauliflower, carrots, beets, pumpkin, squash, berries, figs, kiwi, pineapple, walnuts, chia seeds, flaxseed and hemp seeds, bone broth, salmon and other wild-caught fish, grass-fed beef, avocado, olive oil, coconut, green tea, turmeric, galangal, ginger, rosemary

Top 5 ancient prescriptions:
1. Turmeric. A potent anti-inflammatory herb. Take 1,000 to 3,000 mg daily.
2. Bone broth or collagen powder. Has anti-inflammatory properties and supports connective tissue regeneration. Take 10 to 40 grams daily.
3. Boswellia. High in antioxidants and other anti-inflammatory chemicals. Take 600 to 700 mg several times daily.
4. CBD. Reduces inflammation and pain. Take 20 to 100 mg daily.
5. Fish oil. High in EPA/DHA, which reduce inflammation. Take 1,000 to 3,000 mg daily.

Other remedies: Try acupuncture and/or chiropractic; get 8 to 10 hours of sleep a night; practice yoga and reduce stress by walking in nature, spiritual growth reading, and carving out time to examine thoughts and beliefs that are contributing to unhealthy emotions.

Essential oils: Diffuse 3 drops of frankincense, rosemary, ginger, holy basil, lemongrass, wintergreen, or turmeric oil, all of which are anti-inflammatory.

INFLAMMATORY BOWEL DISEASE (CROHN'S AND COLITIS). Gut-lining inflammation impairs nutrient absorption and immune function. It causes diarrhea, nausea, fatigue, and weight loss.

Ancient perspective: In TCM, inflammatory bowel disease is caused by spleen qi deficiency and dampness. When the digestive system becomes weak, it can't nourish the immune system and intestines. Worry, grief, and past trauma increase risk. For diet, combine earth element and metal element plans.

Foods That Harm	Foods That Heal
Fried food, spicy food, refined carbs, wheat, gluten, dairy products, high-fiber food, soda, caffeine	Cooked cauliflower, carrots, pumpkin, butternut squash, bone broth, miso soup, organic meat, fish, chicken, baked pears, applesauce, blueberries, coconut, avocado, tahini, rice congee, turmeric, ginger

Top 5 ancient prescriptions:

1. Probiotics. Reduces the incidence of diarrhea and supports digestion. Take 50 billion units once or twice daily.
2. Slippery elm. Contains mucilage, which relieves irritation of mucus membranes. Take as a tea or in capsule form twice daily.
3. Astragalus. Strengthens digestion. Take 1,000 mg daily.
4. Turmeric. Reduces inflammation. Take 1,000 to 3,000 mg daily.
5. Bone broth or collagen protein. Helps renew gut lining. Consume 20 g daily.

Other remedies: Try acupuncture. Take omega-3s, glutamine, and a multivitamin. Reduce stress through prayer, meditation, spiritual growth reading, nature walks, and spending time with positive friends to heal from past emotional trauma and build hope in the future.

Essential oils: Dilute 1 or 2 drops each of chamomile, frankincense, ginger, and peppermint oil with 1 teaspoon of coconut oil and rub over the abdomen twice daily.

INSOMNIA. Persistent inability to fall asleep or stay asleep can impair immunity, cause weight gain and moodiness, and increase the risk of relationship problems and car accidents.

Ancient perspective: In TCM, the cause of insomnia is a heart imbalance, with the heart and liver wrestling. Worry and lack of joy contribute.

Foods That Harm	Foods That Heal
Gluten, simple carbs, conventional dairy, sugar, spicy food, fried food, alcohol, caffeine after noon, solid food within 2 hours of bedtime	Omega-3-rich wild-caught fish (salmon, tuna), walnuts, almonds, seeds, turkey, chicken, grass-fed beef, organic fermented dairy, eggs, spinach, chard, kale, broccoli, asparagus, beets, pumpkin, tart cherry juice, kiwis, apples, peaches, passion fruit, beans, sprouted rice congee, oats, coconut, avocados, olives, tahini, mushrooms

Top 5 ancient prescriptions:
1. CBD oil. Reduces anxiety and pain and aids sleep. Take 40 to 160 mg before bed.
2. Valerian root. Promotes sleep. Take 300 to 900 mg before bed.
3. Chamomile. Reduces anxiety. Take 220 to 1,600 mg, or a cup of tea, before bed.
4. Melatonin. Best for those who wake up in the night. Take 0.3 to 3 g before bed.
5. Magnesium. Supports relaxation and sleep. Take 300 to 600 mg in the evening.

Other remedies: Try acupuncture and/or chiropractic; get morning sunlight to reset circadian clock; get daily exercise; reduce stress with prayer, meditation, spiritual reading, yoga, digital fasting (no screen time within 3 hours of bed), and gratitude practice; keep noise and light out of the bedroom; and maintain a regular sleep/wake schedule.

Essential oils: Diffuse 5 drops of lavender or chamomile oil in your bedroom.

IRRITABLE BOWEL SYNDROME. Caused by abnormal nerve, enzyme, and muscle function in the gut, IBS is worsened by food sensitivities, stress, and poor sleep. Symptoms include weekly bouts of constipation, bloating, diarrhea, gas, and abdominal cramps.

Ancient perspective: In TCM, IBS is caused by a pattern of spleen qi deficiency and dampness, with the root cause being stress, overwork, worry, lack of hope, and holding on to hurts from the past.

Foods That Harm	Foods That Heal
Gluten, grains, conventional dairy, sugar, refined flour, spicy food, ice-cold drinks, ice cream, hydrogenated oils, excessive omega-6 fats, caffeine	Cooked cauliflower, carrots, pumpkin, butternut squash, bone broth, miso, organic meat, fish, chicken, baked pears, applesauce, blueberries, coconut, avocados, tahini, rice congee, turmeric, galangal, and ginger

Top 5 ancient prescriptions:
1. Probiotics. Reduces pain and symptoms.[14] Take up to 100 billion units daily.
2. Astragalus. Strengthens digestion and immunity. Take 1,000 mg once or twice daily.
3. Ginger. Reduces gut inflammation. Take 1 to 3 g daily as a capsule or tea.
4. Bone broth protein. It's high in collagen, glucosamine, chondroitin, and hyaluronic acid, which regenerate the gut lining. Consume 20 g daily.
5. Aloe vera juice. A natural laxative for constipation. Good for IBS-C but not IBS-D.[15] Drink ½ cup 3 times daily.

Other remedies: Get exercise; try acupuncture; reduce stress through prayer, spiritual reading, scheduling more downtime, and positive relationships. Take fish oil, and digestive bitters with gentian, pau d'arco, or slippery elm before meals.

Essential oils: Add 1 drop each of peppermint and ginger oil to water and take 3 times daily.

LEAKY GUT. Bad bacteria damages the gut lining, allowing food molecules and microbes to leak into the blood, resulting in inflammation. Signs include food sensitivities, digestive issues, IBS, autoimmune disease, headaches, joint pain, fatigue, and mood changes.

Ancient perspective: In TCM, leaky gut is caused by spleen qi deficiency and dampness. Stress, worry, and overwork, along with eating the wrong diet for your element, contribute.

Foods That Harm	Foods That Heal
Sugar, grain, conventional meat and dairy, hydrogenated oils, ice-cold drinks, gluten, processed food, produce with pesticides	Bone broth, collagen, wild-caught salmon, grass-fed beef, chicken, fermented vegetables, cooked celery, cauliflower, asparagus, carrots, squash, pumpkin, blueberries, stewed pears, coconut, sprouted rice congee, oats, shiitake, cinnamon, ginger, bitter foods, herbs

Top 5 ancient prescriptions:
1. Probiotics. Helps maintain a healthy gut lining and protects it from toxins, allergens, and pathogens.[16] Take 50 billion units daily.
2. Astragalus. Strengthens digestion and immunity. Take 1,000 mg once or twice daily.
3. Bone broth or collagen powder. Heals gut lining. Have 1 cup bone broth daily, or 1 or 2 scoops powdered supplement.
4. Ginger. Take as a tea or in capsules (as directed on the package) 1 to 3 times daily.
5. Licorice root (DGL licorice). Improves acid production in the stomach and supports the gut's mucosal lining.[17] Take 500 to 1,000 mg daily.

Other remedies: Control stress with prayer, spiritual growth reading, exercise, and at least 8 hours of sleep a night; take nature walks; schedule downtime; and build positive relationships.

Essential oils: Diffuse 1 drop of peppermint or ginger oil daily, or add to water and drink.

LIVER DISEASE. Liver disease can be caused by hepatitis, cancer, genetic diseases, alcohol abuse, and poor diet. Symptoms include yellowish skin and eyes, abdominal pain, swollen ankles, and fatigue.

Ancient perspective: In TCM, liver disease is the result of liver qi deficiency, qi stagnation, blood stagnation, and damp heat. Irritability and anger make it worse.

Foods That Harm	Foods That Heal
Spicy food, garlic, pepper, high-fat food, hydrogenated oils, fast food, fried food, dairy, butter, chocolate, peanuts, shrimp, pork, red meat, vinegar, citrus fruits, coffee, alcohol	Organic artichokes, asparagus, beets, broccoli, celery, cauliflower, carrots, radish, zucchini, pumpkin, cilantro, apples, berries, goji, plums, beans, rice, oatmeal, quinoa, liver, bone broth, chicken, wild-caught fish, matcha

Top 5 ancient prescriptions:
1. Milk thistle. Supports liver regeneration and detoxification. Take 50 to 150 mg daily.
2. Bupleurum. Moves liver qi and protects liver on a cellular level. Take as directed.
3. Skullcap. Calms liver heat and qi stagnation. Take as directed.
4. Schisandra. Strengthens qi and improves liver function. Take 1 to 3 g daily, with meals.
5. Turmeric. Reduces inflammation. Take 500 to 2,000 mg daily.

Other remedies: Do a juice fast with nutritious green juices to give your liver a rest; reduce stress with meditation, yoga, tai chi, prayer, nature walks, and daily downtime; and find ways to cope with irritation, whether through exercise, talking to a therapist or minister, rabbi, or spiritual guide, or spending time with supportive friends.

Essential oils: Add 1 or 2 drops of lemon oil to a glass of water and drink once daily for a week.

LUPUS. In this autoimmune disease, the immune system attacks healthy tissue. Symptoms include inflammation, swelling, and damage to joints, skin, and organs.

Ancient perspective: In TCM, the cause of lupus is lung qi deficiency, linked to worrying about the past, and liver qi deficiency, related to chronic stress and toxic emotions, as well as environmental toxins.

Foods That Harm	Foods That Heal
Gluten, sugar, salt, alcohol, garlic, alfalfa, nightshades, commercial baked goods, creamed soups, processed meat	Leafy greens, asparagus, broccoli, cauliflower, carrots, pumpkin, squash, berries, figs, kiwi, mulberries, pears, walnuts, chia seeds, flaxseed and hemp seeds, bone broth, salmon and other wild-caught fish, grass-fed beef, rice congee, oats, coconut, honey, green tea, turmeric, galangal, ginger

Top 5 ancient prescriptions:
1. Bone broth (or powder). Supports gut health and reduces inflammation. Drink 2 cups or take 20 to 40 g daily.
2. Holy basil. Modulates stress. Take 250 mg once or twice daily.
3. Astragalus. Supports immune health and inflammation. Take 1,000 mg daily.
4. Rehmannia. Builds qi and energy. Take 1,000 mg daily.
5. Vitamin D3. Supports immune health. Take 2,000 to 5,000 mg daily.

Other remedies: Try acupuncture; reduce stress through prayer, meditation, yoga, walking in nature, walking barefoot on the grass, digital fasting, and building downtime into your day. To heal past hurts and focus on the future, practice gratitude, affirmations, and spiritual growth reading.

Essential oils: Apply 3 drops of frankincense and helichrysum oil topically to the neck.

LYME DISEASE. This infection is caused by bacteria transmitted by a tick bite. Early signs include flulike symptoms, headache, muscle and joint pain, and, in some cases, a bull's-eye-shaped rash. Over time it can cause neurological problems.

Ancient perspective: In TCM, weak lung qi causes liver qi and blood qi deficiency. Unhealthy emotions including lack of hope, guilt, and grief inhibit healing.

Foods That Harm	Foods That Heal
Grains, gluten, high-sugar fruit, sugar, processed and packaged foods, produce with pesticides, food with dyes and additives	Leafy greens, asparagus, broccoli, cauliflower, carrots, celery, pumpkin, squash, fermented foods, berries, figs, mulberries, pears, chestnuts, chia, and pumpkin seeds, bone broth, salmon and other wild-caught fish, chicken, beef, rice, oats, coconut, garlic, cinnamon, turmeric, ginger

Top 5 ancient prescriptions:

1. Astragalus. Strengthens the immune system. Take 1,000 to 2,000 mg daily.
2. Probiotics. Builds good bacteria. Take 50 to 100 billion IU daily.
3. Sarsaparilla (smilax). Cleanses blood. Take as directed.
4. Rehmannia. Builds lung qi and energy. Take up to 350 mg daily.
5. Schisandra. Strengthens immunity and liver. Take as directed.

Other remedies: Try acupuncture; exercise; get 8 to 10 hours of sleep a night; reduce stress through spiritual growth reading, nature walks, daily downtime, and relaxing with friends and family; practice gratitude and forgiveness to heal past emotional trauma; and reduce mold exposure. Dong quai, Japanese knotweed, reishi, turmeric, burdock, cat's claw, and vitamin D can also help.

Essential oils: Diffuse frankincense, myrrh, holy basil, ylang-ylang, and chamomile oil.

MENOPAUSE SYMPTOMS. Menopause begins 12 months after the last menstrual period, when the ovaries' egg reserves are depleted. The hormonal shift can cause mood swings, hot flashes, low libido, fatigue, weight gain, and insomnia.

Ancient perspective: In TCM, the symptoms are related to a kidney yin qi deficiency.

Foods That Harm	Foods That Heal
Processed meat, meat with hormones or antibiotics, packaged food, processed carbs, sugar, soda, alcohol, caffeine, spicy food	Leafy greens, broccoli, cauliflower, asparagus, seaweed, pumpkin, squash, sweet potatoes, blueberries, goji, apples, bananas, blackberries, peaches, mango, bone broth, eggs, beef, chicken, omega-3-rich foods (salmon, tuna, flaxseed), coconut, olive oil, fermented soy (miso, natto), oats, rice, beans, shiitake

Top 5 ancient prescriptions:
1. Black cohosh. Can ease hot flashes. Take 160 to 200 mg daily.
2. Vitex. Alleviates menopause symptoms. Take 160 to 240 mg daily.
3. Rehmannia. Strengthens reproductive organs. Take up to 350 mg daily.
4. Panax ginseng. Increases energy levels. Take 500 mg twice daily.
5. Maca. Can improve menopause symptoms. Take 1,000 to 2,000 mg daily.

Other remedies: Try acupuncture; exercise; reduce stress through aromatherapy, yoga, walks in nature, fostering close relationships, and spiritual growth reading.

Essential oils: Rub 3 drops of clary sage oil (to reduce anxiety and relieve symptoms), chamomile oil (to reduce stress), peppermint oil (to cool hot flashes), and/or thyme oil (to balance hormones) on the tops of the feet and back of the neck 1 to 3 times daily.

MIGRAINES. These headaches are triggered by stress, food sensitivities, fatigue, hormone imbalance, and dehydration. Symptoms include throbbing pain, commonly on one side of the head, nausea, and sensitivity to light.

Ancient perspective: According to TCM, migraines are caused by liver yang excess. Overwork, anger, frustration, little downtime, and lack of relaxation are root causes.

Foods That Harm	Foods That Heal
Gluten, caffeine, alcohol, sugar, sugary drinks, dairy, hydrogenated oils, high-fat diet, processed carbs, food additives, spicy food, red meat, shrimp, garlic, chiles, cinnamon, vinegar, coffee	Leafy greens, asparagus, broccoli, cauliflower, celery, green beans, carrots, pumpkin, squash, pears, mulberries, blueberries, blackberries, black beans, kidney beans, oats, rice, millet, bone broth, wild-caught fish, eggs, chicken, duck, mushrooms, coconut, seaweed

Top 5 ancient prescriptions:
1. Feverfew. Reduces frequency and symptoms. Take 100 to 300 mg up to 4 times daily.
2. Butterbur. Lowers inflammation and restores normal blood flow in the brain. Take 50 to 75 mg twice daily.
3. CBD oil. Proven pain reliever. Take 100 mg at the first sign of headache.
4. Magnesium. Relaxes muscles to ease pain. Take 500 mg daily.
5. TCM Liver Fire formula. Includes skullcap, gentian, bupleurum, and rehmannia, which calm the liver and reduce migraines. Take as directed.

Other remedies: Try chiropractic, acupuncture, digital fasting, walking in nature, yoga, a consistent sleep schedule, and spiritual growth reading to reduce frustration and anger, boost hope and faith, and counteract liver yang excess.

Essential oils: Rub 3 drops each of lavender and peppermint oil on the neck and temples.

MULTIPLE SCLEROSIS. This disabling autoimmune disease causes central nervous system inflammation, and the immune system attacks the protective fat surrounding nerves, destroying nerve function. Triggers include infections, toxic mold, and food allergies.

Ancient perspective: In TCM, the root cause is spleen qi deficiency and sometimes blood deficiency. Past trauma, or a loss of meaning or purpose, can contribute.

Foods That Harm	Foods That Heal
Sugar, grains, conventional meat and dairy, hydrogenated oils, gluten, processed food, produce with pesticides	Bone broth, grass-fed beef, chicken, omega-3-rich foods (salmon, walnuts, chia seeds, hemp seeds, coconut, avocados), tahini, cooked asparagus, beets, broccoli, cauliflower, celery, carrots, pumpkin, squash, berries, goji, beans, fermented foods, cinnamon, ginger

Top 5 ancient prescriptions:
1. Astragalus. Strengthens the spleen, immune system, and blood. Take 2 to 4 g daily.
2. Ginseng. Boosts the body's qi, blood, and energy. Take as directed.
3. Ginkgo biloba. Reduces inflammation and fatigue.[18] Take 120 mg daily.
4. Turmeric. Inhibits pro-inflammatory cytokines.[19] Take up to 3,000 mg daily.
5. Fish oil. Reduces inflammation and supports brain health. Take 1,000 to 3,000 mg daily.

Other remedies: Vitamin B12 and vitamin D3 have been shown to improve symptoms. Counteract worry and anxiety with meditation, prayer, acupuncture, yoga, and spiritual growth reading to find meaning, purpose, and hope. Also seek therapy for trauma, nurture close relationships, and practice gratitude.

Essential oils: Diffuse a few drops of frankincense, cypress, or helichrysum oil daily.

OSTEOPOROSIS. In this age-related condition, bones become weak and brittle, leading to increased fracture risk and stooped posture. Inactivity and low vitamin D increase risk.

Ancient perspective: In TCM, kidney qi deficiency is the root cause.

Foods That Harm	Foods That Heal
Alcohol, sugar, processed meats, caffeine, high-sodium food	Spinach, kale, broccoli, celery, watercress, green beans, seaweed, bone broth, wild-caught fish (salmon and sardines), eggs, poultry, raw cheese, yogurt, chestnuts, flaxseed, blueberries, goji, figs, grapefruit, avocados, coconut, tahini, rice, oats, kidney beans, chickpeas, miso, natto, shiitake, fermented foods, sage, thyme, matcha

Top 5 ancient prescriptions:
1. Bone broth or collagen protein. High in collagen. Take 20 to 40 mg daily.
2. Calcium, magnesium, and vitamins D3 and K2. Critical nutrients for strong bones. Take together in a formula as directed.
3. Spirulina and algae. High in minerals that help form bone. Take as directed.
4. Rehmannia. Builds kidney qi and yin. Take up to 350 mg daily. (Avoid if pregnant or breastfeeding.)
5. Black cohosh. Boosts bone density. Take 40 mg daily.

Other remedies: Do low-impact exercise, strength training, yoga, and walking in nature. Get 8 hours of sleep a night and reduce stress with prayer, meditation, and spiritual growth reading. Other bone strengtheners: horsetail, dong quai, and fish oil.

Essential oils: Mix 2 or 3 drops of cypress, helichrysum, or fir needle oil with ¼ teaspoon coconut oil and apply to the spine and hip 3 times daily.

PAIN (CHRONIC). Most pain starts with an acute injury, but when it lasts for more than 3 months, it's considered chronic—and it can impair your mood, relationships, sleep, sex drive, mobility, and ability to function. Inflammation almost always plays a role.

Ancient perspective: In TCM, chronic pain is caused by qi stagnation, blood stagnation, and weak kidney qi.

Foods That Harm	Foods That Heal
Gluten, packaged and processed foods, fast food, sugar and artificial sweeteners, produce with pesticides, dairy and meat with hormones and antibiotics, alcohol	Leafy greens, asparagus, broccoli, cauliflower, carrots, beets, pumpkin, squash, berries, figs, kiwi, pineapple, walnuts, chia seeds, flaxseed and hemp seeds, bone broth, salmon and other wild-caught fish, grass-fed beef, avocados, olive oil, coconut, green tea, turmeric, galangal, ginger, rosemary

Top 5 ancient prescriptions:
1. CBD oil. Alters pain pathways. Take 10 to 100 mg daily.
2. Turmeric. Reduces inflammation. Take 1,000 to 3,000 mg daily.
3. Bone broth. Collagen builds connective tissue in joints. Drink 1 or 2 cups daily.
4. Fish oil. Reduces inflammation and pain. Take 1,000 to 3,000 mg daily.
5. Capsaicin cream. Reduces substance P, a chemical pain messenger. Rub a small amount on the painful area up to 4 times daily.

Other remedies: Try acupuncture, cupping, chiropractic, massage, dry needling, and functional movement training, which uses common movements you might do as part of your daily activity (Egoscue can be particularly helpful). Get 8 to 10 hours of sleep a night. Cultivate joy by spending time with supportive friends and doing activities you love.

Essential oils: Rub 5 drops of wintergreen, peppermint, and/or rosemary oil mixed with ½ teaspoon of coconut oil on the affected area.

PARASITES. Tapeworms, pinworms, roundworms, and protozoa can live in the intestines, where they cause abdominal pain, fatigue, dysentery, loss of appetite, and fever.

Ancient perspective: In TCM, the underlying vulnerabilities are spleen qi deficiency, liver blood stagnation with dampness, and lung qi deficiency. The goal of treatment is to make the intestines uninhabitable for parasites.

Foods That Harm	Foods That Heal
Packaged food, sugar, fruit, refined carbs, wheat products, alcohol, shellfish, processed meat, pork	Leafy greens, cooked cruciferous vegetables, pumpkin, carrots, asparagus, rhubarb, coconut oil, bone broth, sauerkraut and other fermented foods, papaya, berries, sunflower seeds, sesame seeds, pumpkin seeds, manuka honey, miso, ginger, garlic, onions, clove, thyme

Top 5 ancient prescriptions:

1. Black walnut extract. Used for centuries to treat intestinal parasites. Put 3 to 5 drops in water and take 3 times daily.
2. Wormwood tea. Research shows it kills tapeworms.[21] Steep ½ teaspoon dried wormwood in 1 cup boiling water for 15 minutes, then drink.
3. Probiotics. Strengthens immunity and gut health. Take 50 billion IU daily.
4. Pau d'arco. Has anti-parasitic and antimicrobial properties. Take as directed.
5. Grapefruit seed extract. An effective antimicrobial. Take 250 to 500 mg twice daily.

Other remedies: Reduce stress with prayer, meditation, 8 to 10 hours of sleep a night, and walking outside. Consider a cleanse, consuming soups and the foods listed above.

Essential oils: Take 2 drops of oregano or clove oil 3 times daily, for no more than 10 days.

PARKINSON'S DISEASE. This degenerative disorder of the central nervous system affects movement, causing tremors, stiffness, and loss of balance. Pesticide exposure, inflammation, poor diet, free radicals, and food allergies can contribute.

Ancient perspective: In TCM, it is linked to excess wind, which generates movement, as well as kidney yin deficiency, which impairs liver function.

Foods That Harm	Foods That Heal
Processed food, artificial sweeteners, alcohol, food allergens, dairy (If you're on medication, protein-rich meals may interfere.)	Leafy greens, asparagus, beets, berries, beans, healthy fats (ghee, coconut oil, avocados), tahini, bone broth, eggs, omega-3-rich food (wild-caught salmon, sardines), walnuts, hemp seeds, miso, honey, turmeric

Top 5 ancient prescriptions:
1. Turmeric. Reduces inflammation. Take 2,000 to 3,000 mg daily.
2. Lion's mane mushrooms. Support brain health and slow the disease's progression.[22] Start with 300 mg 1 to 3 times daily, and increase gradually, up to 3,000 mg.
3. Ginkgo biloba. A potent antioxidant that's great for the brain. Take 40 mg daily.
4. CBD. Supports the brain and nervous system. Take 20 to 100 mg daily.
5. Rehmannia. Strengthens kidney qi and yin. Take up to 350 mg daily. (Avoid if pregnant or breastfeeding.)

Other remedies: Do gentle exercise like yoga or swimming. Reduce stress with meditation, spiritual triathlon (see page 167), and nature walks. CoQ10, fish oil, matcha green tea, and milk thistle can also help.

Essential oils: Diffuse 3 drops each of frankincense, helichrysum, and rosemary oil to reduce brain inflammation, and diffuse 3 drops of vetiver to reduce tremors.

PNEUMONIA. This viral or bacterial lung infection causes coughing, mucus, shortness of breath, wheezing, fever, body aches, and loss of appetite—and can be deadly.

Ancient perspective: The root cause of pneumonia is lung qi and blood deficiency, with dampness. Unprocessed grief, the emotion most associated with lungs, can play a role.

Foods That Harm	Foods That Heal
Gluten and wheat, refined grains, conventional dairy, lactose, sugar, processed food, fast food, bread, egg whites, chips	Bone broth soup, chicken, cooked celery, carrots, asparagus, cauliflower, beets, radishes, squash, peas, pumpkin, chickpeas, rice congee, pears, parsley, garlic, onions, miso, shiitake mushrooms, ginger, thyme

Top 5 ancient prescriptions:

1. Echinacea. Has antiviral properties. Take 5 ml twice daily for 10 days.
2. Elderberry. Fights bacteria and viruses. Take as directed.
3. Probiotics. Decrease the incidence of pneumonia.[23] Take 50 to 100 billion IU daily.
4. Astragalus. Strengthens the immune defenses. Take 2,000 to 4,000 mg daily.
5. Mullein. Natural expectorant and virus fighter. Take 1,000 mg 3 times daily.

Other remedies: Try acupuncture, prayer, 9 to 10 hours of sleep a night, ginger tea to limit inflammation (mince a 2-inch knob and steep in 3 cups of boiling water), letting go of grief or past hurts (a therapist can help), and focusing on future plans that instill hope. The nutrients zinc, vitamin C, NAC, and cordyceps can also help.

Essential oils: Diffuse 5 drops of eucalyptus or tea tree oil, or take 1 or 2 drops of oregano oil each day for no more than 10 days.

POLYCYSTIC OVARIAN SYNDROME (PCOS). A cause of infertility, PCOS occurs when ovaries form small cysts, causing irregular periods, pain, facial hair, acne, and weight gain.

Ancient perspective: In TCM, the underlying causes are deficient kidney qi, often due to overwork, and damp heat in the spleen.

Foods That Harm	Foods That Heal
Processed food, artificial sweeteners, food allergens including gluten and lactose, refined vegetable oils, alcohol, caffeine	Omega-3-rich fish, bone broth, grass-fed beef, chicken, walnuts, tahini, coconut, olives, kombu, asparagus, broccoli, cauliflower, spinach, celery, carrots, pumpkin, squash, beans, rice, mushrooms, blueberries, raspberries, goji, cherries, onions, parsley, garlic, cinnamon, ginger

Top 5 ancient prescriptions:

1. Vitex. Balances estrogen and progesterone. Take 800 to 2,000 mg daily.
2. Holy basil. Balances blood sugar and reduces stress. Take 800 to 2,000 mg daily.
3. TCM Free and Easy Wanderer formula. Studies show that this blend of bupleurum, dong quai, peony, atractylodes, and poria improves PCOS symptoms. Take as directed.
4. TCM Liver formula. Contains milk thistle and dandelion, which support the liver and hormone balance by eliminating xeno-estrogens. Take as directed.
5. Dong quai. Balances hormones. Take 1,000 mg daily.

Other remedies: Try acupuncture; do weight training and cardio exercise; reduce stress with spiritual growth reading, nature walks, and daily downtime; and get 8 to 9 hours of sleep a night. Chromium, vitamin B-complex, and vitamin D can also help.

Essential oils: Diffuse 3 drops each of clary sage oil, which reduces cortisol and balances estrogen, and thyme oil, which supports healthy progesterone production.

PREGNANCY. Supporting your health and your baby's development requires a healthy diet and some key nutrients. Ancient remedies can help.

Ancient perspective: In TCM, the goal is to strengthen kidney and spleen qi.

Foods That Harm	Foods That Heal
Packaged and processed foods, sugar, artificial sweeteners, produce with pesticides, fish high in mercury (swordfish, albacore tuna), raw or undercooked fish or meat or eggs, deli meat, refined vegetable oils, alcohol, caffeine	Organic leafy greens, cooked vegetables, broccoli, pumpkin, carrots, squash, sweet potatoes, berries, grapefruit, fermented foods, wild-caught fatty fish, poultry, grass-fed beef, eggs, healthy fats (coconut oil, olives, avocados, nuts, seeds), rice, oats, beans, dates, cinnamon, ginger

Top 5 ancient prescriptions:

1. Prenatal multivitamin. Contains the nutrients your baby needs to thrive. Buy one with nutrients from real food and methylated B vitamins. Take as directed.
2. Omega-3s. A high-DHA supplement supports neurological and visual development. Take 300 mg of DHA daily.
3. Red raspberry leaf tea. Strengthens the uterus and shortens labor. Drink 1 or 2 cups daily during the last trimester.
4. Ginger tea. Can reduce nausea and vomiting in the first trimester. Steep 1 teaspoon grated root in 3 cups of water and sip throughout the day.
5. Chamomile. Can promote sleep during the last trimester. Drink 1 cup before bed.

Other remedies: Magnesium and vitamin B6 can ease morning sickness. Relieve stress with meditation, spiritual triathlon (page 167), nature walks, yoga, and daily downtime. Consider working with a doula and/or midwife, who can offer additional support and suggestions.

PREMENSTRUAL SYNDROME (PMS). Changing hormone levels a week or two before menstruation can cause cramps, bloating, acne, mood swings, and breast tenderness.

Ancient perspective: In TCM, PMS is caused by liver qi stagnation and blood deficiency.

Foods That Harm	Foods That Heal
Sugar, salt, hydrogenated fats, gluten and other food allergens, caffeine, fatty meat, greasy or fried food, processed grains	Spinach, kale, chard, asparagus, artichokes, brussels sprouts, broccoli, cauliflower, celery, onions, cilantro, parsley, beets, pumpkin, squash, sweet potatoes, grapes, goji, figs, cherries, citrus, coconut, olives, liver, bone broth, omega-3-rich foods (salmon, tuna, flaxseed), beans, rice, oats, mushrooms, miso, turmeric, fennel

Top 5 ancient prescriptions:
1. Vitex. Reduced symptoms by 93 percent according to one study.[24] Take 400 mg at breakfast.
2. Dong quai. Strengthens blood. Take 2 to 4 g, divided into 3 doses, daily.
3. TCM Liver Cleanse formula. Bupleurum, milk thistle, and dandelion cleanse the body of xeno-estrogens. Take as directed.
4. Crampbark. Relieves cramps and PMS symptoms. Take 500 mg 2 to 4 times daily.
5. Magnesium and vitamin B6. Together they balance estrogen and reduce PMS symptoms. Take 250 mg magnesium and 50 mg B6 twice daily.

Other remedies: Try acupuncture, exercise, get at least 8 hours of sleep a night, and reduce stress with meditation, spiritual triathlon (see page 167), yoga, walking in nature, practicing gratitude, affirmations, and making time to do things that bring you joy.

Essential oils: For cramps, rub 3 drops each of clary sage and peppermint oil on the abdomen, then apply warm compress.

PROSTATITIS. Inflammation or infection of the prostate can cause difficulty urinating, painful urination, frequent urination, cloudy or bloody urine, groin pain, and painful ejaculation.

Ancient perspective: In TCM, the root cause is kidney yang excess. Emotionally, it is associated with feeling stuck, unfulfilled, bored, or uninspired.

Foods That Harm	Foods That Heal
Dairy, red meat, processed and packaged foods, spicy food, acidic food, refined carbs, sugar, artificial sweeteners, alcohol, caffeine	Omega-3-rich foods (wild-caught salmon, sardines, walnuts, flaxseed, pumpkin seeds), eggs, chicken, bone broth, blueberries, blackberries, mulberries, goji, figs, spinach, kale, broccoli, cauliflower, green beans, zucchini, beets, pumpkin, sweet potatoes, squash, coconut, rice, oats, beans, mushrooms, matcha green tea, spirulina

Top 5 ancient prescriptions:
1. Bee pollen. Reduces symptoms. Take 1 teaspoon 3 times daily.
2. Saw palmetto. Improves prostate health. Take as directed.
3. Echinacea. Boosts immune function. Take 5 ml twice daily for 10 days.
4. Probiotics. Boost immunity and fight infections. Take 50 billion IU daily.
5. Zinc. Strengthens the immune system to fight infections. Take 30 mg twice daily.

Other remedies: Drink 8 to 10 glasses of water daily; get 8 or more hours of sleep a night; reduce stress with spiritual growth reading; create a vision board and bucket list, then take action; connect with a group of close friends and schedule fun activities together.

Essential oils: Add 2 drops each of frankincense, thyme, and sandal-wood oil to ¼ teaspoon coconut oil and apply to the area just in front of the rectum twice daily.

PSORIASIS. An autoimmune disease that causes red plaques on the skin, it flares with stress and immune impairment. Poor diet, impaired gut health, hormonal changes, impaired liver function, nutrient deficiencies, and difficulty digesting fat and protein contribute.

Ancient perspective: In TCM, the cause is lung qi and lung yin deficiency, often triggered by an unhealed emotional wound.

Foods That Harm	Foods That Heal
Meat and dairy with hormones and antibiotics, processed meat and other foods, gluten and other food allergens, sugar, hydrogenated oils, alcohol	Leafy greens, asparagus, broccoli, cauliflower, carrots, celery, pumpkin, squash, fermented foods, spirulina, berries, mulberries, pears, walnuts, flaxseed, bone broth, wild-caught fish, vegan protein, rice congee, oats, shiitake, coconut, honey, green tea, turmeric, galangal

Top 5 ancient prescriptions:

1. CBD oil. Research shows it can help.[25] Dab ¼ teaspoon on plaques twice daily.
2. Sarsaparilla (smilax). Clears damp inflammation. Take 500 mg 2 or 3 times daily.
3. Marshmallow root. Moistens lung and colon. Take 500 to 2,000 mg daily.
4. Turmeric. Reduces inflammation. Take 1,000 mg twice daily.
5. Vitamin D3. Strengthens immunity. Take 5,000 IU daily.

Other remedies: Try acupuncture; exercise; get 20 minutes of sunshine 3 to 4 days a week to bolster vitamin D; reduce stress with prayer, meditation, spiritual growth reading, walking in nature, and digital fasting; rub Dead Sea mud on the affected area; and see a therapist to work through past hurts. Fish oil, milk thistle, and bone broth protein can also help.

Essential oils: Mix 3 drops of geranium oil, along with 1 drop each of lavender or frankincense oil, with ¼ teaspoon coconut oil and rub onto affected areas once or twice daily.

RESTLESS LEG SYNDROME. This is a jittery feeling that you need to move your legs, mostly at night. It's a common cause of insomnia tied to poor diet, stress, pregnancy, and immobility.

Ancient perspective: In TCM, it's linked to heat in the heart and kidney yin deficiency.

Foods That Harm	Foods That Heal
Sugar, artificial sweeteners, soda, refined oils, processed carbs and grains, fried food, gluten, caffeine, chocolate, spicy food, alcohol	Iron-rich foods, grass-fed beef, organ meats, chicken, bone broth, wild-caught fish, leafy greens, asparagus, beets, brussels sprouts, carrots, parsley, zucchini, beans, lentils, seeds, prunes, apples, pears, almonds, avocados, olives, coconut, barley, millet

Top 5 ancient prescriptions:
1. CBD oil. Calms nerves and relaxes muscles. Take 40 to 100 mg daily.
2. Magnesium. Relaxes nervous system and muscles. Take as an Epsom salt bath for 20 minutes daily or take 300 to 600 mg daily.
3. TCM Blood Builder formula. Treats symptoms. Take as directed.
4. Rehmannia. Treats yin deficiency and heart heat. Take 55 to 350 mg daily. (Avoid if pregnant or breastfeeding.)
5. Vegetable juice. Make juice from parsley, celery, and beets. Drink a cup daily.

Other remedies: Try chiropractic, acupuncture, exercise, yoga, and stretching. Reduce stress with spiritual triathlon (see page 167), gratitude journal, and walking in nature. Use red light therapy for 10 to 20 minutes daily, which is relaxing and improves sleep.

Essential oils: Add 5 drops each of cypress, rosemary, and lavender oil to 1 teaspoon coconut oil and massage into your low back and legs before bed. Then apply very warm and cold compress for 10 minutes each.

ROSACEA. This skin condition, more common in fair-skinned people, causes visible blood vessels, redness, and, sometimes small pus-filled bumps, often occurring in cycles. Stress, genetics, and poor digestive health contribute.

Ancient perspective: In TCM, rosacea is caused by liver and lung heat and dampness. Stress, overwork, anger, and frustration also contribute.

Foods That Harm	Foods That Heal
Citrus, spicy food, sugar, processed food, red meat, fried food, hydrogenated oils, conventional dairy, cheese, nuts, soy sauce, gluten, vinegar, alcohol, caffeine, chocolate, hot beverages	Spinach, celery, chard, cucumber, radish, asparagus, broccoli, cauliflower, zucchini, carrots, pumpkin, apples, pears, plums, mung beans, rice, millet, bone broth, wild-caught fish, chicken, miso, seaweed, peppermint

Top 5 ancient prescriptions:
1. Gentian. Clears heat from the liver and skin. Take 300 mg before meals.
2. Burdock. Supports liver and lung cleansing. Take 300 mg 3 times daily.
3. Chamomile. Reduces stress and anger. Take as directed as a tea or capsule.
4. Probiotics. Gut health plays a role in skin health. Take 25 to 50 billion IU daily.
5. Skullcap. Reduces inflammation in lung and liver. Take as directed.

Other remedies: Try acupuncture. Use red light therapy to limit redness. Reduce stress with meditation, spiritual growth reading, yoga, exercise, walking in nature, digital fasting, and daily downtime. If anger is a problem, talking to a therapist can provide tools for staying calm. B-complex vitamins, fish oil, spirulina, and milk thistle can also help.

Essential oils: Mix 3 drops of tea tree oil with 3 drops of lavender, geranium, or chamomile oil, plus ½ teaspoon manuka honey and ½ teaspoon aloe vera gel, then rub on the affected area once daily.

SHINGLES. This herpes infection affects the skin, causing intense, stabbing pain, a blistering rash, fatigue, flu-like achiness, and appetite changes.

Ancient perspective: In TCM, shingles results when toxic heat builds up, causing liver qi stagnation and lung qi deficiency. Stress is a major causative factor in shingles.

Foods That Harm	Foods That Heal
Processed food, sugar, artificial sweeteners, fried food, alcohol, food allergens, caffeine, fruit juices, carbonated beverages	Leafy greens, asparagus, broccoli, cauliflower, carrots, celery, onions, garlic, pumpkin, squash, fermented foods, spirulina, berries, mulberries, pears, citrus, walnuts, bone broth, wild-caught fish, chicken, rice congee, oats, shiitake, coconut, honey, ginger, thyme

Top 5 ancient prescriptions:
1. Echinacea. Has antiviral properties. Take 1,000 mg 2 or 3 times daily.
2. Astragalus. Strengthens immunity and reduces stress. Take 2,000 mg twice daily.
3. Olive leaf. Has antiviral properties. Take 500 mg 4 times daily.
4. Vitamin B12. Speeds recovery. Take as directed.
5. Vitamin C and zinc. Boosts immunity. Take 1,000 mg vitamin C 3 or 4 times daily and 30 mg zinc twice daily.

Other remedies: Try acupuncture, colloidal oatmeal baths, and stress-reducing activities, including prayer, meditation, spiritual reading, yoga, walking in nature, digital fasting, and building downtime into your day. Schisandra, licorice, andrographis, reishi, and cordyceps can also help.

Essential oils: Combine 3 drops of myrrh, oregano, thyme, or geranium oil with ¼ teaspoon coconut oil and rub onto the affected areas.

SINUS INFECTION. An inflammation of the tissue lining the sinuses can lead to mucus buildup, pain, and pressure in the forehead and cheeks; it sometimes causes infection as well.

Ancient perspective: In TCM, it's caused by lung dampness, which often stems from weak digestion.

Foods That Harm	Foods That Heal
Sugar, fruit juices, dairy products, egg whites, high-fat food, refined flour and grains, bananas, dried fruit, avocados, tofu, pork, raw vegetables	Leafy greens, asparagus, broccoli, carrots, celery, squash, pumpkin, vitamin C–rich fruits (citrus, kiwi, goji, pineapple), fermented foods, miso, chickpeas, rice congee, bone broth, chicken, wild-caught fish, garlic, onions, thyme, sage, oregano, ginger

Top 5 ancient prescriptions:
1. Grapefruit seed extract nasal spray. Fights infection. Use according to package directions 4 times daily.
2. Echinacea. Clears mucus and strengthens immunity. Take 1,000 mg twice daily.
3. Homeopathic formula. Belladonna and other homeopathic ingredients relieve sinus infection symptoms. Take as directed.
4. Stinging nettle. Acts as a natural antihistamine. Take 300 to 500 mg 3 times daily.
5. Bromelain and quercetin. Natural anti-inflammatories that improve sinusitis. Take as directed.

Other remedies: Clear sinus passages with a neti pot; get 9 to 10 hours of sleep a night; use a humidifier to reduce congestion; do gentle exercise. Astragalus and probiotics strengthen digestion, which can prevent chronic problems.

Essential oils: Diffuse 5 drops of eucalyptus or peppermint oil to open sinuses.

SLEEP APNEA. Characterized by pauses in breathing, it impairs sleep quality and quantity, causing daytime sleepiness, and increases risk for heart disease, stroke, diabetes, obesity, depression, memory problems, impaired immunity, and low libido.

Ancient perspective: In TCM, it's caused by lung qi deficiency, spleen qi deficiency, and excess phlegm. Worry and ruminating about the past add to the problem.

Foods That Harm	Foods That Heal
Sugar, fruit juices, soda, dairy products, egg whites, high-fat food, refined flour and grains, bananas, dried fruit, avocados, tofu, pork, raw vegetables, caffeine, alcohol	Leafy greens, asparagus, broccoli, carrots, celery, squash, pumpkin, peas, citrus, kiwi, plantain, plums, grapes, coconut, olives, walnuts, miso, kidney beans, rice, barley, bone broth, chicken, wild-caught fish, garlic, onions, thyme, sage, mustard

Top 5 ancient prescriptions:
1. Chamomile. Improves sleep quality and quantity. Drink a cup of tea before bed or, for greater effect, take 220 to 1,600 mg of a supplement daily.
2. Thyme. Strengthens lungs, curbs phlegm. Take as directed.
3. Astragalus. Boosts lung, spleen qi. Take 500 to 2,000 mg daily.
4. Melatonin. Helps you fall asleep and stay asleep. Take as directed.
5. Vitamin D. Levels are often low in those with sleep apnea. Take 1,000 IU daily.

Other remedies: Exercise 4 times a week for 30 minutes, combining strength training and high-intensity intervals, and go for a brisk walk twice daily. Reduce stress with spiritual growth reading, meditation, and yoga. Turn your mind toward the future by scheduling things you love to do.

Essential oils: Diffuse 3 to 5 drops of clary sage, lavender, or vetiver oil in the bedroom at night.

SMALL INTESTINAL BACTERIAL OVERGROWTH (SIBO). SIBO occurs when bacteria from other parts of the gut migrate to the small intestine, causing gut pain and diarrhea.

Ancient perspective: In TCM, SIBO is caused by small intestine qi stagnation and spleen qi deficiency and dampness. Stress, worry, and working while eating contribute.

Foods That Harm	Foods That Heal
Sugar, high-fructose corn syrup, agave nectar, honey, soda, dried fruit, flavored yogurt, dairy with lactose, barley, rye, grains, garlic, onions, asparagus, butternut squash	Bone broth, collagen, wild-caught salmon, grass-fed beef, chicken, cooked vegetables, leafy greens, celery, cauliflower, carrots, pumpkin, squash, blueberries, stewed pears, grapes, goji, coconut oil, olives, sprouted rice congee, oatmeal, shiitake, ginger, bitter herbs

Top 5 ancient prescriptions:

1. TCM Four Gentlemen formula. Contains codonopsis, atractylodes, poria, and licorice, which bolster spleen qi and counteract stress. Take as directed.
2. Astragalus. Strengthens the digestive system. Take 1,000 mg once or twice daily.
3. SBO probiotic. Ones with *Lactobacillus casei, Lactobacillus plantarum,* and *Bifidobacterium brevis* have been shown to help. Take 50 to 100 billion IU daily.
4. Herbal antimicrobials. Olive leaf, pau d'arco, oregano, and grapefruit seed can keep bacteria in check. Take as directed.
5. Triphala. Heals and repairs the intestine. Take as directed.

Other remedies: Eat 5 to 6 small meals daily to help food digest more quickly. Reduce stress with yoga, tai chi, nature walks, spiritual triathlon (see page 167), and daily downtime. Acupuncture helps, too.

Essential oils: Add 1 or 2 drops of peppermint, oregano, frankincense, or clove oil to water and drink before meals.

SPRAIN OR STRAIN. Both involve stretching or tearing connective tissue. Sprains affect ligaments (which hold joints together); strains affect muscles or tendons (which connect muscle to bone). They limit motion and cause pain, swelling, and stiffness.

Ancient perspective: In TCM, the cause is excess heat in a localized area.

Foods That Harm	Foods That Heal
Sugar, artificial sweeteners, salt, refined grains, packaged food, fast food, hydrogenated oils, fried food, caffeine, soda, alcohol	Leafy greens, asparagus, broccoli, cauliflower, carrots, beets, pumpkin, squash, berries, figs, kiwi, pineapple, walnuts, chia seeds, flaxseed, bone broth, salmon and other wild-caught fish, grass-fed beef, avocados, olive oil, coconut, green tea, turmeric, galangal, ginger, rosemary

Top 5 ancient prescriptions:
1. Arnica. Reduces pain, bruising, and swelling. Use as directed.
2. Ice. Eases pain and inflammation. Wrap an ice pack in a thin towel and apply to the area for 20 minutes 3 times daily for the first 2 days. On day 3, alternate hot and cold for 10 minutes each 3 times daily.
3. Bone broth. Contains collagen, which builds connective tissue. Drink 2 or 3 cups daily.
4. Turmeric. Reduces inflammation. Take 1,000 to 3,000 mg daily.
5. Epsom salt bath. The magnesium in Epsom salt is healing. Follow the package directions and soak for 20 to 30 minutes once or twice daily.

Other remedies: Try acupuncture. Take a break from activity and let pain dictate when you return. For the first 48 hours, elevate the injured area and wrap it with an athletic bandage.

Essential oils: Add 3 drops of peppermint, helichrysum, or marjoram oil to ½ teaspoon coconut oil and massage into the injured area.

ULCERS. Gastric acids, bacteria (*H. pylori* is the most common), over-use of over-the-counter painkillers, or other toxins can damage the tissue lining the stomach, causing dull pain, weight loss, loss of appetite, nausea, vomiting, bloating, and burping.

Ancient perspective: In TCM, the root cause is stomach heat caused by excess worry and stress.

Foods That Harm	Foods That Heal
Sugar, soda, processed food, packaged food, conventional dairy and meat, alcohol, chocolate, citrus, fried food, tomatoes, peppermint, spicy food (black pepper, hot pepper, chili powder)	Cabbage juice, bone broth, wild-caught fish, chicken, cooked asparagus, broccoli, cabbage, cauliflower, carrots, celery, fennel, leafy greens, pumpkin, squash, parsley, avocados, coconut, red grapes, apples, berries, goji, rice congee, oatmeal, miso, shiitake

Top 5 ancient prescriptions:
1. Licorice root. Impairs *H. pylori* growth. Take 500 to 1,000 mg daily.
2. Probiotics. Balances gut bacteria. Take 25 to 50 billion IU daily.
3. Aloe vera juice. Promotes healing. Take 100 to 200 mg daily.
4. Zinc. Strengthens the gut and stomach lining. Take 30 mg once or twice daily.
5. Bone broth and collagen protein. Repairs the gut lining. Take 10 to 40 mg of a powdered supplement or drink 2 cups of broth daily.

Other remedies: Try acupuncture; exercise; reduce stress with spiritual growth reading, yoga, walking in nature, and gratitude practice; work less and talk with friends or a therapist; eat mostly cooked foods; drink 1 cup of chamomile and/or slippery elm tea 3 times daily; and don't eat after 7 p.m. to give your body plenty of time to digest.

Essential oils: Diffuse 5 drops of lavender, frankincense, clary sage, holy basil, or chamomile oil to reduce stress and promote calm.

URINARY TRACT INFECTION. Caused by bacteria, it leads to painful, frequent urination, fatigue, low-back pain, and, if it has reached the kidneys, fever and chills.

Ancient perspective: In TCM, the root cause is damp heat in the kidney and liver.

Foods That Harm	Foods That Heal
Sugar, caffeine, soda, alcohol, spicy food	Bone broth, wild-caught salmon, chicken, cranberries, blueberries, coconut, olive, leafy greens, asparagus, broccoli, cauliflower, celery, carrots, pumpkin, radishes, parsley, beans, lentils, rice, rye, seaweed

Top 5 ancient prescriptions:
1. Cranberry juice (sugar-free). Prevents bacteria from sticking to the bladder walls. Drink 2 or 3 cups daily.
2. Probiotics. Good bacteria helps get rid of the bad. Take 50 billion IU daily.
3. Uva ursi. Studies show it kills bad bacteria in the urinary tract. Take as directed.
4. D-mannose. Prevents bacteria from attaching to the bladder walls. Take 500 mg 4 times daily.
5. Echinacea. Enhances immune function and fights infection. Take 1,000 mg twice daily.

Other remedies: Drink 8 to 10 glasses of water daily; drink dandelion tea; get 8 to 10 hours of sleep a night; reduce stress with spiritual growth reading and walks in nature. Wear cotton underwear (or no underwear) and loose-fitting pants. Daily exercise and remedies such as garlic and bearberry also help.

Essential oils: Take 1 or 2 drops of oregano, clove, or myrrh oil each day for 10 days to fight infection.

VARICOSE VEINS. These bulging blue veins, mostly in the legs, cause achy legs, particularly after standing for a long time. Being overweight and sedentary increases the risk, as does age, family history, pregnancy, oral contraceptives, and skin damage from the sun.

Ancient perspective: In TCM, the root cause is blood stasis and spleen qi deficiency, since the spleen governs smooth muscle, including that in blood vessels and veins.

Foods That Harm	Foods That Heal
Hydrogenated oils, sugar, processed food, alcohol, caffeine	Spinach, kale, asparagus, artichokes, broccoli, cauliflower, celery, cilantro, parsley, beets, pumpkin, squash, citrus, peaches, plums, bone broth, liver, omega-3-rich foods (salmon, flaxseed), beans, rice, oats, mushrooms, turmeric

Top 5 ancient prescriptions:
1. Butcher's broom. Helps veins contract. Take 200 mg 2 or 3 times daily.
2. Horse chestnut. Promotes blood flow and reduces swelling. Take 100 to 150 mg of aescin (the active ingredient) daily. Most extracts are 20% aescin.
3. Bilberry. Strengthens veins and increases circulation. Take as directed.
4. Ginkgo biloba. It's a potent antioxidant. Take 60 to 120 mg twice daily.
5. Bone broth powder or collagen powder. Collagen lines the veins' cell walls and strengthens the veins' ability to pump blood. Take 10 to 40 mg daily.

Other remedies: Try acupuncture; exercise, such as yoga, walking in nature, cycling, and swimming; and do things that bring you joy, since poor mood can contribute.

Essential oils: Rub 5 drops of cypress or thyme oil mixed with witch hazel on the affected veins twice daily.

Warts. Caused by the human papilloma virus, these benign, grainy growths occur most often on the hands, legs, soles of the feet, and genitals.

Ancient perspective: In TCM, the root cause is blood stasis and damp heat in the blood.

Foods That Harm	Foods That Heal
Sugar, artificial sweeteners, packaged and processed foods, spicy food, fast food, ice cream	Kale, spinach, broccoli, cabbage, carrots, red bell peppers, celery, cilantro, parsley, beets, radish, onion, pumpkin, squash, citrus, peachs, plums, mangos, papaya, bone broth, liver, wild-caught fish, brazil nuts, chestnuts, chickpeas, rice, oats, mushrooms, seaweed, turmeric, green tea

Top 5 ancient prescriptions:
1. Thuja oil. Made from the leaf of the thuja tree, it's an effective homeopathic treatment for warts. Take thuja occidentalis or apply topically as directed.
2. Olive leaf. Has antiviral properties. Take 500 mg twice daily.
3. Echinacea and astragalus. Strengthens the immune system. Take 1,000 mg of each daily.
4. Dong quai and rehmannia. Together, they move blood. Take as directed. (Avoid rehmannia if pregnant or breastfeeding.)
5. Selenium and zinc. Strengthen the immune system. Take 200 mcg of selenium and 30 mg of zinc daily.

Other remedies: Try acupuncture; reduce stress through prayer, meditation, and spiritual growth reading; address depression, hurt, grief, grudges, or regrets that might be leading to blood stasis (talking to a therapist can help). Before bed, cut a small piece of raw potato, tape it over the wart, and wear overnight. Practice gratitude and schedule fun activities.

Essential oils: Mix 1 drop each of oregano and frankincense oil with 1 teaspoon coconut oil; apply 2 or 3 times daily till the wart is gone.

WEIGHT GAIN. Weight gain can be caused by a diet high in refined carbs, sugar, and hydrogenated oils; a sedentary lifestyle (which causes a loss of calorie-burning muscle tissue); genetics; stress; lack of sleep; insulin resistance; environmental toxins; and some medications.

Ancient perspective: In TCM, the root cause is damp phlegm accumulation with spleen qi deficiency and kidney yang deficiency.

Foods That Harm	Foods That Heal
Sugar, refined carbs, processed and packaged foods, produce with pesticides, soda and other sugar-sweetened beverages, alcohol	Leafy greens, cruciferous vegetables, pumpkin, carrots, squash, berries, wild-caught fatty fish (salmon, sardines), poultry, grass-fed beef, eggs, coconut oil, olive oil, avocados, seeds, nuts, dark chocolate, stevia, asparagus, liver, monk fruit

Top 5 ancient prescriptions:
1. Collagen protein powder. Supports muscle growth and metabolism. Take 10 to 40 mg daily.
2. Matcha green tea. Promotes healthy metabolism. Drink 2 cups daily.
3. Digestive bitters. Reduces dampness and phlegm. Take as directed.
4. Ashwagandha. Supports thyroid health and hormone balance. Start with 500 mg daily, and increase gradually, up to 1,250 mg.
5. Astragalus. Supports spleen qi and digestion. Take 1,000 mg once or twice daily.

Other remedies: To boost metabolism, do high-intensity interval training and strength training. Reduce stress with meditation, yoga, spiritual triathlon, daily downtime, and digital fasting. Bolster joy by spending time with people you love.

Essential oils: Diffuse 3 drops each of peppermint, lemon, or grapefruit oil, or take 1 drop of each in water orally.

PART IV

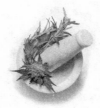

Recipes for Ancient Nutrition

Food Purchasing Advice

- For produce, buy local and organic whenever possible.
- For meats, try to select antibiotic-free, grass-fed, and pasture-raised.
- For fish, go with wild-caught.

Diet Types

- Dairy Free
- Gluten Free
- Keto
- Low Carb

- Paleo
- Vegan
- Vegetarian

BEVERAGES

VANILLA CHERRY SMOOTHIE

SERVES: 1 OR 2
TOTAL TIME: 2 MINUTES

Ingredients

1 cup frozen cherries
1 tablespoon chia seeds
1/2 cup unsweetened almond milk

1 scoop vanilla-flavored
collagen protein powder

Directions

Combine all the ingredients in a high-speed blender. Blend until smooth, adding water to reduce the thickness, if desired.

VANILLA BLUEBERRY SMOOTHIE

SERVES: 1 OR 2
TIME: 2 MINUTES

Ingredients

1 cup frozen blueberries
1/2 banana
1 cup unsweetened canned
coconut milk

1 scoop vanilla-flavored
collagen protein powder

Directions

Combine all the ingredients in a high-speed blender. Blend until smooth, adding water to reduce the thickness, if desired.

PUMPKIN SMOOTHIE

SERVES: 1

TOTAL TIME: 5 MINUTES

   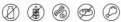

Ingredients

1 cup unsweetened almond milk or canned coconut milk

1/2 cup canned pumpkin puree

1 scoop vanilla-flavored collagen protein powder

1/4 teaspoon pumpkin pie spice

Directions

Combine all the ingredients in a high-speed blender. Blend until smooth, adding water to reduce the thickness, if desired.

CHOCOLATE CHERRY SHAKE

SERVES: 1

TOTAL TIME: 5 MINUTES

   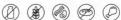

Ingredients

1 cup canned coconut milk

1 cup frozen cherries

1 scoop chocolate-flavored collagen protein powder

3 or 4 ice cubes

Directions

Combine all the ingredients in a high-speed blender. Blend until smooth, adding water to reduce the thickness, if desired.

GOJI COLLAGEN SMOOTHIE

SERVES: I

TOTAL TIME: 5 MINUTES

  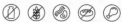

Ingredients

I cup unsweetened almond milk

2 tablespoons goji berry powder

¾ cup blueberries

I scoop vanilla-flavored
  collagen protein powder

Directions

Combine all the ingredients in a high-speed blender. Blend until smooth, adding water to reduce the thickness, if desired.

DETOX SHAKE

SERVES: I

TOTAL TIME: I5 MINUTES

Ingredients

½ cup chopped carrots

½ apple, chopped

I½ cups water, plus more if
  needed

Handful of spinach leaves

I tablespoon matcha green tea
  powder

3 or 4 ice cubes

Directions

Put a steamer basket in a small saucepan and pour in about an inch of water. Bring to a boil over medium-high heat. Add the carrots and apple, cover, and steam for 10 minutes. Drain the carrots and apple in a colander and rinse with cold water to cool down.

Transfer the carrots and apple to a high-speed blender and add the water, spinach, matcha, and ice cubes. Blend until smooth, adding more water to reduce the thickness, if desired.

BANANA-VANILLA CLEANSING SHAKE

SERVES: 1

TOTAL TIME: 5 MINUTES

Ingredients

1¼ cups water

½ cup diced pineapple

1 cup spinach

½ banana

1 scoop vanilla-flavored
collagen protein powder

Directions

Combine all the ingredients in a high-speed blender. Blend until smooth, adding water to reduce the thickness, if desired.

MATCHA LATTE

SERVES: 1

TOTAL TIME: 10 MINUTES

Ingredients

1½ cups unsweetened almond
milk or canned coconut milk

1 scoop unflavored collagen
protein powder

1 teaspoon matcha green tea
powder

1 teaspoon coconut oil

1 teaspoon maple syrup
(optional; this will make it
non-keto, non-Paleo, and
higher-carb)

Pinch ground cinnamon
(optional)

Directions

Warm the milk in a tea kettle or small pot.

Transfer the milk to a blender and add the protein powder, matcha powder, coconut oil, and maple syrup (if using). Blend until smooth.

Top with cinnamon, if desired.

TURMERIC GOLDEN MILK

SERVES: 2
TOTAL TIME: 10 MINUTES

   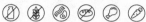

Ingredients

2 cups unsweetened almond milk or canned coconut milk

1 tablespoon coconut oil

1 tablespoon ground turmeric

1 teaspoon maple syrup (optional; this will make it non-keto, non-Paleo, and higher-carb)

½ teaspoon vanilla extract

⅛ to ¼ teaspoon ground cinnamon

⅛ to ¼ teaspoon ground ginger

⅛ teaspoon ground black pepper

Pinch ground cinnamon (optional)

Directions

Combine the nut milk, coconut oil, and turmeric in a small saucepan. Stir the mixture over medium heat until it is hot and the ingredients are well combined.

Add the maple syrup (if using), vanilla, cinnamon, ginger, and pepper. Stir until blended.

Top with cinnamon, if desired.

BREAKFAST

CONGEE 5 WAYS

SERVES: 4

PREP TIME: 5 MINUTES   TOTAL TIME: 1¼ HOURS

IMMUNE BOOSTING

Ingredients

I cup white basmati rice

4 cups chicken broth or water

I teaspoon sea salt

Optional garnishes:

Sliced shiitake mushrooms

Chopped scallions

Shredded nori seaweed

Chopped fresh parsley

Directions

Rinse and drain the rice, then put it in a medium saucepan. Add the broth and salt.

Bring to a boil over medium-high heat, then reduce to a simmer. Cook for at least I hour, stirring occasionally, until the mixture becomes porridge-like.

Divide into 4 bowls and add your garnishes of choice.

ANTI-INFLAMMATORY

Ingredients

I cup brown jasmine rice

6 cups mushroom broth

2 teaspoons ground turmeric

I teaspoon sea salt

Optional garnishes:

Grated fresh ginger

Chopped scallions

Coconut aminos or tamari

Chopped fresh cilantro

Directions

Rinse and drain the rice, then put it in a medium saucepan. Add the broth, turmeric, and salt.

Bring to a boil over medium-high heat, then reduce to a simmer. Cook for at least 1 hour, stirring occasionally, until the mixture becomes porridge-like.

Divide into 4 bowls and add your garnishes of choice.

DIGESTION

Ingredients

2 cups cauliflower rice or finely chopped cauliflower

2 tablespoons coconut oil

4 cups chicken broth (or canned coconut milk, for a sweet version)

1 teaspoon sea salt

Optional garnishes:

Chopped mushrooms

Minced garlic

Grated fresh ginger

Shredded cooked chicken

Honey or vanilla-flavored collagen protein powder, plus ground cinnamon or pumpkin pie spice (for the sweet version)

Directions

Rinse and drain the cauliflower, then put it in a medium saucepan. Add the coconut oil, broth, and salt.

Bring to a boil over medium-high heat, then reduce to a simmer. Cook for at least 30 minutes, stirring occasionally, until the mixture becomes porridge-like.

Divide into 4 bowls and add your garnishes of choice.

ENERGIZING

Ingredients

1 cup steel-cut oats

4 cups water

2 scoops unflavored collagen protein powder

1 teaspoon sea salt

Optional garnishes:

Blueberries	Raw honey
Hemp seeds	Bee pollen

Directions

Rinse and drain the oats, then put them in a medium saucepan. Add the water, collagen powder, and salt.

Bring to a boil over medium-high heat, then reduce to a simmer. Cook for at least 1 hour, stirring occasionally, until the mixture becomes porridge-like.

Divide into 4 bowls and add your garnishes of choice.

STRENGTHENING

Ingredients

1 cup quinoa	1 teaspoon sea salt
6 cups chicken broth	

Garnishes:

Poached eggs	Chopped spinach or kale
Chopped scallions	Tamari

Directions

Rinse and drain the quinoa, then put it in a medium saucepan. Add the broth and salt.

Bring to a boil over medium-high heat, then reduce to a simmer. Cook for at least 1 hour, stirring occasionally, until the mixture becomes porridge-like.

Divide into 4 bowls and add your garnishes of choice.

SWEET POTATO HASH BOWL

SERVES: 4

TOTAL TIME: 25 MINUTES

Ingredients

4 tablespoons coconut oil, divided

3 medium sweet potatoes, peeled and grated

3 cups stemmed and chopped kale

½ medium onion, finely diced

2 garlic cloves, minced

1 teaspoon sea salt

1 teaspoon ground black pepper

1 pound chicken breakfast sausage, removed from its casings

Chopped fresh parsley, for garnish

Directions

Heat 2 tablespoons of the coconut oil in a medium skillet over medium-high heat. Add the sweet potatoes, kale, onion, garlic, salt, and pepper and cook, stirring occasionally, until the sweet potatoes are tender, about 20 minutes.

Heat the remaining 2 tablespoons coconut oil in another medium-size skillet over medium heat. Add the chicken sausage and cook, breaking up the meat with a wooden spoon, until fully cooked, about 5 minutes. Add the sausage to the vegetables and stir to combine.

Divide onto 4 plates and garnish with fresh parsley.

MUSHROOM AND KALE FRITTATA

SERVES: 4

TOTAL TIME: 25 MINUTES

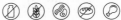

Ingredients

1 cup water

1 scoop unflavored collagen or bone broth protein powder

½ teaspoon sea salt

3 cups stemmed and chopped kale

1 cup sliced mushrooms

½ red onion, diced

½ red bell pepper, seeded and diced

8 large eggs

1 tablespoon minced fresh basil

¼ teaspoon crushed red pepper (optional)

Directions

Turn on the broiler.

In a large oven-safe skillet, combine the water, protein powder, and salt and bring to a boil over medium-high heat, then reduce to a simmer.

Add the kale, mushrooms, onion, and bell pepper and simmer for 8 minutes.

In a medium bowl, whisk together the eggs, basil, and crushed red pepper (if using). Add the egg mixture to the pan and stir to combine.

Turn the heat to medium, cover, and cook for 4 to 6 minutes, until the eggs are beginning to firm up.

Uncover and put the skillet under the broiler for 4 to 6 minutes, until the eggs are set and just beginning to brown. Watch carefully so it doesn't burn.

Cut the frittata into wedges to serve.

BLUEBERRY PUMPKIN PANCAKES

SERVES: 2
TOTAL TIME: 30 MINUTES

Ingredients

2 large eggs

½ cup canned coconut milk

½ cup canned pumpkin puree

2 tablespoons unsalted grass-
fed butter, melted

1 teaspoon vanilla extract

1 cup gluten-free pancake mix

1 teaspoon ground cinnamon

½ cup fresh or frozen blueberries

1 teaspoon coconut oil

Directions

In a medium bowl, whisk together the eggs, coconut milk, pumpkin puree, melted butter, and vanilla until smooth.

Add the pancake mix and cinnamon and mix well. Fold in the blueberries, using a silicone spatula to spread them throughout the mixture without crushing them.

Heat a griddle pan over medium-low heat and coat with the coconut oil. Pour ¼ cup of the batter on the hot griddle to form each pancake. Cook for a few minutes, until bubbles form on top, then flip and cook for an additional 1 to 2 minutes, until the underside is cooked. Transfer to a plate and continue with the remaining batter.

BERRY SCONES

SERVES: 6

PREP TIME: 25 MINUTES   TOTAL TIME: I HOUR

Ingredients

SCONES

2½ cups oat flour

¼ cup coconut sugar

I tablespoon baking powder

I teaspoon ground cinnamon

½ teaspoon sea salt

I teaspoon vanilla extract

I teaspoon fresh lemon juice

⅓ cup coconut butter

⅓ cup unsweetened almond milk

I cup fresh blueberries

LEMON CASHEW GLAZE (optional)

I cup cashews, soaked for 4 to I2 hours in water in the refrigerator, then drained

½ cup unsweetened almond milk, plus more if needed

¼ cup maple syrup

3 tablespoons fresh lemon juice

I teaspoon vanilla extract

¼ teaspoon sea salt

Directions

Preheat the oven to 375°F. Line a rimmed baking sheet with parchment paper.

In a large bowl, whisk together the oat flour, coconut sugar, baking powder, cinnamon, salt, vanilla, and lemon juice.

Heat the coconut butter in a small saucepan over medium-low heat, so it is easy to scoop out and not dry or crumbly.

Add the coconut butter to the bowl, then use your hands or a pastry cutter to incorporate it until the mixture crumbles easily into pebble-size pieces.

Add the almond milk, using your hands to knead the dough. Do not overwork the dough; just knead until combined. Gently fold in the blueberries.

If the dough feels wet, place it in the freezer for I5 minutes to firm up.

Shape the dough into a disk about 8 inches in diameter. Cut into 6 wedges and transfer to the prepared baking sheet.

Bake for 15 to 18 minutes, until golden brown on the edges.

Let the scones cool briefly before serving. If topping with the lemon cashew glaze, allow to cool completely.

To make the glaze, combine the drained cashews, almond milk, maple syrup, lemon juice, vanilla, and salt in a food processor or blender. Blend until smooth. If the mixture is too thick, add more almond milk, 1 tablespoon at a time, until a thick but pourable consistency is reached.

Drizzle the glaze over the scones, then let it set for about 10 minutes before serving.

APPLE PIE SAUCE

SERVES: 2

TOTAL TIME: 15 MINUTES

Ingredients

2 apples, cored, peeled, and chopped

Juice of ½ lemon

2 cups water

2 tablespoons coconut oil

2 tablespoons almond butter

2 Medjool dates, pitted and finely chopped

¼ teaspoon ground cinnamon

Pinch sea salt

Directions

Combine all the ingredients in a medium saucepan and mix well. Bring to a boil over medium heat, stirring often. Boil for 2 minutes, then reduce the heat to a simmer. Cook for 5 minutes, stirring occasionally.

Pour the applesauce into one or more mason jars and let cool to room temperature, then cover and store in the refrigerator.

OVERNIGHT PEAR OATMEAL

SERVES: 4

PREP TIME: 5 MINUTES   TOTAL TIME: OVERNIGHT

Ingredients

1 cup steel-cut oats

4 cups water

2 Asian pears, cored and chopped

1 tablespoon coconut butter

½ cup chopped walnuts

1 teaspoon ground cinnamon

Directions

The evening before serving, combine the oats, water, pears, and coconut butter in a medium saucepan. Bring to a boil over medium heat, then turn off the heat. Cover and let sit overnight at room temperature.

In the morning, heat over medium-high heat for 5 to 10 minutes, stirring occasionally.

Divide into 4 bowls and top each serving with some walnuts and cinnamon.

COCONUT YOGURT PARFAIT

SERVES: 1

TOTAL TIME: 5 MINUTES

Ingredients

1 cup unsweetened coconut milk yogurt

2 tablespoons hemp seeds

1 cup mixed berries

½ cup Baked Granola (page 324) or store-bought granola

Directions

Scoop half of the yogurt into a wide glass. Layer on half of the hemp seeds, half of the berries, and half of the granola. Repeat the layers.

ELEMENTS TOAST

SERVES: 2
TOTAL TIME: 10 MINUTES

Ingredients

1 medium avocado, peeled and
  pitted
½ onion, diced
2 slices sprouted wheat berry
  bread, toasted

6 thin slices smoked salmon
2 teaspoons capers
Juice of ½ lemon
Sea salt and ground black pepper,
  to taste

Directions

Mash the avocado in a small bowl and mix in the onion. Spread the mixture evenly on the toast slices. Lay the salmon on top. Add the capers and lemon juice. Season with salt and pepper.

SOUPS

HEALING CHICKEN SOUP

SERVES: 4
PREP TIME: 10 MINUTES   TOTAL TIME: 40 MINUTES

Ingredients

1 tablespoon coconut oil
4 cups peeled and chopped
  butternut squash
½ cup diced red onion
3 cups shredded cooked chicken
8 cups chicken bone broth (or 8
  scoops unflavored collagen or

bone broth protein powder
  mixed with 8 cups water)
2 tablespoons chopped garlic
1 teaspoon sea salt
1 teaspoon ground black pepper
½ teaspoon ground turmeric

Directions

Heat the coconut oil in a large soup pot over medium-high heat. Add the squash and onion and cook, stirring often, for 3 to 4 minutes, until tender.

Stir in the chicken, broth, garlic, salt, pepper, and turmeric. Bring to a boil, then turn the heat to medium-low.

Cover the pot and let the soup simmer for 25 to 30 minutes, until the squash is cooked through.

DR. AXE IMMUNITY BOWL

SERVES: 8

PREP TIME: 15 MINUTES   TOTAL TIME: 45 MINUTES

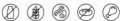

Ingredients

1 tablespoon coconut oil

½ onion, diced

2 pounds boneless, skinless chicken thighs, cut into bite-size pieces

8 cups chicken broth (or 8 scoops unflavored collagen or bone broth protein powder mixed with 8 cups water)

1 head cauliflower, cored and chopped

3 cups stemmed and chopped kale

2 cups chopped shiitake mushrooms

¼ cup white miso paste (chickpea or soybean)

Directions

Heat the coconut oil in a large soup pot over medium heat. Add the onion and chicken thighs and cook, stirring frequently, until browned, about 10 minutes.

Stir in the broth, cauliflower, kale, mushrooms, and miso. Bring to a boil then turn the heat to medium-low.

Cover the pot and let the soup simmer for 20 to 25 minutes, until the cauliflower is cooked through.

BEEF STEW

SERVES: 6

PREP TIME: 20 MINUTES   TOTAL TIME: 6 TO 8 HOURS

Ingredients

2 pounds grass-fed beef stew
  meat

4 carrots, peeled and coarsely
  chopped

2 parsnips, peeled and coarsely
  chopped

2 cups beef broth

2 tablespoons Worcestershire
  sauce

2 tablespoons balsamic vinegar

1 (6-ounce) can tomato paste

1 (14.5-ounce) can fire-roasted
  tomatoes

1 cup sliced mushrooms, such as
  cremini or oyster

1 onion, sliced

1 teaspoon garlic powder

1 teaspoon onion powder

1 teaspoon smoked paprika

2 tablespoons chopped fresh dill

¼ cup arrowroot starch

1 teaspoon sea salt

1 teaspoon ground black pepper

Chopped fresh parsley, for
  garnish

Directions

Combine all the ingredients (except the parsley) in a slow cooker. Cover and cook on low for 6 to 8 hours. Top with chopped parsley to serve.

BUTTERNUT SQUASH BISQUE

SERVES: 6-8

PREP TIME: 20 MINUTES   TOTAL TIME: I HOUR

Ingredients

I tablespoon coconut oil

I large or 2 small butternut squash, halved lengthwise and seeded

Sea salt and ground black pepper, to taste

3 carrots, chopped

½ white onion, sliced

2 garlic cloves, chopped

I green apple, peeled, cored, and sliced

I tablespoon unsalted grass-fed butter

I teaspoon ground ginger

½ teaspoon ground cinnamon

½ teaspoon ground nutmeg

5 cups vegetable broth

Directions

Preheat the oven to 425°F. Grease two rimmed baking sheets with the coconut oil.

Season the cut sides of the squash with salt and pepper. Place the squash halves, cut-side down, on the baking sheets.

Scatter the carrots, onion, garlic, and apple around the squash halves. Bake for 40 minutes, until the squash is tender.

Allow the squash to cool slightly, then scoop the flesh into a high-speed blender, along with the carrots, onion, garlic, apple, butter, ginger, cinnamon, and nutmeg. Blend until smooth.

In a large soup pot, bring the vegetable broth to a boil over medium-high heat. Reduce the heat to medium and stir in the blended squash mixture until well incorporated. Cook for 5 minutes, then reduce the heat and simmer for 10 minutes. Season with salt and pepper.

CARROT GINGER SOUP

SERVES: 8

PREP TIME: 20 MINUTES   TOTAL TIME: 1 HOUR

Ingredients

2 pounds carrots, peeled and chopped

3 tablespoons grated fresh ginger

3 garlic cloves, chopped

6 cups vegetable broth

1 tablespoon coconut oil

2 onions, chopped

1 cup canned coconut milk

Sea salt, ground black pepper, and onion powder, to taste

Directions

Combine the carrots, ginger, garlic, and broth in a large soup pot. Bring to a boil over medium–high heat. Reduce the heat and simmer until the carrots are soft when pierced, about 20 minutes. Set aside to cool slightly.

Meanwhile, heat the coconut oil in a skillet over medium-high heat. Add the onions and cook, stirring occasionally, about 10 minutes.

Working in batches if necessary, transfer the broth mixture and onions to a blender and blend until smooth.

Return the blended mixture to the pot and stir in the coconut milk and seasonings. Rewarm over medium heat.

CAULIFLOWER SOUP

SERVES: 8

PREP TIME: 20 MINUTES   TOTAL TIME: 40 MINUTES

Ingredients

1 tablespoon coconut oil or unsalted grass-fed butter

1 head cauliflower, cored and cut into bite-size pieces

2 turnips, peeled and diced

1 onion, chopped

5 garlic cloves, minced

4 cups chicken broth (or 4 scoops unflavored collagen or bone broth protein powder mixed with 4 cups water)

1 teaspoon grated fresh ginger or ½ teaspoon ground ginger

2 teaspoons ground turmeric

1 teaspoon ground cumin

½ teaspoon sea salt

Juice of ½ lemon

2 (14-ounce) cans coconut milk

Directions

Heat the coconut oil in a large soup pot over medium heat until shimmering. Add the cauliflower, turnips, onion, and garlic and cook, stirring often, for 5 to 8 minutes, until the vegetables are tender.

Increase the heat to medium-high. Add the chicken broth, ginger, turmeric, cumin, and salt. Cover and bring the soup to a boil. Stir in the lemon juice and coconut milk. Reduce the heat and simmer for 10 minutes.

DETOX SOUP

SERVES: 4

PREP TIME: 20 MINUTES   TOTAL TIME: 40 MINUTES

Ingredients

1 tablespoon extra virgin olive oil

1 onion, chopped

3 celery stalks, chopped

3 carrots, peeled and chopped

1 pound boneless, skinless chicken breasts, cut into bite-size pieces

4 cups chicken broth (or 4 scoops unflavored collagen or bone broth protein powder mixed with 4 cups water)

2 tablespoons grated fresh ginger

1 tablespoon white miso paste (chickpea or soybean)

1 tablespoon apple cider vinegar

1 teaspoon ground turmeric

1 teaspoon sea salt

2 cups frozen peas

Directions

Heat the oil in a large soup pot over medium heat. Add the onion, celery, carrots, and chicken and cook, stirring often, for 5 to 8 minutes, until the chicken is cooked through.

Add the broth, ginger, miso, vinegar, turmeric, and salt and stir well. Cover, increase the heat to medium-high, and bring the soup to a boil. Stir in the peas. Reduce the heat to low and simmer for 10 minutes.

TURKEY MEATBALL SOUP

SERVES: 8

PREP TIME: 20 MINUTES   TOTAL TIME: 45 MINUTES

Ingredients

2 large eggs

1½ pounds ground turkey or ground chicken

1 teaspoon smoked paprika

1½ teaspoons sea salt, divided

2 tablespoons coconut oil

4 cups chicken bone broth (or 4 scoops unflavored collagen or bone broth protein powder mixed with 4 cups water)

4 carrots, peeled and chopped

1 large sweet potato, peeled and chopped

2 bay leaves

1 cup green beans, cut in half

1 cup frozen peas

2 tomatoes, chopped

Directions

Whisk the eggs in a large bowl. Add the ground turkey, paprika, and ¾ teaspoon of the salt. Mix the ingredients together with your hand and form into 1- to 1½-inch meatballs.

In a large soup pot, heat the oil over medium heat. Add the meatballs and cook for 5 to 8 minutes, until they're brown on all sides.

Add the broth, carrots, sweet potato, bay leaves, and remaining ¾ teaspoon salt and bring to a boil. Add the green beans, peas, and tomatoes, reduce the heat, and simmer for 20 minutes, or until the sweet potato is tender.

LENTIL SOUP

SERVES: 8

PREP TIME: 20 MINUTES   TOTAL TIME: 45 MINUTES

Ingredients

1 tablespoon coconut oil or
   unsalted grass-fed butter

3 carrots, peeled and chopped

3 celery stalks, chopped

1 onion, chopped

2 garlic cloves, minced

5 cups vegetable broth

1 cup green or brown lentils

1 teaspoon dried thyme

2 cups stemmed and chopped
   kale or Swiss chard

Sea salt and ground black pepper,
   to taste

Directions

Heat the oil in a large soup pot over medium heat. Add the carrots, celery, onion, and garlic and cook, stirring often, for 5 to 8 minutes, until the vegetables are tender.

Add the broth, lentils, and thyme. Bring the soup to a boil. Cover, reduce the heat to a simmer, and cook for 20 minutes, or until the lentils are tender.

Add the kale and cook for 3 to 4 more minutes to wilt the kale. Season with salt and pepper.

WHITE BEAN SOUP

SERVES: 8

PREP TIME: 10 MINUTES   TOTAL TIME: 40 MINUTES

Ingredients

2 tablespoons avocado oil

3 celery stalks, chopped

3 carrots, peeled and chopped

1 onion, chopped

3 garlic cloves, minced

6 cups vegetable broth or chicken bone broth (or 6 scoops unflavored collagen or bone broth protein powder broth mixed with 6 cups water)

2 (15.5-ounce) cans cannellini beans, rinsed and drained

2 yellow squash, diced

1 Roma tomato, diced

1½ cups stemmed and chopped kale

Sea salt and ground black pepper, to taste

Crumbled goat cheese or vegan cheese, for topping (optional)

Directions

Heat the avocado oil in a large soup pot over medium heat. Add the celery, carrots, onion, and garlic and cook, stirring often, for 5 to 8 minutes, until tender.

Add the broth and bring to a boil. Add the beans, squash, tomato, and kale, reduce the heat to a simmer, and cook for 30 minutes.

Season with salt and pepper, and top individual servings with crumbled cheese, if desired.

BISON CHILI

SERVES: 8

PREP TIME: 20 MINUTES   TOTAL TIME: 8 HOURS

Ingredients

1½ teaspoons coconut oil

2 pounds ground bison

1 onion, chopped

4 garlic cloves, chopped

1 cup chopped red bell pepper

1 cup chopped carrot

1 cup chopped celery

1 jalapeño, seeded and chopped

1 (28-ounce) can crushed tomatoes

1 (14-ounce) can fire-roasted diced tomatoes, with their juice

1 (15-ounce) can tomato sauce

1 (15.5-ounce) can black beans, rinsed and drained

1 (15.5-ounce) can kidney beans, rinsed and drained

2 tablespoons chili powder

1 tablespoon dried oregano

1 tablespoon dried basil

1 tablespoon ground cumin

1 teaspoon adobo sauce (from a can of chipotles in adobo sauce)

½ teaspoon cayenne pepper

Sea salt and ground black pepper, to taste

Directions

Heat the oil in a large skillet over medium heat. Add the bison, onion, and garlic and cook, breaking up the meat with a wooden spoon, until no longer pink, 5 to 8 minutes. Transfer the contents of the skillet to a slow cooker.

Add all of the remaining ingredients and mix well. Cover and cook on low for 8 to 10 hours.

SALADS

ARUGULA SALAD WITH BEETS AND GOAT CHEESE

SERVES: 2
TOTAL TIME: 15 MINUTES

Ingredients

½ cup walnuts

1 tablespoon coconut oil

1 onion, minced

1 medium red beet, scrubbed and shredded

1 tablespoon balsamic vinegar

5 cups loosely packed arugula

½ cup crumbled goat cheese

Cracked black pepper, to taste

Directions

Heat a skillet over medium-low heat. Add the walnuts and toast in the dry skillet for 4 minutes, swirling and tossing often. Transfer the walnuts to a plate and set aside.

Add the coconut oil to the same skillet and heat over medium heat. Add the onion and beet and cook, stirring occasionally, for 5 minutes. Increase the heat to medium-high and add the vinegar. Cook, stirring often for another 3 minutes.

Put the arugula on a serving plate and top with the warm beet mixture. Garnish with the toasted walnuts, goat cheese, and black pepper.

SPINACH SALAD WITH TAHINI DRESSING

SERVES: 2
TOTAL TIME: 20 MINUTES

Ingredients

SALAD

5 cups baby spinach

½ cucumber, sliced

½ cup canned chickpeas, rinsed
and drained

4 radishes, thinly sliced

2 tablespoons sunflower seeds,
unsalted

10 cherry tomatoes, cut in half

DRESSING

½ cup fresh lemon juice

½ cup extra virgin olive oil

⅓ cup tahini

2 tablespoons maple syrup or
honey

2 garlic cloves, minced

Sea salt and ground black pepper,
to taste

Directions

Combine all the salad ingredients in a salad bowl.

For the dressing, combine the lemon juice, olive oil, tahini, maple syrup, and garlic in a blender or bowl. Blend, shake, or whisk until smooth. Season with sea salt and pepper.

Pour the dressing over the salad and toss to coat well.

CHICKPEA SALAD

SERVES: 6

TOTAL TIME: 25 MINUTES

Ingredients

SALAD

2 (15.5-ounce) cans chickpeas, rinsed and drained

1/2 red onion, thinly sliced

1 small tomato, diced

1 medium English cucumber, diced

1/2 cup chopped fresh parsley

1 teaspoon sea salt

1/2 teaspoon black pepper

DRESSING

1/4 cup extra virgin olive oil

2 tablespoons red wine vinegar

2 garlic cloves, minced

2 tablespoons Dijon mustard

1 teaspoon fresh lemon juice

1 teaspoon sea salt

1/2 teaspoon ground black pepper

Directions

Combine all the salad ingredients in a salad bowl.

For the dressing, whisk together all the ingredients in a small bowl.

Pour the dressing over the salad and toss to coat well.

ARUGULA SALAD WITH BAKED PEAR AND GOAT CHEESE

SERVES: 4

TOTAL TIME: 1 HOUR

Ingredients

Juice of 1 lemon

1 tablespoon apple cider vinegar

1/3 cup raw honey

4 tablespoons extra virgin olive oil, divided

4 ripe pears, cored and quartered

1 teaspoon coconut oil

6 cups arugula

1/2 cup crumbled goat cheese

1/2 cup walnuts, chopped

Sea salt and ground black pepper, to taste

Directions

Preheat the oven to 375°F.

In a medium bowl, whisk together the lemon juice, vinegar, honey, and 2 tablespoons of the olive oil. Add the pears and allow them to marinate in the mixture for 15 minutes.

Transfer the pears to an 8-inch baking pan, reserving the marinade. Bake, basting every 10 minutes with the reserved marinade, for 40 to 50 minutes, until the pears are fork-tender.

For the dressing, whisk together the remaining 2 tablespoons olive oil and remaining marinade and set aside.

Heat the coconut oil in a large skillet over medium heat. Add the arugula and cook, stirring often, for 2 to 4 minutes, until wilted.

Divide the arugula, goat cheese, and walnuts onto 4 plates. Top each with 4 roasted pear quarters and drizzle with the dressing. Season with salt and pepper.

AHI TUNA SALAD

SERVES: 8

TOTAL TIME: 15 MINUTES

Ingredients

1 (12-ounce) box brown rice macaroni

2 (5-ounce) cans wild-caught ahi tuna

1/2 red onion, chopped

1/2 cup pitted kalamata olives

1/2 cup chopped red bell pepper

2 tablespoons capers

1 cup cherry tomatoes, sliced

1/3 cup mayonnaise (made from olive, avocado, or coconut oil)

1/3 cup Dijon mustard

1/2 teaspoon sea salt

1/2 teaspoon ground black pepper

1/2 cup chopped scallions

Directions

Bring a large pot of salted water to a boil over medium-high heat. Add the pasta and cook until al dente, then drain in a colander and rinse under cold water.

Combine the remaining ingredients, except for the scallions, in a large bowl and mix until well combined. Add the pasta and mix again. Top with the scallions.

KALE SALAD WITH CRANBERRIES AND PINE NUTS

SERVES: 4

TOTAL TIME: 10 MINUTES

Ingredients

12 ounces kale, stemmed and chopped

2 tablespoons extra virgin olive oil

2 tablespoons lemon juice

1/3 cup pine nuts

1/3 cup dried cranberries

Sea salt, to taste

Directions

Put the kale in a large bowl. Add the oil, lemon juice, and salt and massage the kale with your hands until it becomes shiny. Divide onto plates and top with the pine nuts and cranberries. Season with salt.

SNACKS

FIG BARS

SERVES: 4

PREP TIME: 10 MINUTES   TOTAL TIME: 4 HOURS

Ingredients

1 cup dried figs

1 cup almond butter

1 tablespoon flax meal

3 tablespoons unflavored collagen or bone broth protein powder

Directions

Line an 8-inch baking pan with parchment paper.

Combine all the ingredients in a food processor and pulse until the dough starts to form a ball.

Press the dough evenly into the prepared pan and refrigerate for 3 to 4 hours, until the mixture sets.

Cut into squares and store in an airtight container.

BLUEBERRY MUFFINS

MAKES: 12 MUFFINS

PREP TIME: 15 MINUTES   TOTAL TIME: 45 MINUTES

Ingredients

2 tablespoons coconut oil, melted, plus more for greasing pan

1 cup gluten-free oat flour

½ cup almond flour

½ teaspoon baking powder

¼ teaspoon sea salt

6 scoops unflavored collagen protein powder

3 large eggs

½ cup applesauce

½ cup raw honey

1 teaspoon vanilla extract

1 teaspoon apple cider vinegar

1 cup fresh or frozen blueberries

Directions

Preheat the oven to 350°F. Grease a standard muffin tin with oil.

In a large bowl, whisk together the oat flour, almond flour, baking powder, salt, and collagen powder.

In a separate bowl, whisk together the eggs, applesauce, honey, vanilla, vinegar, and melted coconut oil.

Gradually add the dry mixture to the wet mixture and stir until smooth. Fold the blueberries into the batter. Divide the dough evenly among the cups of the prepared muffin tin.

Bake for 30 minutes, or until golden brown on top.

COFFEE CAKE

SERVES: 8

PREP TIME: 20 MINUTES   TOTAL TIME: I HOUR I0 MINUTES

Ingredients

CAKE

2 tablespoons coconut oil, melted, plus more for greasing pan

I large egg

½ cup canned coconut milk

¼ cup raw honey

I teaspoon vanilla extract

I½ cups almond flour

2 teaspoons baking powder

I teaspoon ground cinnamon

½ teaspoon sea salt

TOPPING

½ cup almond flour

I½ tablespoons coconut oil, melted

I tablespoon raw honey

2 teaspoons ground cinnamon

Directions

Preheat the oven to 350°F. Grease an 8-inch baking pan or loaf pan.

In a large bowl, whisk together the melted coconut oil, egg, coconut milk, honey, and vanilla.

In a separate bowl, whisk together the almond flour, baking powder, cinnamon, and sea salt. Gradually add the dry mixture to the wet mixture and stir until smooth. Pour the batter into the prepared baking pan.

For the topping, mix the almond flour, coconut oil, honey, and cinnamon in a small bowl. Crumble the topping over the cake.

Bake for 45 to 50 minutes, until golden brown on top.

PUMPKIN BREAD

SERVES: 8

PREP TIME: 20 MINUTES   TOTAL TIME: 1 HOUR 40 MINUTES

Ingredients

1/2 cup coconut oil, melted, plus
   more for greasing pan
1 cup canned pumpkin puree
1/2 cup maple syrup or raw honey
2 large eggs
1/4 cup unsweetened almond milk
1 teaspoon vanilla extract

2 1/2 cups gluten-free oat flour
1 cup almond flour
3/4 teaspoon baking soda
1/2 teaspoon baking powder
1/2 teaspoon sea salt
2 teaspoons pumpkin pie spice
Ground cinnamon (optional)

Directions

Preheat the oven to 350°F. Grease a loaf pan.

In a large bowl, whisk together the pumpkin puree, coconut oil, maple syrup, eggs, almond milk, and vanilla.

In a separate bowl, whisk together the oat flour, almond flour, baking soda, baking powder, salt and pumpkin pie spice.

Gradually add the dry mixture to the wet mixture and stir until smooth. Pour the batter into the prepared loaf pan and, if desired, sprinkle the top lightly with cinnamon.

Bake for 55 to 60 minutes, until a toothpick inserted in the center comes out clean.

Let the loaf cool for 10 minutes, then remove it from the pan, transfer it to a cooling rack, and let it continue to cool for 20 minutes before slicing.

OATMEAL ALMOND BUTTER BARS

SERVES: 12

PREP TIME: 10 MINUTES   TOTAL TIME: 2 HOURS

Ingredients

- 1½ cups old-fashioned rolled oats
- ¼ cup unsalted roasted almonds, chopped
- 1 cup almond butter
- ⅓ cup maple syrup
- ¼ cup vanilla-flavored collagen or bone broth protein powder
- ⅛ teaspoon sea salt

Directions

In a medium bowl, mix together the ingredients until well combined.

Pour mixture into a greased loaf pan.

Refrigerate for 1 to 2 hours, and then cut into bar or cookie shapes.

Store in the refrigerator or freezer.

BLUEBERRY-MACADAMIA COLLAGEN BARS

SERVES: 8

PREP TIME: 25 MINUTES   TOTAL TIME: 2 HOURS

Ingredients

- ½ cup coconut butter, melted, plus more for pan
- ¼ cup raw honey
- 1 teaspoon vanilla extract
- ⅛ teaspoon sea salt
- 4 scoops vanilla-flavored collagen protein powder
- ½ cup dried blueberries
- ½ cup raw macadamia nuts, chopped
- 3 tablespoons water

Directions

Grease a loaf pan.

In a medium bowl, whisk together the coconut butter, honey, vanilla, and salt. Add the protein powder and whisk to combine. Add the blueberries, macadamia nuts, and water and mix well.

Pour the mixture into the prepared pan. Refrigerate for 1 to 2 hours, until set, then cut into bars. Store in the refrigerator or freezer.

BAKED GRANOLA

SERVES: 8

PREP TIME: 10 MINUTES   TOTAL TIME: 25 MINUTES

Ingredients

2 tablespoons coconut oil, plus more for greasing pan

4 cups gluten-free old-fashioned rolled oats

1 cup raw pecans, chopped

1 cup dried cranberries or dried blueberries

1/2 cup coconut flakes

1/2 teaspoon sea salt

1/2 cup maple syrup or raw honey

1/2 teaspoon ground cinnamon

Directions

Preheat the oven to 350°F. Grease a rimmed baking sheet.

Combine all the ingredients in a bowl and mix well. Spread the mixture in a single layer on the prepared baking sheet.

Bake for 12 to 15 minutes, until golden brown. Let cool, then store in an airtight container at room temperature.

APPLE CHIPS

SERVES: 4

PREP TIME: 10 MINUTES   TOTAL TIME: 1 HOUR 10 MINUTES

Ingredients

6 large apples, cored and thinly
   sliced
1 teaspoon ground cinnamon,
   plus more for topping
   (optional)

1 teaspoon ground ginger
1 teaspoon ground nutmeg

Directions

Preheat oven to 200°F. Line a rimmed baking sheet with parchment paper.

Toss the apple slices with the spices, then place them on the prepared baking sheet. Bake for 1 hour. Sprinkle with additional cinnamon, if desired.

ISRAELI HUMMUS

SERVES: 8

TOTAL TIME: 5 MINUTES

Ingredients

1 (15.5-ounce) can chickpeas,
   rinsed and drained
2 garlic cloves, roughly chopped
1/3 cup tahini
1/4 cup fresh lemon juice

1 tablespoon extra virgin olive
   oil
1 teaspoon sea salt
1/2 teaspoon baking soda
Paprika, to taste

Directions

Combine the chickpeas, garlic, tahini, lemon juice, olive oil, salt, and baking soda in a food processor and blend until smooth. Sprinkle paprika on top before serving.

TAHINI DIPPING SAUCE

SERVES: 8
TOTAL TIME: 10 MINUTES

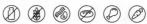

Ingredients

½ cup lemon juice
½ cup extra virgin olive oil
⅓ cup tahini
2 garlic cloves, minced
2 tablespoons raw honey or
    maple syrup (optional)

Sea salt and ground black pepper,
    to taste
Cut-up cauliflower, carrots,
    cucumbers, and/or bell
    peppers, for serving (optional)

Directions

Combine the lemon juice, olive oil, tahini, garlic, and honey (if using) in a blender or bowl. Blend, shake, or whisk until smooth. Season with salt and pepper. Serve with cut-up vegetables, if desired.

CAULIFLOWER HUMMUS

SERVES: 12
PREP TIME: 10 MINUTES   TOTAL TIME: 50 MINUTES

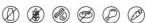

Ingredients

3½ cups cauliflower florets
2 tablespoons extra virgin olive
    oil, divided
3 garlic cloves, roughly chopped
½ cup tahini

¼ cup water
2 tablespoons fresh lemon juice
1 teaspoon sea salt
1 teaspoon ground cumin
½ teaspoon paprika

Directions

Preheat the oven to 375°F.

Put the cauliflower on a rimmed baking sheet, drizzle with 1 tablespoon of the olive oil, and spread out in a single layer. Roast for 40 minutes, or until tender.

Transfer the cauliflower to a food processor and add the garlic, tahini, water, lemon juice, remaining 1 tablespoon olive oil, salt, cumin, and paprika. Blend until smooth.

MAIN DISHES

SPAGHETTI SQUASH WITH GRASS-FED BEEF MEATBALLS

SERVES: 4

PREP TIME: 25 MINUTES   TOTAL TIME: 1 HOUR

Ingredients

SQUASH

2 tablespoons extra virgin olive oil, divided

1 large spaghetti squash, halved lengthwise and seeded

½ teaspoon sea salt

½ teaspoon ground black pepper

MEATBALLS

2 large eggs

1 pound ground grass-fed beef

1 (10-ounce) package frozen spinach, thawed and drained

¼ cup finely grated raw sheep milk cheese, such as Pecorino or Zamorano

¼ teaspoon sea salt

½ teaspoon ground black pepper

1 tablespoon olive oil

Directions

Preheat the oven to 375°F. Line a rimmed baking sheet with parchment paper and drizzle with 1 tablespoon of the olive oil.

Sprinkle the cut sides of the spaghetti squash with the salt and pepper, then place the halves, cut-side down, on the prepared baking sheet. Roast for 30 to 40 minutes, until easily pierced with a fork.

Meanwhile, for the meatballs, whisk the eggs in a large bowl. Add the beef, spinach, cheese, salt, and pepper. Mix the ingredients together with your hands and form into 1- to 1½-inch meatballs.

Heat the oil in a large skillet over medium-high heat. Add the meatballs and cook for 5 to 8 minutes, until they're browned on all sides. Transfer to a plate.

When the squash is done, let it cool for 5 minutes. Scrape the spaghetti strands into a large bowl. Add the meatballs and remaining 1 tablespoon olive oil, then toss well.

SALMON TERIYAKI

SERVES: 4

PREP TIME: 20 MINUTES   TOTAL TIME: 40 MINUTES

Ingredients

⅓ cup tamari or coconut aminos

2 tablespoons coconut sugar or raw honey

¼ cup sesame oil or coconut oil, plus more for brushing

3 tablespoons fresh lemon juice

3 garlic cloves, minced

1 teaspoon ground mustard

Sea salt and ground black pepper, to taste

4 (6-ounce) skin-on, boneless wild-caught Alaskan salmon fillets

Directions

Preheat the oven to 375°F. Line a rimmed baking sheet with a large sheet of aluminum foil.

In a small bowl, whisk together the tamari, coconut sugar, sesame oil, lemon juice, garlic, mustard, sea salt, and pepper.

Place the salmon on the prepared baking sheet and fold up all 4 sides of the foil. Brush each fillet with coconut oil, then spoon the tamari mixture over the salmon.

Fold the sides of the foil over the salmon, sealing the packet completely.

Bake until the salmon is cooked through, 15 to 20 minutes.

COCONUT CHICKEN TENDERS WITH HONEY MUSTARD SAUCE

SERVES: 4

TOTAL TIME: 25 MINUTES

Ingredients

SAUCE

¼ cup Dijon mustard

3 tablespoons raw honey

Pinch sea salt

TENDERS

2 large eggs

4 boneless, skinless chicken breasts, sliced into thin strips

1 cup gluten-free rice flour

Italian seasoning and sea salt, to taste

1 tablespoon coconut oil

Directions

In a small bowl, whisk together all of the sauce ingredients until smooth. Set aside.

For the tenders, whisk the eggs in a medium bowl.

Put the rice flour in another medium bowl and season with Italian seasoning and salt.

Dip each chicken strip in the egg mixture and let the excess drip off, then coat it in the flour.

Melt the coconut oil in a large skillet over medium heat. Add the chicken tenders and cook until golden brown on both sides, about 15 minutes.

Serve the chicken tenders with the honey mustard sauce on the side.

SWEET AND SOUR CHICKEN

SERVES: 4

TOTAL TIME: 45 MINUTES

Ingredients

CHICKEN

1 cup tapioca flour

2 large eggs

1 pound boneless, skinless
chicken breasts, cut into bite–
size pieces

1 teaspoon sea salt

1/2 teaspoon ground black pepper

1 tablespoon extra virgin olive oil

Cooked brown rice or
cauliflower rice, for serving

2 to 3 tablespoons sesame
seeds, for garnish

Sliced scallions, for garnish
(optional)

SAUCE

1 tablespoon extra virgin
olive oil

2 red bell peppers, seeded and
sliced

1/2 yellow onion, diced

2 garlic cloves, minced

1/2 cup pineapple juice

1/2 cup apple cider vinegar

1/3 cup ketchup

1/4 cup coconut sugar

1 teaspoon sea salt

Directions

Put the tapioca flour in a shallow bowl and whisk the eggs in another
shallow bowl.

Season the chicken with the salt and pepper. Dip each piece of chicken
in the tapioca flour, then dip it in the egg and let the excess drip off, then
dredge it again in the flour to evenly coat.

Heat the olive oil in a large skillet over medium-high heat. Working in
batches, add the chicken and cook for 3 to 4 minutes, then flip the chicken
and cook for another 3 to 4 minutes, until cooked through. Transfer to a
plate.

Wipe the skillet clean. For the sauce, heat the olive oil over medium-
high heat. Add the bell peppers, onion, and garlic and sauté until tender,
3 to 4 minutes. Add the pineapple juice, vinegar, ketchup, coconut sugar,

and salt and bring to a boil. Reduce the heat and simmer for 5 to 7 minutes, until thickened. Add the chicken and stir until the chicken is coated with the sauce.

Serve over rice, and garnish with sesame seeds and scallions, if desired.

LENTIL-STUFFED SWEET POTATOES

SERVES: 4

TOTAL TIME: I HOUR

Ingredients

4 medium sweet potatoes, well scrubbed

I cup green lentils

2 cups water

I tablespoon extra virgin olive oil

I red bell pepper, seeded and diced

I onion, diced

2 garlic cloves, minced

I (15-ounce) can tomato sauce

2 tablespoons tomato paste

¼ cup coconut aminos

2 tablespoons coconut sugar

I teaspoon sea salt

Directions

Preheat the oven to 425°F.

Put the sweet potatoes on a rimmed baking sheet and bake for 50 minutes, or until tender.

Meanwhile, combine the lentils and water in a small saucepan and bring to a boil over medium-high heat. Reduce the heat to a simmer and cook for about 18 minutes, until tender. Drain the lentils and set aside.

In a large skillet, heat the olive oil over medium-high heat. Add the bell pepper, onion, and garlic and cook, stirring often, until tender, 4 to 5 minutes.

Add the tomato sauce, tomato paste, coconut aminos, coconut sugar, and salt and bring to a boil. Reduce the heat to a simmer and cook for 15 minutes. Add the lentils and continue cooking over low heat.

When the sweet potatoes are ready, slice them in half and top them with the lentil mixture.

ANCIENT GRAINS BOWL

SERVES: 4

PREP TIME: 20 MINUTES   TOTAL TIME: 50 MINUTES

Ingredients

2 teaspoons coconut oil, divided

2 cups whole grains (such as quinoa or brown rice)

2 cups cubed sweet potatoes

Sea salt and ground black pepper, to taste

½ onion, diced

1 cup sliced mushrooms

1 cup stemmed and chopped kale

½ cup shredded carrot

¼ cup dairy-free pesto

¼ cup pine nuts, for garnish

Directions

Preheat the oven to 400°F. Grease a rimmed baking sheet with 1 teaspoon of the coconut oil.

Spread the sweet potatoes in a single layer on the prepared baking sheet and season with salt and pepper. Bake, for 30 minutes, turning once, or until browned on both sides.

While the sweet potatoes are in the oven, cook the whole grains according to the package directions.

Heat the remaining 1 teaspoon coconut oil in a large skillet over medium-high heat. Add the onion, mushrooms, and kale and cook, stirring often, until tender, about 5 minutes.

Combine the sweet potatoes, whole grains, vegetable mixture, and pesto in a large bowl and toss to mix. Divide among 4 bowls and garnish with the pine nuts.

SALMON CAKES

SERVES: 2
TOTAL TIME: 15 MINUTES

Ingredients

2 large eggs
1 (6-ounce) can wild-caught
   Alaskan salmon
¼ onion, chopped
¼ cup almond flour or crushed
   gluten-free crackers

½ teaspoon sea salt
½ teaspoon ground black pepper
1 tablespoon extra virgin
   olive oil

Directions

Whisk the eggs in a large bowl. Add the salmon, onion, almond flour, salt, and pepper and mix together with your hands. Form into 2 patties.

Heat the olive oil over medium heat. Add the salmon cakes and cook until well browned, 5 to 8 minutes on each side.

CHICKEN CURRY

SERVES: 4
TOTAL TIME: 35 MINUTES

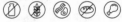

Ingredients

1 tablespoon coconut oil
1 onion, chopped
2 boneless, skinless chicken
   breasts, cut into bite-size
   pieces
1 (14-ounce) can coconut milk
2 cups chopped broccoli
4 garlic cloves, minced

1 teaspoon grated fresh ginger
1 (8-ounce) can sliced water
   chestnuts, drained
2 tablespoons curry powder
1 teaspoon ground cinnamon
Sea salt, to taste
Cooked brown rice, for serving

Directions

Heat the oil in a large skillet over medium heat. Add the onion and chicken and cook, stirring often, for 5 to 8 minutes, until the chicken is browned.

Add the coconut milk, broccoli, garlic, ginger, water chestnuts, curry powder, and cinnamon and cook for 5 minutes. Cover, reduce the heat to low, and cook for 10 more minutes.

Serve over brown rice.

MUSHROOM AND ONION PIZZA

SERVES: 2

PREP TIME: 20 MINUTES   TOTAL TIME: 1 HOUR 20 MINUTES

Ingredients

PIZZA CRUST

1 cup chickpea flour

1 cup water

¼ cup extra virgin olive oil or avocado oil

1 teaspoon dried oregano

1 teaspoon dried basil

½ teaspoon garlic powder

½ teaspoon sea salt

½ teaspoon ground black pepper

TOPPINGS

1 tablespoon extra virgin olive oil or avocado oil

1 cup sliced button, cremini, or wild mushrooms

1 onion, sliced

¼ cup pizza sauce

1 cup crumbled vegan goat or feta cheese

Fresh basil leaves

Directions

In a medium bowl, combine all the crust ingredients and mix well. Set aside the mixture for 1 hour.

Preheat the oven to 425°F, and put a large cast-iron skillet in the oven to preheat at the same time.

Remove the skillet from the oven, pour in the crust mixture, and bake for 5 to 8 minutes, until browned.

Meanwhile, for the toppings, heat the oil in a large skillet over medium heat. Add the mushrooms and onion and cook, stirring often, until tender, 5 to 8 minutes.

Spread the sauce on the pizza crust, then scatter the mushrooms, onion, cheese, and basil leaves evenly on top. Return the pizza to the oven and bake for 10 minutes.

Allow the pizza to cool for 2 minutes before slicing.

SHEPHERD'S PIE

SERVES: 8

PREP TIME: 30 MINUTES   TOTAL TIME: 1 HOUR 15 MINUTES

Ingredients

FILLING

1½ teaspoons coconut oil

1 pound ground grass-fed beef or lamb

2 large carrots, peeled and thinly sliced

1 onion, diced

1½ cups frozen green peas

MASHED FAUX-TATO TOPPING

2 medium heads cauliflower

8 tablespoons (1 stick) unsalted grass-fed butter

½ cup minced fresh chives

4 roasted garlic cloves, chopped

½ teaspoon sea salt

½ teaspoon ground black pepper

GRAVY

2 cups beef or lamb broth

1 cup chopped cauliflower

1 onion, chopped

½ teaspoon sea salt

½ teaspoon ground black pepper

3 garlic cloves, minced

2 tablespoons chopped fresh thyme

2 tablespoons chopped fresh rosemary

1½ teaspoons Worcestershire sauce

4 tablespoons (½ stick) unsalted grass-fed butter, melted

½ cup arrowroot starch

Directions

Preheat the oven to 400°F.

For the filling, heat the oil in a large skillet over medium-high heat. Add the meat, carrots, and onion and cook, breaking up the meat with a wooden spoon, until the meat is browned and the vegetables have begun to soften, 10 to 15 minutes. Pour off any excess fat. Add the peas and stir to combine. Pour the filling into an 8-inch baking pan and set aside.

Meanwhile, for the topping, put a steamer basket in a large saucepan and pour in about an inch of water. Bring to a boil over medium-high heat. Add the cauliflower, cover, and boil for 7 to 10 minutes, until tender. Drain. Transfer the cauliflower to a food processor and add the butter, chives, garlic, salt, and pepper. Blend until smooth, then set aside.

For the gravy, combine the broth, cauliflower, onion, salt, and pepper in a medium pot. Bring to a boil over medium-high heat. Reduce the heat and simmer for 10 minutes, then stir in the garlic, thyme, and rosemary. Transfer the contents of the pot to a high-speed blender, add the Worcestershire and butter, and blend until smooth. Add the arrowroot starch and blend again.

Pour the gravy evenly over the filling in the baking pan. Then spread the mashed faux-tato topping on top. Bake for 30 minutes, or until the topping begins to brown and the gravy is bubbling. Cool for 10 minutes before serving.

PALEO MEATLOAF

SERVES: 4

PREP TIME: 15 MINUTES   TOTAL TIME: 1 HOUR 15 MINUTES

Ingredients

Coconut oil, for greasing pan

3 tablespoons coconut flour

2 tablespoons almond flour

1 teaspoon cayenne pepper

1 teaspoon dried thyme

1 teaspoon ground cumin

1/2 teaspoon sea salt

1/2 teaspoon ground black pepper

1 1/2 pounds ground grass-fed beef

1 large egg, whisked

1 medium onion, chopped

2 garlic cloves, minced

1/2 cup ketchup

1 tablespoon maple syrup

Directions

Preheat the oven to 350°F. Grease a loaf pan.

In a large bowl, combine all the ingredients and mix well with your hands.

Transfer the mixture to the prepared loaf pan and pack lightly. Bake for 1 hour, or until cooked through.

SHORT RIB TACOS

SERVES: 4

PREP TIME: 15 MINUTES   TOTAL TIME: 8 HOURS

Ingredients

2 tablespoons extra virgin olive oil or avocado oil

6 to 8 grass-fed beef short ribs

½ teaspoon sea salt

½ teaspoon ground black pepper

5 cups beef bone broth

1 (15-ounce) can tomato sauce

1 onion, chopped

4 garlic cloves, minced

2 bay leaves

2 tablespoons coconut sugar

1 tablespoon dried oregano

1 tablespoon ground cumin

½ teaspoon ground cinnamon

Corn tortillas, for serving (optional)

Chopped fresh cilantro, for garnish (optional)

Crumbled goat cheese, for garnish (optional)

Directions

Heat the oil in a large skillet over medium heat. Sprinkle the ribs with the salt and pepper on both sides and add them to the pan. Cook for 4 to 5 minutes, until lightly browned on both sides. Transfer to a plate.

In a slow cooker, combine the broth, tomato sauce, onion, garlic, bay leaves, coconut sugar, oregano, cumin, and cinnamon and mix well. Add the ribs and toss to coat. Cover and cook on low for 8 hours.

Remove the ribs and shred the meat from the bones. Serve in corn tortillas (if using), topped with the sauce from the slow cooker. Garnish with cilantro and goat cheese, if desired.

EGGPLANT LASAGNA

SERVES: 8

PREP TIME: 25 MINUTES   TOTAL TIME: 1 HOUR 20 MINUTES

Ingredients

MEAT SAUCE

2 tablespoons extra virgin olive oil

1 onion, chopped

2 garlic cloves, minced

1½ pounds ground grass-fed beef

Sea salt and ground black pepper, to taste

½ cup tomato paste

½ cup tomato sauce

1 cup dry red wine

1 bay leaf

3 thyme sprigs

LASAGNA

1 large eggplant, trimmed and cut lengthwise into ¼-inch-thick slices

2 tablespoons extra virgin olive oil

Sea salt and ground black pepper, to taste

1 cup shredded Pecorino cheese

2 cups shredded buffalo mozzarella cheese, divided

½ cup chopped fresh basil

1 tablespoon dried oregano

Directions

For the meat sauce, heat the olive oil in a large pot over medium heat. Add the onion and garlic and cook, stirring often, for 2 minutes, then add the ground beef. Season with salt and pepper and cook, breaking up the meat with a wooden spoon, until brown, 10 to 15 minutes.

Stir in the tomato paste and tomato sauce and cook for 5 minutes. Add the red wine, stir, and cook for 2 more minutes.

Add the bay leaf and thyme sprigs to the pan. Reduce the heat to low and cook, stirring occasionally, for 45 minutes. Add water if the sauce is too thick. Remove and discard the bay leaf and thyme sprigs.

Meanwhile, preheat the oven to 400°F. Line a rimmed baking sheet with aluminum foil.

For the lasagna, spread out the eggplant slices in a single layer on the prepared baking sheet. Brush both sides with olive oil and season with salt and pepper. Bake for 7 minutes, then flip the eggplant slices and bake for another 7 minutes.

In a large bowl, combine the Pecorino, 1 cup of the mozzarella, and the basil and mix well.

Pour 2 cups of the meat sauce into a 9 × 13-inch baking dish and spread it in an even layer. Lay half of the eggplant slices on top. Cover the eggplant slices with half of the cheese mixture, spreading it evenly. Repeat the layers with another 2 cups meat sauce, the remaining eggplant slices, and the remaining cheese mixture. Sprinkle another ½ cup of the mozzarella cheese on top.

Pour the remaining meat sauce on top of the mozzarella and spread in an even layer across the entire dish. Sprinkle the remaining ½ cup mozzarella and the oregano evenly over the dish.

Cover with aluminum foil and bake at 400 degrees for 30 minutes. Turn on the broiler. Remove the foil and broil for 5 minutes. Let stand for at least 10 minutes before slicing.

VEGAN MAC AND CHEESE

SERVES: 6
TOTAL TIME: 45 MINUTES

Ingredients

VEGAN CHEESE SAUCE

2 cups peeled and chopped russet potatoes (3 to 4 potatoes)

1 carrot, peeled and chopped

1 red bell pepper, seeded and chopped

1/2 onion, chopped

1/2 cup canned coconut milk

1/4 cup water

1/4 cup nutritional yeast

1 tablespoon chickpea miso paste (optional)

1 tablespoon sea salt

1/2 teaspoon garlic powder

1/2 teaspoon paprika, plus more for garnish (optional)

1/2 teaspoon ground mustard

Crushed red pepper (optional)

PASTA

12 ounces rice macaroni (or pasta of choice)

Directions

Fill a medium pot with water and bring to a boil over medium-high heat. Add the potatoes, carrot, bell pepper, and onion and cook until fork-tender, about 15 minutes. Drain.

Transfer the vegetables to a blender and add the remaining cheese sauce ingredients (add the miso paste for more umami flavor). Puree until smooth. If the sauce is too thick, add water, 1 tablespoon at a time, until the desired consistency is reached.

While the vegetables are cooking, bring a large pot of salted water to a boil over medium-high heat. Add the pasta and cook until al dente, then drain.

Transfer the pasta to a large bowl, pour in the cheese sauce, and mix well. Divide into bowls and serve. Garnish with additional paprika or crushed red pepper, if desired.

QUINOA, BLACK BEAN, AND MUSHROOM BURGERS

SERVES: 6
TOTAL TIME: 45 MINUTES

Ingredients

½ red onion, sliced

2 carrots, peeled and chopped

1 red bell pepper, seeded and chopped

1 jalapeño, seeded and chopped

1 cup chopped fresh cilantro

2 (15.5-ounce) cans black beans, rinsed and drained

1 cup chopped button or cremini mushrooms

½ cup almond flour

2 teaspoons sea salt

1 teaspoon ground black pepper

1 teaspoon chili powder

1 teaspoon ground cumin

¼ teaspoon smoked paprika

¾ cup quinoa flour

½ teaspoon coconut oil

Burger toppings, for serving (optional)

Gluten-free buns or lettuce wraps, for serving (optional)

Directions

Preheat the oven to 350°F. Line a rimmed baking sheet with parchment paper.

In a food processor, blend the onion, carrots, bell pepper, jalapeño, and cilantro until smooth. Add the black beans, mushrooms, flour, salt, pepper, chili powder, cumin, and smoked paprika and blend until smooth.

Transfer the mixture to a large bowl. With your hands, form 6 equal patties, about ¼ inch thick. (Add more quinoa flour to thicken the mixture if necessary.)

Melt the coconut oil in a large skillet over medium heat. Working in batches if necessary, add the patties and cook for 8 minutes on each side, until browned. Transfer the burgers to the prepared baking sheet and bake for 10 minutes, then flip the burgers and bake for another 10 minutes.

Top with your favorite burger toppings and enjoy on a gluten-free bun or lettuce wrap.

RICE NOODLES WITH MISO PESTO

SERVES: 2

TOTAL TIME: 30 MINUTES

Ingredients

4 cups baby kale

1 cup chopped fresh cilantro

¼ onion, roughly chopped

1 garlic clove, roughly chopped

1 tablespoon white miso

½ cup extra virgin olive oil or avocado oil

1 teaspoon toasted sesame oil

1 teaspoon fresh lemon juice

Sea salt, to taste

4 ounces brown rice noodles

1 tablespoon unsalted grass-fed butter, cut into small pieces

Toasted sesame seeds, for garnish

Directions

In a food processor or high-speed blender, blend the kale, cilantro, onion, garlic, miso, olive oil, sesame oil, and lemon juice until smooth. Season with salt, then pour the pesto mixture into a medium bowl.

Bring a large pot of water to a boil over medium-high heat. Cook the noodles until al dente, then drain.

Add the noodles to the pesto bowl. Add the butter and toss until the butter is melted and the noodles are evenly coated in pesto. Divide between 2 bowls and garnish with sesame seeds.

SESAME-GINGER NOODLE BOWL

SERVES: 4

PREP TIME: 25 MINUTES   TOTAL TIME: 45 MINUTES

  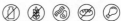

Ingredients

SAUCE

½ cup creamy almond butter
2 garlic cloves, minced
½ teaspoon grated fresh ginger
¼ cup tamari or coconut aminos
Juice of ½ lime
½ teaspoon sea salt

ZOODLE BOWL

1 tablespoon extra virgin olive oil
1 pound boneless, skinless chicken breasts, cut into bite-size pieces, or 1 (15-ounce) block extra firm sprouted tofu, drained and cubed
1 teaspoon sea salt, divided
1 teaspoon ground black pepper
1 cup shaved purple cabbage
Juice of ½ lime
4 zucchini, spiralized
2 medium carrots, peeled and spiralized
2 tablespoons minced fresh cilantro
2 scallions, sliced
2 to 3 tablespoons black sesame seeds
Chopped cashews, almonds, or peanuts, for topping (optional)

Directions

Preheat the oven to 425°F. Line a rimmed baking sheet with parchment paper.

For the sauce, in a medium bowl or food processor, combine the almond butter, garlic, ginger, tamari, lime juice, and salt. Thin the mixture by adding water, 1 tablespoon at a time, until pourable but not watery. Transfer ¼ cup of the sauce to a shallow bowl and reserve the rest for serving.

Season the chicken pieces with ¾ teaspoon of the salt and the black pepper, then add them to the bowl of sauce and turn to coat. Marinate for 15 minutes.

In a medium bowl, combine the shaved cabbage, lime juice, and remaining ¼ teaspoon salt. Massage the cabbage until softened—the cabbage should look almost pickled.

Transfer the chicken to the prepared baking sheet. Bake for 25 minutes.

In a large bowl, combine the zucchini, carrot, and cabbage and toss with the reserved sauce. Top with the chicken, cilantro, scallions, black sesame seeds, and nuts (if using).

STUFFED BELL PEPPERS

SERVES: 6

PREP TIME: 25 MINUTES   TOTAL TIME: I HOUR

Ingredients

3 cups quinoa

I tablespoon coconut oil

I pound ground grass-fed beef

½ onion, chopped

½ cup canned diced fire-roasted tomatoes

½ cup crumbled goat's milk feta cheese

3 tablespoons chopped fresh cilantro

I teaspoon ground cumin

I teaspoon garlic powder

½ teaspoon chili powder

½ teaspoon smoked paprika

½ teaspoon sea salt

½ teaspoon ground black pepper

6 bell peppers (any color), tops sliced off, seeds and ribs removed

Plain goat's milk yogurt, for serving (optional)

Salsa, for serving (optional)

Chopped scallions, for serving (optional)

Directions

Preheat the oven to 350°F. Line a 9 × 13-inch baking pan with parchment paper.

Cook the quinoa according to the package directions.

Meanwhile, heat the coconut oil in a large skillet over medium heat. Add the beef and onion and cook, breaking up the meat with a wooden spoon, until browned, 10 to 15 minutes.

Transfer the meat mixture to a large bowl and add the quinoa, tomatoes, cheese, cilantro, cumin, garlic powder, chili powder, paprika, salt, and pepper. Mix well.

Spoon the filling into each bell pepper. Place the stuffed peppers in the prepared baking pan. Bake for 25 to 30 minutes, or until the peppers are tender. If desired, serve topped with yogurt, salsa, and chopped scallions.

BEEF AND BROCCOLI BOWLS

SERVES: 2
TOTAL TIME: 25 MINUTES

Ingredients

½ cup brown rice

1 tablespoon coconut oil

1 pound ribeye steak, thinly sliced

1 onion, sliced

1 cup chopped carrots

1 head broccoli, cut into florets

2 garlic cloves, chopped

¼ cup tamari or coconut aminos

1 tablespoon white rice vinegar

1 tablespoon apple cider vinegar

½ teaspoon crushed red pepper

1 tablespoon sesame seeds

Directions

Cook the brown rice according to the package directions.

Heat the coconut oil in a large skillet or wok over medium-high heat. Add the beef, onion, and carrots and cook, stirring continuously, for 2 to 3 minutes, until the onion begins to soften.

Add the broccoli, garlic, tamari, vinegars, and crushed red pepper flakes. Stir and cook until the beef is just cooked through.

Serve immediately on top of the brown rice and garnish with the sesame seeds.

SIDES

CAULIFLOWER RICE

SERVES: 6

PREP TIME: 10 MINUTES   TOTAL TIME: 20 MINUTES

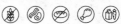

Ingredients

2 tablespoons ghee

4 cups grated cauliflower

3 garlic cloves, minced

Juice of 1 lime

½ cup chopped fresh cilantro

Sea salt and ground black pepper, to taste

Directions

In a large skillet, melt the ghee over medium-high heat. Add the cauliflower and garlic and cook, stirring occasionally, until tender, 8 to 10 minutes.

Transfer the cauliflower to a large bowl and add the lime juice and cilantro. Mix well. Season with salt and pepper.

BAKED BRUSSELS SPROUTS WITH HONEY GLAZE

SERVES: 4

PREP TIME: 15 MINUTES   TOTAL TIME: 50 MINUTES

Ingredients

BRUSSELS SPROUTS

15 to 20 brussels sprouts, halved

1 small red onion, halved lengthwise and thinly sliced crosswise

½ cup walnuts, chopped

2 tablespoons coconut oil, melted

Sea salt and ground black pepper, to taste

SAUCE

¼ cup raw honey

⅓ cup red wine vinegar

Juice of ½ lemon

2 tablespoons unsalted grass-fed butter

3 scallions, chopped

Directions

Preheat the oven to 425°F.

Combine the brussels sprouts, red onion, walnuts, and oil in a large bowl. Mix until the oil is evenly distributed. Spread the brussels sprouts in a single layer on a rimmed baking sheet. Season with salt and pepper. Roast until the brussels sprouts are slightly browned, 25 to 40 minutes.

For the sauce, bring the honey to a simmer in a small saucepan over medium-high heat, then remove the pan from the heat. Add the vinegar and lemon juice to the hot honey and whisk until smooth. Return the pan to medium heat and add the butter. Cook while whisking for 3 minutes.

Transfer the brussels sprouts to a serving bowl and add the sauce and scallions. Toss to mix well.

ROASTED CAULIFLOWER WITH PINE NUTS

SERVES: 4

PREP TIME: 10 MINUTES   TOTAL TIME: 50 MINUTES

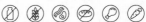

Ingredients

2 tablespoons coconut oil, plus more for pan

1 large head cauliflower, cut into florets

1 garlic clove, minced

1/2 teaspoon sea salt

Juice of 1/2 lemon

1/2 cup pine nuts

1/2 cup cranberries

1/2 cup chopped fresh parsley, for garnish

Directions

Preheat the oven to 425°F. Grease a rimmed baking sheet with oil.

In a large bowl, combine the cauliflower, garlic, oil, and sea salt. Spread out on the prepared baking sheet and roast for 30 to 40 minutes, until slightly browned.

Transfer the cauliflower to a bowl. Add the lemon juice, pine nuts, and cranberries and mix well. Garnish with the parsley.

QUINOA TABBOULEH

SERVES: 8

PREP TIME: 10 MINUTES   TOTAL TIME: 30 MINUTES

Ingredients

1 cup quinoa

1 cup chopped scallions

3 medium tomatoes, diced

1 cucumber, diced

1 cup chopped fresh parsley

2 garlic cloves, minced

1/4 cup extra virgin olive oil

Juice of 1 lemon

Sea salt and ground black pepper, to taste

Directions

Cook the quinoa according to the package directions. Transfer the quinoa to a large bowl and add the scallions, tomatoes, cucumber, parsley, and garlic.

In a small bowl, whisk together the olive oil and lemon juice and add it to the quinoa bowl. Stir to combine thoroughly. Season with salt and pepper. Serve at room temperature or, even better, cover and refrigerate. Serve the next day, when the flavors are more fully expressed.

OVEN-ROASTED VEGETABLES

SERVES: 4

PREP TIME: 15 MINUTES   TOTAL TIME: 40 MINUTES

Ingredients

6 medium yellow squash, peeled and cut into ½-inch-thick slices

3 medium beets, peeled and cut into ½-inch-thick slices

4 medium sweet potatoes, peeled and cut into ½-inch-thick slices

1 medium onion, thinly sliced

2 tablespoons olive oil

2 teaspoons herbes de Provence

1 teaspoon sea salt, plus more to taste

1 teaspoon ground black pepper, plus more to taste

Directions

Preheat the oven to 350°F.

Combine the squash, beets, sweet potatoes, and onion in a casserole dish. Drizzle with the olive oil, add the herbes de Provence, salt, and pepper, and mix well.

Bake for 20 to 25 minutes, until the sweet potatoes are tender. Taste and add more salt and pepper if needed.

ZUCCHINI SQUASH BAKE

SERVES: 6

PREP TIME: 15 MINUTES   TOTAL TIME: 45 MINUTES

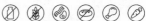

Ingredients

3 tablespoons extra virgin olive oil

1¼ teaspoons dried oregano

2 yellow squash, cut into ½-inch-thick slices

2 zucchini, cut into ½-inch-thick slices

10 ounces cherry tomatoes, cut in half

½ red onion, sliced

1 teaspoon sea salt

½ teaspoon ground black pepper

1 cup shredded vegan parmesan cheese (optional)

Directions

Preheat the oven to 425°F. Line a rimmed baking sheet with parchment paper or aluminum foil.

In a small bowl, whisk together the olive oil and oregano, then let it rest for about 5 minutes to infuse the flavor.

Combine the yellow squash, zucchini, tomatoes, and onion in a large bowl. Pour the olive oil mixture over the top and toss to coat evenly. Dump the vegetables onto the prepared baking sheet and spread them into an even layer. If you're using the parmesan, sprinkle it on top.

Roast for 30 minutes, or until vegetables are slightly golden and tender.

SAUTÉED SPINACH

SERVES: 4
TOTAL TIME: 10 MINUTES

  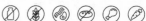

Ingredients

1 tablespoon coconut oil
3 garlic cloves, minced
8 to 10 cups spinach

Sea salt and ground black pepper,
to taste

Directions

Melt the coconut oil in a large skillet over medium heat. Add the garlic and cook, stirring, for 1 minute. Add the spinach, season with salt and pepper, and cook, stirring, until the spinach wilts, about 5 minutes. Taste and add more salt and pepper if needed.

SWEET POTATO MASH

SERVES: 4
PREP TIME: 10 MINUTES   TOTAL TIME: 40 MINUTES

Ingredients

1 tablespoon coconut oil,
melted
4 medium sweet potatoes,
peeled and chopped
½ cup canned coconut milk
2 tablespoons unsalted grass-
fed butter or ghee

1 teaspoon ground cinnamon
2 teaspoons dried or minced
fresh rosemary
1 teaspoon sea salt
Ground black pepper, to taste

Directions

Preheat the oven to 350°F. Line a rimmed baking sheet with parchment paper.

Put the sweet potatoes on the prepared baking sheet and toss with the melted coconut oil. Spread out in a single layer. Roast for 30 minutes, or until the sweet potatoes are fork tender.

Transfer the sweet potatoes to a food processor. Add the coconut milk, butter, cinnamon, rosemary, salt, and pepper and blend until smooth.

SWEET POTATO AND RUTABAGA FRIES

SERVES: 4

PREP TIME: 10 MINUTES   TOTAL TIME: 50 MINUTES

Ingredients

3 rutabagas, peeled and cut into long, thin strips

4 medium sweet potatoes, peeled and cut into long, thin strips

2 tablespoons coconut oil or ghee, melted

1 teaspoon onion powder

1 teaspoon garlic powder

1 teaspoon sea salt

1 teaspoon ground black pepper

Directions

Preheat the oven to 425°F.

Put the rutabagas and sweet potatoes on a rimmed baking sheet, drizzle with the melted coconut oil, and sprinkle them with the onion powder, garlic powder, salt, and pepper. Spread the fries out in a single layer. Bake for 40 minutes, or until golden brown and crisp.

EGGPLANT AND ZUCCHINI FRIES

SERVES: 4

PREP TIME: 15 MINUTES   TOTAL TIME: 35 MINUTES

Ingredients

3 medium eggplants, cut into long, thin strips

5 medium zucchinis, cut into long, thin strips

1 cup gluten-free panko bread crumbs

1 tablespoon Italian seasoning

1 teaspoon sea salt

1 teaspoon ground black pepper

2 large eggs

½ cup gluten-free flour

Directions

Preheat the oven to 425°F.

Put the flour in a large bowl. In another bowl, whisk the eggs. In a third bowl, combine the panko, Italian seasoning, salt, and pepper.

Working in batches, first dredge the fries in the flour, then dip them into the eggs, then dredge them in the panko mixture, pressing to coat.

Spread out the fries in a single layer on a rimmed baking sheet. Bake for 20 minutes, or until golden brown and crisp.

DESSERTS

CHOCOLATE CHIP COOKIES

MAKES: 12 COOKIES
PREP TIME: 15 MINUTES   TOTAL TIME: 30 MINUTES

Ingredients

1 cup almond flour
1 cup gluten-free oat flour
1/2 teaspoon baking soda
1/2 teaspoon sea salt
2 large eggs
1/4 cup coconut oil, melted

1/4 cup maple syrup
2 tablespoons unsweetened
    almond milk or canned
    coconut milk
2 teaspoons vanilla extract
1/2 cup dark chocolate chips

Directions

Preheat the oven to 375°F. Line a rimmed baking sheet with parchment paper.

Combine the flours, baking soda, and salt in a large bowl.

In a separate bowl, whisk together the eggs, melted coconut oil, maple syrup, milk, and vanilla.

Gradually add the dry mixture to the wet mixture and stir until smooth. Fold in the chocolate chips.

Put the dough in the freezer for 10 minutes, until the dough is slightly firm.

Scoop out the dough with a tablespoon and roll it into balls, then place them on the prepared baking sheet about 2 inches apart. Press each dough ball with a fork to flatten it somewhat.

Bake for 12 to 15 minutes, until the edges are golden brown. Let the cookies cool on the baking sheet for 3 minutes, then transfer to a cooling rack to cool completely.

BETTER BROWNIES

SERVES: 12

PREP TIME: 10 MINUTES   TOTAL TIME: 55 MINUTES

Ingredients

½ cup coconut oil, plus more for greasing pan

⅓ cup dark chocolate chips

2 large eggs

½ cup maple syrup

2 teaspoons vanilla extract

1½ cups almond flour

¼ cup cocoa or cacao powder

1 teaspoon baking powder

1 teaspoon sea salt

Directions

Preheat the oven to 350°F. Grease an 8-inch baking pan.

Heat the coconut oil and chocolate chips in a small saucepan over medium heat, stirring constantly, until thoroughly melted and combined. Remove from the heat and set aside to cool slightly.

In a medium bowl, whisk the eggs. Add the maple syrup, vanilla, flour, cocoa powder, baking powder, and salt and mix well until the batter is thick. Fold in the melted oil and chocolate until combined. Pour the batter into the prepared pan.

Bake for 30 to 35 minutes, until a toothpick inserted in the center comes out clean. Let cool for 15 minutes before slicing.

MATCHA ICE CREAM

SERVES: 8

PREP TIME: 10 MINUTES   TOTAL TIME: 1 HOUR

Ingredients

1 (14-ounce) can full-fat coconut milk

1 cup unsweetened vanilla almond milk

¼ cup pitted Medjool dates

¼ cup maple syrup

3 tablespoons matcha green tea powder

¼ teaspoon xanthan gum

Directions

Combine the coconut milk, almond milk, dates, maple syrup, and matcha in a high-speed blender and blend until well combined. Add the xanthan gum and blend again. Pour the mixture into a bowl and refrigerate for 3 hours.

Pour into a chilled ice cream maker and use according to the manufacturer's instructions. (If you don't have an ice cream maker, pour the ice cream base into a freezer container, cover, and place it in the freezer, stirring thoroughly every hour in order to aerate.)

Eat as soft serve or store in a container in the freezer. Before eating, set the ice cream out at room temperature for 30 minutes to allow it to soften.

APPLE CRISP

SERVES: 8

PREP TIME: 10 MINUTES   TOTAL TIME: 55 MINUTES

Ingredients

Coconut oil, for greasing pan
6 to 8 apples, peeled, cored, and
    chopped
¼ cup maple syrup
2 tablespoons fresh lemon juice
½ cup coconut oil, melted
2½ cups gluten-free rolled oats

2 cups gluten-free all-purpose
    flour
¼ cup coconut sugar
2 teaspoons ground cinnamon
¼ teaspoon ground nutmeg
½ teaspoon sea salt

Directions

Preheat the oven to 350°F. Lightly grease a casserole dish.

In a large bowl, toss the apples with the maple syrup and lemon juice to coat evenly. Mix in the melted coconut oil and toss again.

In a separate bowl, whisk together the oats, flour, coconut sugar, cinnamon, nutmeg, and salt together in a separate bowl.

Transfer the apple mixture to the prepared casserole dish. Scatter the oat mixture evenly over the top. Bake for 45 minutes, or until lightly browned

BLUEBERRY PIE

SERVES: 8

PREP TIME: 20 MINUTES   TOTAL TIME: 1 HOUR

Ingredients

Coconut oil, for greasing pan

2 large eggs

3 tablespoons raw honey

2 teaspoons fresh lemon juice

1 to 2 tablespoons almond or other nut butter

2 tablespoons fruit-only blueberry jam

2 cups gluten-free old-fashioned rolled oats

2 tablespoons chia seeds

2 teaspoons ground cinnamon

1 teaspoon baking powder

½ teaspoon sea salt

3 cups frozen blueberries, thawed

Directions

Preheat the oven to 400°F. Grease an 8-inch baking pan.

Beat the eggs in a small bowl, then whisk in the honey and lemon juice. Stir in the almond butter and blueberry jam.

In a separate bowl, combine the rolled oats, chia seeds, cinnamon, baking powder, and salt.

Pour the oat mixture into the prepared pan and spread evenly. Add the blueberries in an even layer, then pour the jam mixture on top.

Bake for 40 minutes.

PUMPKIN PIE

SERVES: 12

PREP TIME: 25 MINUTES   TOTAL TIME: 2 HOURS

Ingredients

CRUST

¼ cup coconut oil, melted, plus more for greasing pan

2½ cups almond flour

⅓ cup coconut sugar

¼ teaspoon sea salt

1 large egg

½ teaspoon vanilla extract

PIE FILLING

1 (15-ounce) can pumpkin puree

3 large eggs

¼ cup maple syrup

¼ cup unsweetened almond milk or canned coconut milk

1 teaspoon vanilla extract

¼ cup coconut sugar

1½ teaspoons ground cinnamon

½ teaspoon ground nutmeg

½ teaspoon ground ginger

½ teaspoon ground allspice

¼ teaspoon sea salt

Directions

Preheat the oven to 350°F. Grease a pie pan.

For the crust, in a large bowl, whisk together the almond flour, coconut sugar, and salt. Stir in the melted coconut oil, egg, and vanilla until well combined. The dough will be dry and crumbly. Just keep mixing, pressing, and stirring until it's uniform and there is no almond flour powder left. (Alternatively, you can use a food processor to mix it all together.) Press the dough into the bottom of the prepared pan and bake for 10 to 12 minutes, until golden.

For the filling, in a large bowl, whisk together the pumpkin puree, eggs, maple syrup, almond milk, vanilla, coconut sugar, cinnamon, nutmeg, ginger, allspice, and salt until smooth. Pour the mixture into the pie pan, on top of the crust.

Bake for 50 to 60 minutes, until the filling is no longer jiggly in the middle. Let the pie cool for at least 30 minutes before slicing.

CARROT CAKE

SERVES: 8

PREP TIME: 30 MINUTES   TOTAL TIME: I HOUR

Ingredients

CAKE

I cup coconut oil, plus more for greasing pan

2 cups gluten-free all-purpose flour

1½ cups maple sugar

2 teaspoons baking soda

2 teaspoons baking powder

I teaspoon sea salt

I teaspoon ground nutmeg

3 cups grated carrots

4 large eggs, whisked

2 teaspoons vanilla extract

½ cup raisins

FROSTING

2 (8-ounce) packages organic grass-fed cream cheese

½ cup evaporated coconut milk or canned coconut milk

¼ cup maple sugar

I cup unsweetened shredded coconut flakes

Directions

Preheat the oven to 350°F. Grease a 9-inch cake pan.

For the cake, in a large bowl, whisk together the flour, maple sugar, baking soda, baking powder, salt, and nutmeg. Add the carrots, eggs, vanilla, and raisins and mix well. Pour the carrot cake batter into the prepared pan and bake for 40 minutes, or until the top is golden.

While the cake is baking, blend all the frosting ingredients together in an electric mixer until smooth.

Let the cake cool, then top with the frosting.

HALVAH

SERVES: 8

PREP TIME: 15 MINUTES   TOTAL TIME: 3 HOURS

Ingredients

Coconut oil, for greasing pan

1/2 cup tahini

1 teaspoon vanilla extract

1/3 cup roasted pistachios

1/4 cup raw honey

Directions

Grease a small glass baking dish.

Warm the tahini, vanilla, and pistachios in a small saucepan over low heat.

In a separate saucepan, heat the honey until it almost boils. Remove from the heat and add the warm tahini mixture to the hot honey. Stir with a wooden spoon until the mixture starts to thicken. Pour immediately into the prepared baking dish and use a silicone spatula to spread it into an even layer.

Let the halvah cool at room temperature for at least 3 hours before removing it from the baking dish. Cut into small squares.

AVOCADO CHOCOLATE MOUSSE

SERVES: 10

TOTAL TIME: 15 MINUTES

Ingredients

1/2 cup pitted Medjool dates, soaked for 4 to 6 hours, then drained

1/2 cup maple syrup

1 teaspoon vanilla extract

3 medium avocados, peeled and pitted

3/4 cup raw cacao powder

1/2 cup water

Directions

Combine the dates, maple syrup, and vanilla in a food processor and process until smooth. Add the avocado and cacao powder and process until creamy, stopping periodically to scrape down the sides of the bowl with a silicone spatula if needed. Add the water and process again, until smooth.

Serve at room temperature, or transfer to an airtight container and store in the refrigerator for up to 3 days or in the freezer for up to 2 weeks.

RICE PUDDING

SERVES: 8

TOTAL TIME: 30 MINUTES

Ingredients

3 cups unsweetened almond milk

1 (14-ounce) can full-fat coconut milk

2 tablespoons unsalted grass-fed butter

1 cup brown rice

½ cup raisins

¼ cup raw honey

1 teaspoon vanilla extract

1 teaspoon ground cinnamon

½ teaspoon sea salt

Directions

Combine all the ingredients in a large pot and stir well. Bring to a boil over medium heat. Reduce the heat to a simmer and cook for 20 minutes, or until thickened. Stir occasionally to prevent the bottom from burning. Serve warm, or let cool, then transfer to an airtight container and refrigerate to serve chilled.

COCONUT CHIA SEED PUDDING

SERVES: 6

PREP TIME: 10 MINUTES   TOTAL TIME: 35 MINUTES

Ingredients

1 (14-ounce) can full-fat coconut milk

1 tablespoon maple syrup

1 teaspoon vanilla extract

1 scoop vanilla-flavored collagen protein powder

1/2 teaspoon ground cinnamon

1/2 teaspoon sea salt

1/2 cup chia seeds

1/2 cup fresh blueberries (optional)

Directions

In a large bowl, whisk together the coconut milk, maple syrup, vanilla extract, collagen powder, cinnamon, and salt until thoroughly combined. Add the chia seeds and stir well. Allow the mixture to soak until thickened, about 30 minutes, or cover the bowl and refrigerate overnight.

Stir the pudding well before dividing it into bowls to serve. Garnish with blueberries if desired.

PEPPERMINT PATTIES

MAKES: 12 PATTIES

TOTAL TIME: 30 MINUTES

Ingredients

2 1/2 cups coconut oil, divided

1/2 cup raw honey

1 teaspoon peppermint extract

3 (3.5-ounce) bars dark chocolate (at least 72% cacao)

Directions

Line a plate with parchment paper.

Mix 2 cups of the coconut oil, honey, and peppermint extract in a bowl. Form the mixture into 12 patties and place them on the prepared plate. Transfer to the freezer to harden, about 30 minutes.

Meanwhile, melt the chocolate bars with the remaining ½ cup coconut oil in a saucepan over medium-low heat. Remove from the heat and let cool for 5 to 10 minutes.

One at a time, dip the hardened patties in the chocolate until evenly covered and return them to the plate. Return the chocolate-covered patties to the freezer until the chocolate has hardened, about 15 minutes. Serve frozen.

SUNFLOWER SEED BUTTER CUPS

SERVES: 12

PREP TIME: 25 MINUTES TOTAL TIME: 1 HOUR

Ingredients

CHOCOLATE SHELL

3 cups dark chocolate chips (70 to 85% cacao)

1 tablespoon coconut oil
1 teaspoon vanilla extract

FILLING

3 tablespoons sunflower seed butter
¼ cup pitted Medjool dates
1 teaspoon coconut oil

1 teaspoon sea salt
Pink Himalayan salt, for sprinkling

Directions

Line two mini-muffin tins with mini-muffin liners.

Pour an inch of water into a small saucepan and bring to a gentle simmer. Combine the chocolate chips, coconut oil, and vanilla in a heat-resistant bowl and set it over the saucepan. (Alternatively, use a double boiler.) Melt them together, stirring gently, until well incorporated.

Fill the bottom of each muffin liner with 1 to 2 teaspoons of the chocolate mixture. Reserve the leftover chocolate.

Put the muffin tins in the freezer for 30 minutes.

For the filling, in a food processor or high-speed blender, combine the sunflower seed butter, dates, coconut oil, and salt. Blend or pulse until smooth and creamy.

Remove the muffin tins from the freezer. Spoon 1 teaspoon of the sunflower seed butter mixture into each chocolate-filled muffin liner. Spoon another 1 to 2 tablespoons of the remaining melted chocolate (re-melt if needed) on top of the sunflower seed butter layer. Lightly sprinkle Himalayan salt on top. Return the muffin tins to the freezer for another 30 minutes, or until set. Serve frozen.

DARK CHOCOLATE-COVERED BERRIES

SERVES: 8

PREP TIME: 10 MINUTES   TOTAL TIME: 25 MINUTES

Ingredients

2 (3.5-ounce) bars dark chocolate (at least 72% cacao)

2 tablespoons toasted flaxseed

2 cups fresh blueberries

Directions

Pour an inch of water into a small saucepan and bring to a gentle simmer. Put the chocolate chips in a heat-resistant bowl and set it over the saucepan. (Alternatively, use a double boiler.) Melt the chocolate, stirring frequently, until smooth. Stir in the flaxseed and then remove from the heat.

Line a rimmed baking sheet with parchment paper.

Pat the blueberries dry and add them to the melted chocolate. Stir gently to coat. Spoon small clumps of blueberries onto the prepared baking sheet.

Refrigerate until firm, about 10 minutes. Store in an airtight container in the refrigerator for up to 2 days.

DARK CHOCOLATE TURTLES

SERVES: 8

PREP TIME: 10 MINUTES   TOTAL TIME: 25 MINUTES

Ingredients

2 (3.5-ounce) bars dark chocolate (at least 72% cacao)

16 pecan halves

8 Medjool dates, pitted and halved

Pink Himalayan salt, for sprinkling

Directions

Pour an inch of water into a small saucepan and bring to a gentle simmer. Put the chocolate chips in a heat-resistant bowl and set it over the saucepan. (Alternatively, use a double boiler.) Melt the chocolate, stirring frequently, until smooth. Remove from the heat.

Line a rimmed baking sheet with parchment paper.

Press a pecan half into each date half, then dip in the melted chocolate. Spoon onto the prepared baking sheet. Lightly sprinkle each "turtle" with Himalayan salt.

Refrigerate until firm, about 10 minutes. Store in an airtight container in the refrigerator for up to 1 week.

MOCHI CAKE

SERVES: 10

PREP TIME: 20 MINUTES   TOTAL TIME: 1 HOUR 30 MINUTES

Ingredients

6 tablespoons coconut oil, melted, plus more for greasing pan

1 (14-ounce) can full-fat coconut milk

2 cups maple syrup or raw honey

2 large eggs

2 teaspoons vanilla extract

1 teaspoon sea salt

2 cups Mochiko or other rice flour

3 tablespoons matcha green tea powder

1 teaspoon ground cinnamon

1 teaspoon baking powder

¼ cup unsweetened shredded coconut

Directions

Preheat the oven to 350°F. Grease a 9-inch cake pan.

In a small saucepan, warm the coconut oil, coconut milk, and honey over medium-high heat, whisking until smooth. Remove from the heat, then slowly add the eggs, vanilla, and salt, whisking to combine.

In a medium bowl, whisk together rice flour, matcha, cinnamon, and baking powder. Mix well, then pour it into the egg mixture and whisk again until everything is incorporated. Pour the batter into the prepared pan and sprinkle with the shredded coconut.

Bake for 55 to 60 minutes, until the surface is golden and the cake springs back when gently pressed, and a toothpick inserted into the center of the cake comes out clean.

Transfer the cake pan to a wire rack and let cool for at least 10 minutes. Run a knife around the perimeter of the cake, then place a plate over the pan and invert the cake so it falls gently onto the plate.

Acknowledgments

I want to thank the brilliant Ginny Graves for helping me bring this book to life. Also, my sincere thanks to the entire Little, Brown Spark team, especially Tracy Behar, Ian Straus, Betsy Uhrig, and Karen Wise, for their phenomenal feedback, vision, editing, and guidance. Your enthusiasm for this project made it a joy from start to finish. I am grateful to my literary agent, Bonnie Solow, who is, quite simply, the best in the business. And I owe a debt of gratitude to Jordan Rubin, my great friend and business partner, as well as Gil Ben-Ami, my Chinese medicine mentor and dear friend, and Dr. Anis Khalaf and Dr. Christopher Motley, for their help and guidance. To my rock star team at Ancient Nutrition: Thank you for all your hard work and for your dedication to our mission: improving the health of our country and our world. Finally, I'm deeply grateful to those of you who follow me on social media and visit my website—and who bought this book. May you all achieve greater health and well-being by utilizing ancient remedies.

Big blessings to all!

Notes

Introduction

1. Centers for Disease Control and Prevention, "Outpatient Antibiotic Prescriptions: United States, 2017," last reviewed October 22, 2019. http://www.cdc.gov/antibiotic -use/community/programs-measurment/state-local-activities/outpatient -antibiotic-prescriptions-US-2017.html

Chapter 1: Ancient Medicine for a Modern World

1. Centers for Disease Control and Prevention, "Therapeutic Drug Use," last reviewed January 19, 2017. https://www.cdc.gov/nchs/fastats/drug-use-therapeutic.htm
2. Ashley Kirzinger, Tricia Neuman, Juliette Cubanski, and Mollyann Brodie, "Data Note: Prescription Drugs and Older Adults," *Kaiser Family Foundation Heath Reform*, August 9, 2019.
3. Ben Boursi, Ronac Mamtani, Kevin Haynes, et al., "Recurrent Antibiotic Exposure May Promote Cancer Formation: Another Step in Understanding the Role of the Human Microbiota?" *European Journal of Cancer* 17 (November 2016): 2655–64.
4. Centers for Disease Control and Prevention, "Outpatient Antibiotic Prescriptions: United States, 2017," last reviewed October 22, 2019. https://www.cdc.gov /antibiotic-use/community/programs-measurement/state-local-activities /outpatient-antibiotic-prescriptions-US-2017.html
5. Centers for Disease Control and Prevention, "Antibiotic Prescribing and Use in the U.S.," updated August 9, 2019. https://www.cdc.gov/antibiotic-use/stewardship -report/index.html
6. Centers for Disease Control and Prevention, "Be Antibiotics Aware: Smart Use, Best Care," last reviewed November 9, 2018. https://www.cdc.gov/patientsafety /features/be-antibiotics-aware.html
7. Yan Xie, Benjamin Bowe, Yan Yan, et al., "Estimates of All Cause Mortality and Cause Specific Mortality Associated with Proton Pump Inhibitors Among US Veterans: A Cohort Study," *British Medical Journal* 365 (March 2019).

8. Emily S. Mohn, Hua J. Kern, Edward Saltzman, et al., "Evidence of Drug-Nutrient Interactions with Chronic Use of Commonly Prescribed Medications: An Update," *Pharmaceutics* 10 (March 2018).

9. Nadine Shebab, Maribeth C. Lovegrove, Andrew I. Geller, et al., "US Emergency Department Visits for Outpatient Adverse Drug Events, 2013–2014," *Journal of the American Medical Association* 316 (November 2016): 2115–25.

10. Ibid.

11. Ibid.

12. Benedict Carey and Robert Gebeloff, "Many People Taking Antidepressants Discover They Cannot Quit," *New York Times*, April 7, 2018. https://www.nytimes.com/2018/04/07/health/antidepressants-withdrawal-prozac-cymbalta.html

13. Centers for Disease Control and Prevention, "Antidepressant Use Among Persons Aged 12 and Over in the United States, 2011–2014," NCHS Data Brief No. 283, August 2017. https://www.cdc.gov/nchs/products/databriefs/db283.htm

14. Marta M. Maslej, Benjamin M. Bolker, Marley J. Russel, et al., "The Mortality and Myocardial Effects of Antidepressants Are Moderated by Preexisting Cardiovascular Disease: A Meta-Analysis," *Psychotherapy and Psychosomatics* 86 (September 2017): 268–82.

15. Ramin Mojtabai and Mark Olfson, "Proportion of Antidepressants Prescribed without a Psychiatric Diagnosis Is Growing," *Health Affairs* 30 (August 2011): 1434–42.

16. Qin Xiang Ng, Nandini Venkatanarayanan, and Collin Yih Xian Ho, "Clinical Use of Hypericum Perforatum (St. John's Wort) in Depression: A Meta-Analysis," *Journal of Affective Disorders* 210 (March 2017): 211–21.

17. Madhav Goyal, Sonal Singh, Erica M. S. Siginga, et al., "Meditation Program for Psychological Stress and Well-Being: A Systematic Review and Meta-Analysis," *JAMA Internal Medicine* 174 (March 2014): 357–68.

18. Britta K. Holzel, James Carmody, Mark Vangel, et al., "Mindfulness Practice Leads to Increases in Regional Brain Gray Matter Density," *Psychiatric Research: Neuroimaging* 191 (January 2011): 36–43.

19. Nasrin Falsafi and Louisa Leopard, "Pilot Study: Use of Mindfulness, Self-Compassion and Yoga Practices with Low Income and/or Uninsured Patients with Depression and/or Anxiety," *Journal of Holistic Nursing* 33 (December 2015): 289–97.

20. Robin E. Cushing, Kathryn L. Braun, Susan W. Alden, and Alan R. Catz, "Military Tailored Yoga for Veterans with Post-Traumatic Stress Disorder," *Military Medicine* 183 (May 2019): e223–31.

21. Galia Oron, Erica Allnut, Tasha Lackman, et al., "A Prospective Study Using Hatha Yoga for Stress Reduction Among Women Waiting for IVF Treatment," *Reproductive Biomedicine Online* 30 (May 2015): 542–48.

22. Fang Wang, Eun-Kyoung, Othelia Lee, et al., "The Effects of Tai Chi on Depression, Anxiety and Psychological Well-Being: A Systematic Review and Meta-Analysis," *International Journal of Behavioral Medicine* 21 (August 2014): 605–17.

23. Harvard Health Letter, "Exercise Is an All-Natural Treatment to Fight Depression," updated April 30, 2018. https://www.health.harvard.edu/mind-and-mood/exercise -is-an-all-natural-treatment-to-fight-depression

24. Centers for Disease Control and Prevention, "Prevalence of Chronic Pain and High Impact Chronic Pain in the United States, 2016," September 14, 2018. https:// www.cdc.gov/mmwr/volumes/67/wr/mm673a2.htm

25. National Institute on Drug Abuse, "Opioid Overdose Crisis," updated January 2019. https://www.drugabuse.gov/drugs-abuse/opioids/opioid-overdose-crisis

26. Ibid.

27. Centers for Disease Control and Prevention, "Drug Overdose Deaths in the United States, 1999–2016," December 2017. https://www.cdc.gov/nchs/products/databriefs /db294.htm

28. Erin E. Krebs, Amy Gravely, and Sean Nugent, "Effect of Opioid vs Nonopioid Medications on Pain-Related Function in Patients with Chronic Back Pain or Hip or Knee Osteoarthritis Pain," *Journal of the American Medical Association* 319 (March 6, 2018): 872–82.

29. Cochrane, "Acupuncture for Tension-Type Headache," January 2016. https:// www.cochrane.org/CD007587/SYMPT_acupuncture-tension-type-headache

30. Andrew J. Vickers, Angel M. Cronin, Alexandra C. Maschino, "Acupuncture for Chronic Pain Individual Patient Meta-Analysis," *Archives of Internal Medicine* 172 (October 2012): 1444–53.

31. Sonja Vuckovic, Dragan Srebro, Katarina Savic Vujovic, et al., "Cannabinoids and Pain: New Insights from Old Molecules," *Frontiers in Pharmacology* 9 (November 2018).

32. Mario Maresca, Laura Micheli, Lorenzo Cinci, et al., "Pain Relieving and Protective Effects of Astragalus Hydroalcoholic Extract in Rat Arthritis Models," *Journal of Pharmacy and Pharmacology* 69 (December 2017): 1858–70.

33. Jia-Ming Yang, Yan-Fang Xian, Paul S.P. Ip, et al., "Schisandra Chinensis Reverses Visceral Hypersensitivity in Neonatal-Maternal Separated Rat Model," *Phytomedicine* 19 (March 2012): 402–8.

34. European Medicines Agency, "Assessment Report on Angelica Sinensis (Oliv.) Diels, Radix," July 2013. http://www.e-lactancia.org/media/papers/AngelicaSinensis -EMA2013.pdf

35. James W. Daily, Mini Yang, and Sunmin Park, "Efficacy of Turmeric Extracts and Curcumin for Alleviating the Symptoms of Joint Arthritis: A Systematic Review and Meta-Analysis of Randomized Clinical Trials," *Journal of Medicinal Food* 19 (August 2016): 717–29.

36. J. Winter, S. Bevan, and E. A. Campbell, "Capsaicin and Pain Mechanisms," *British Journal of Anesthesia* 75 (1995): 157–68.

37. Mahmood Rafieian-Kopaei, Ali Hasnpour-Dehkordi, Zahra Lorigooini, et al., "Comparing the Effect of Intranasal Lidocaine 4% with Peppermint Essential Oil Drop 1.5% on Migraine Attacks: A Double-Blind Clinical Trial," *International Journal of Preventive Medicine* 10 (July 2019).

38. Ashok Kumar Grover and Sue E. Samson, "Benefits of Antioxidant Supplements for Knee Osteoarthritis: Rationale and Reality," *Nutrition Journal* 15 (January 2016).

39. Shaheen E. Lakhan, Heather Sheafer, and Deborah Tepper, "The Effectiveness of Aromatherapy in Reducing Pain: A Systematic Review and Meta-Analysis," *Pain Research and Treatment* 2016 (December 2016).

40. Ling Jun Kong, Romy Lauche, Petra Close, et al., "Tai Chi for Chronic Pain Conditions: A Systematic Review and Meta-Analysis of Randomized Controlled Trials," *Scientific Reports* 6 (April 2016).

41. Jost Langhorst, Petra Klose, Gustav J. Dobos, et al., "Efficacy and Safety of Meditative Movement Therapies in Fibromyalgia Syndrome: A Systematic Review and Meta-Analysis of Randomized Controlled Trials," *Rheumatology International* 33 (January 2013): 193–207.

42. Sharon L. Kolaninski, Marian Garfinkel, Adam Gilden Tsai, et al., "Iyengar Yoga for Treating Symptoms of Osteoarthritis of the Knees: A Pilot Study," *Journal of Complementary and Alternative Medicine* 11 (2005): 689–93.

43. Erik J. Groessl, Kimberly R. Weingart, Kirsten Aschbacher, et al., "Yoga for Veterans with Chronic Low Back Pain," *Journal of Complementary and Alternative Medicine* 14 (2008): 1123–29.

44. Holger Cramer, Romy Lauche, Heidemarie Haller, et al., "I'm More in Balance: A Qualitative Study of Yoga for Patients with Chronic Neck Pain," *Journal of Complementary and Alternative Medicine* 19 (2013): 536–42.

45. Lara Hilton, Susanne Hempel, Brett A. Ewing, et al., "Mindfulness Meditation for Chronic Pain: Systematic Review and Meta-Analysis," *Annals of Behavioral Medicine* 51 (2017): 199–213.

46. Martins Ekor, "The Growing Use of Herbal Medicine: Issues Relating to Adverse Reactions and Challenges in Monitory Safety," *Frontiers in Pharmacology* 4 (2013).

Chapter 2: Curing the Root Cause

1. Luo Hui, Tang Qiao-ling, Shang Ya-xi, et al., "Can Chinese Medicine Be Used for Prevention of Corona Virus Disease 2019 (COVID-19)? A Review of Historical Classics, Research Evidence and Current Prevention Programs," *Chinese Journal of Integrative Medicine* 26 (April 2020): 243–50.

2. Tanya Lewis, "Mystery Mechanisms," *The Scientist*, July 29, 2016. https://www.the-scientist.com/news-analysis/mystery-mechanisms-33119

Chapter 3: Eat Right for Your Ancient Element

1. The 1000 Genomes Project Consortium, "A Global Reference for Human Genetic Variation," *Nature* 526 (September 2015): 68–74.

Chapter 4: The Ancient Way of Eating

1. Guida Shoba, David Joy, Thangam Joseph, et al., "Influence of Piperine on the Pharmacokinetics of Curcumin in Animals and Human Volunteers," *Planta Medica* 64 (May 1998): 353–56.

2. Yeon Soo Kim, Bong Kil Song, Ji Sun Oh, and Seung Seok Woo, "Aerobic Exercise Improves Gastrointestinal Motility in Psychiatric Inpatients," *World Journal of Gastroenterology* 20 (August 2014): 10577–84.

3. Le Xu, Xi Zhang, Jun Lu, et al., "The Effects of Dinner-to-Bed Time and Post-Dinner Walk on Gastric Cancer across Different Age Groups," *Medicine* 95 (April 2016).

4. Science Daily, "Chew More to Retain More Energy," July 15, 2013. https://www.sciencedaily.com/releases/2013/07/130715134643.htm

5. Yong Zhu and James H. Hollis, "Increasing the Number of Chews before Swallowing Reduces Meal Size in Normal-Weight, Overweight, and Obese Adults," *Journal of the Academy of Nutrition and Dietetics* 114 (June 2014): 926–31.

6. Quanhe Yang, Zefeng Zhang, Edward W. Gregg, et al., "Added Sugar Intake and Cardiovascular Diseases Mortality among US Adults," *JAMA Internal Medicine* 174 (April 2014): 516–24.

7. Michelle A. Zabat, William H. Sano, Jenna I. Wurster, et al., "Microbial Community Analysis of Sauerkraut Fermentation Reveals a Stable and Rapidly Established Community," *Foods* 7 (May 2018).

8. Su-Jin Jung, Soo-Hyun Park, Eun-Kyung Choi, et al., "Beneficial Effects of Korean Traditional Diets in Hypertensive and Type 2 Diabetic Patients," *Journal of Medicinal Food* 17 (January 2014): 161–71.

9. Mengjiao Guo, Fahao Wu, Guangen Hao, et al., "Bacillus subtilis Improves Immunity and Disease Resistance in Rabbits," *Frontiers in Immunology* 8 (March 2017).

10. Mona A. M. Ghoneim, Amal I. Hassan, Manal G. Mahmoud and Mohsen S. Asker, "Effect of Polysaccharide from Bacillus subtillis sp. on Cardiovascular Diseases and Atherogenic Indices in Diabetic Rats," *BMC Complementary and Alternative Medicine* 16 (March 2016).

11. Yoshinori Tsukamoto, Hideyuki Ichise, Hiroyuki Kakuda, and Masayoshi Yamaguchi, "Intake of Fermented Soybean (Natto) Increases Circulating Vitamin K2 (Menaquinone-7) and γ-Carboxylated Osteocalcin Concentration in Normal Individuals," *Journal of Bone and Mineral Metabolism* 18 (June 2000): 216–22.

12. Goro Hori, Shunsuke Kakinuma, Satoshi Nagaoka, Kazuhiro Yamamoto, "The Effects of the Miso Soup Containing Soy Protein Hydrolyzate with Bound Phospholipids on Serum Cholesterol Levels," *Japanese Pharmacology and Therapeutics* 31 (January 2003): 155–61.

13. Hiromitsu Watanabe, "Beneficial Biological Effects of Miso with Reference to Radiation Injury, Cancer and Hypertension," *Journal of Toxicological Pathology* 26 (June 2013): 91–103.

14. Esra Kupeli Akkol, Didem Deliorman Orhan, Ilhan Gurbuz, and Erdem Yesilada, "In Vivo Activity Assessment of a 'Honey-Bee Pollen Mix' Formulation," *Pharmaceutical Biology* 48 (March 2010): 253–59.

15. Eric N. Hammond and Eric S. Donkor, "Antibacterial Effect of Manuka Honey on Clostridium difficile," *BMC Research Notes* 6 (May 2013).

16. Rowena Jenkins, Neil Burton, and Rose A. Cooper, "Manuka Honey Inhibits Cell Division in Methicillin-Resistant Staphylococcus aureus," *Journal of Antimicrobial Chemotherapy* 66 (September 2011): 2536–42.

17. Ganesa Wegienka, Christine Cole Johnson, Suzanne Havstad, et al., "Lifetime Dog and Cat Exposure and Dog and Cat Specific Sensitization at Age 18 Years," *Clinical and Experimental Allergy* 41 (July 2011): 979–86.

Chapter 5: Meals Are Medicine

1. Ashkan Afshin, Patrick John Sur, Kairsten A. Fay, et al., "Health Effects of Dietary Risks in 195 Countries, 1990–2017: A Systematic Analysis For the Global Burden of Disease Study 2017," *The Lancet* 393 (May 2019): 1958–72.

2. Jennifer M. Poti, Michelle A. Mendez, Shu Wen Ng, and Barry M. Popkin, "Is the Degree of Food Processing and Convenience Linked with the Nutritional Quality of Foods Purchased by U.S. Households?" *American Journal of Clinical Nutrition* 101 (June 2015): 1251–62.

3. Euridice Martinez Steele, Barry M. Popkin, Boyd Swinburn, and Carlos A. Monteiro, "The Share of Ultra-Processed Foods and the Overall Nutritional Quality of Diets in the US: Evidence from a Nationally Representative Cross-Sectional Study," *Population Health Metrics* 15 (February 2017).

4. Kristine L. Clark, Wayne Sebstianelli, Klaus R. Flechsenhar, et al., "24-Week Study on the Use of Collagen Hydrolysate as a Dietary Supplement in Athletes with Activity-Related Joint Pain," *Current Medical Research and Opinion* 24 (June 2008): 1485–96.

5. Liane Bolke, Gerrit Schlippe, Joachin Gertz, et al., "A Collagen Supplement Improves Skin Hydration, Elasticity, Roughness, and Density: Results of a Randomized, Placebo-Controlled, Blind Study," *Nutrients* 10 (October 17, 2019): 2494.

6. Barbara Rennard, B. A. Ertl, Ronald Grossman, et al., "Chicken Soup Inhibits Neutrophil Chemotaxis in Vitro," *Chest* 118 (October 2000): 1150–57.

7. Iris Shai, Dan Schwarzfuchs, Yaakov Henkin, et al., "Weight Loss with a Low-Carbohydrate, Mediterranean, or Low-Fat Diet," *New England Journal of Medicine* 359 (July 2008): 229–41.

8. Lukas Schwingshackl and Georg Hoffmann, "Monounsaturated Fatty Acids and Risk of Cardiovascular Disease: Synopsis of the Evidence Available from Systematic Reviews and Meta-Analyses," *Nutrients* 4 (December 2012): 1989–2007.

9. Kathleen A. Page, Anne Williamson, Namyi Yu, et al., "Medium-Chain Fatty Acids Improve Cognitive Function in Intensively Treated Type 1 Diabetic Patients and Support in Vitro Synaptic Transmission During Acute Hypoglycemia," *Diabetes* 58 (May 2009): 1237–44.

10. Sivia Teres, Gwendolyn Barcelo-Coblijn, Regina Alemany, et al., "Oleic Acid Is Responsible for the Blood Pressure Reduction Induced by Olive Oil through Its 'Membrane-Lipid Therapy' Action," *Chemistry and Physics of Lipids* 149 (September 2007): 13811–16.

11. Muhammad Ali Hashmi, Afsar Khan, Muhammed Hanif, et al., "Traditional Uses, Phytochemistry, and Pharmacology of Olea Europaea (Olive)," *Evidence-Based Complementary and Alternative Medicine* (February 2015).

12. Sandra Martin-Pelaez, Juana Ines Mosele, Neus Pizarro, et al., "Effect of Virgin Olive Oil and Thyme Phenolic Compounds on Blood Lipid Profile: Implications of Human Gut Microbiota," *European Journal of Nutrition* 56 (February 2017): 119–31.

13. Pouya Nematolahi, Mitra Mehrabani, Somayyeh Karami-Mohajeri, and Fatemeh Dabaghzadeh, "Effects of Rosmarinus Officinalis L. On Memory Performance, Anxiety, Depression, and Sleep Quality in University Students: A Randomized Clinical Trial," *Complementary Therapy in Clinical Practice* 30 (February 2018): 24–28.

14. Massimo Nabissi, Oliviero Marinelli, Maria Beatric Morelli, et al., "Thyme Extract Increases Mucociliary-Beating Frequency in Primary Cell Lines from Chronic Obstructive Pulmonary Disease Patients," *Biomedicine and Pharmacotherapy* 105 (September 2018): 1248–53.

15. Onder Aybastier, Sam Dawbaa, Cevdet Demir, et al., "Quantification of DNA Damage Products by Gas Chromatography Tandem Mass Spectrometry in Lung Cell Lines and Prevention Effect of Thyme Antioxidants on Oxidative Induced DNA Damage," *Mutation Research* 808 (March 2018): 1–9.

16. Karin Ried, "Garlic Lowers Blood Pressure in Hypertensive Individuals, Regulates Serum Cholesterol, and Stimulates Immunity: An Updated Meta-Analysis and Review," *Journal of Nutrition* 146 (February 2016): 389S–96S.

17. Kyung-Bok Lee, Eun Cho, and Young-Sook Kang, "Changes in 5-Hydroxytryptamine and Cortisol Plasma Levels in Menopausal Women after Inhalation of Clary Sage Oil," *Phytotherapy Research* 28 (November 2014): 1599–605.

18. Afef Bejaoui, Hedia Chaabane, Maroua Jemli, et al., "Essential Oil Composition and Antibacterial Activity of Origanum Vulgare Subsp. Glandulosum Desf. at Different Phenological Stages," *Journal of Medicinal Food* 16 (December 2013): 1115–20.

19. Mehrnaz Nikhah Bodagh, Iradj Maleki, and Azita Hekmatdoost, "Ginger in Gastrointestinal Disorders: A Systematic Review of Clinical Trials," *Food Science and Nutrition* 7 (January 2019): 96–108.

20. Christine M. Kaefer and John A. Milner, "The Role of Herbs and Spices in Cancer Prevention," *The Journal of Nutritional Biochemistry* 19 (June 2008): 347–61.

21. Alan Jiang, "Health Benefits of Culinary Herbs and Spices," *Journal of AOAC International* 102 (March 2019): 395–411.

22. Kiran S. Panickar, "Beneficial Effects of Herbs, Spices and Medicinal Plants on the Metabolic Syndrome, Brain and Cognitive Function," *Central Nervous System Agents in Medicinal Chemistry* 13 (March 2013): 13–29.

23. Mendel Friedman from, "Chemistry, Nutrition, and Health-Promoting Properties of Hericium erinaceus (Lion's Mane) Mushroom Fruiting Bodies and Mycelia and

Their Bioactive Compounds," *Journal of Agricultural and Food Chemistry* 19 (August 2015): 7108–23.

24. Ye Jin, Xue Meng, Zhidong Qiu, et al., "Anti-Tumor and Anti-Metastatic Roles of Cordycepin, One Bioactive Compound of Cordyceps militaris," *Saudi Journal of Biological Sciences* 25 (July 2018): 991–95.

25. Alena G. Guggenheim, Kirsten M. Wright, and Heather L. Zwickey, "Immune Modulation Five Major Mushrooms: Application to Integrative Oncology," *Integrative Medicine* 13 (February 2014): 32–44.

26. Golnoosh Torabian, Peter Valtchev, Qayyum Adil, and Fariba Dehghani, "Anti-Influenza Activity of Elderberry (Sambucus Nigra)," *Journal of Functional Foods* 54 (March 2019): 353–60.

27. Harunobu Amagase and Dwight M. Nance, "A Randomized, Double-Blind, Placebo-Controlled Clinical Study of the General Effects of a Standardized Lycium barbarum (Goji) Juice, GoChi," *Journal of Complementary and Alternative Medicine* 14 (June 2008): 403–12.

28. Peter Bucheli, Qiutao Gao, Robert Redgwell, et al., *Herbal Medicine: Biomolecular and Clinical Aspects,* 2nd ed. (Boca Raton, FL: CRC Press/Taylor & Francis, 2011).

29. Memorial Sloan Kettering Cancer Center, "Triphala," updated November 7, 2019. https://www.mskcc.org/cancer-care/integrative-medicine/herbs/triphala

30. Albert Jacob, Manju Pandey, Sorabh Kapoor, Raghavan Saroja, "Effect of the Indian Gooseberry (Amla) on Serum Cholesterol Levels in Men Aged 35–55 Years," *European Journal of Clinical Nutrition* 42 (November 1988): 939–44.

31. Biswas Gopa, Jagatkumar Bhatt, and Kovur G. Hemavathi, "A Comparative Clinical Study of Hypolipidemia Efficacy of Amla (Emblica officinalis) with 3-Hydroxy-3Methylglutaryl-Coenzyme-A Reductase Inhibitor Simvastatin," *Indian Journal of Pharmacology* 44 (March–April 2012): 238–42.

32. Kerry S. Kuehl, Diane L. Elliot, Adriana E. Sleigh, and Jennifer L. Smith, "Efficacy of Tart Cherry Juice to Reduce Inflammation Biomarkers among Women with Inflammatory Osteoarthritis (OA)," *Journal of Food Studies* 1 (2012).

33. Hsin-Chia Hung, Kaumudi J. Joshipura, Rui Jiang, et al., "Fruit and Vegetable Intake and Risk of Major Chronic Disease," *Journal of the National Cancer Institute* 96 (November 2004): 1577–84.

34. Patricia Matanjun, Suhaila Mohamed, Kharidah Muhammed, and Noordin Mohamed Mustapha, "Comparison of Cardiovascular Protective Effects of Tropical Seaweeds, Kappaphycus Alvarezii, Caulerpa Lentillifera, and Sargassum Plycystum, on High Cholesterol/High-Fat Diet in Rats," *Journal of Medicinal Food* 13 (August 2010): 792–800.

35. Jee Ae Shim, Young Ae Son, Ji Min Park, and Mi Kyung Kim, "Effect of Chlorella Intake on Cadmium Metabolism in Rats," *Nutrition Research and Practice* 3 (Spring 2009): 15–22.

36. Jung Hyun Kwak, Seung Han Baek, Yongje Woo, et al., "Beneficial Immunostimulatory Effect of Short-Term Chlorella Supplementation: Enhancement of Natural Killer Cell Activity and Early Inflammatory Response (Randomized, Double-Blinded, Placebo-Controlled Trial)," *Nutrition Journal* 11 (July 2012).

37. Toru Mizoguchi, Isao Takehara, Tohru Masuzawa, et al., "Nutrigenomic Studies of Effects of Chlorella on Subjects with High-Risk Factors for Lifestyle-Related Disease," *Journal of Medicinal Food* 11 (September 2008): 395–404.

38. S. Sreelatha and R. Inbavalli, "Antioxidant, Antihyperglycemic, and Antihyperlipidemic Effects of Coriandrum Sativum Leaf and Stem in Alloxan-Induced Diabetic Rats," *Journal of Food Science* 77 (July 2012): T119–23.

39. Pascal J. Delaquis, Kareen Stanich, Benoit Girard, and G. Mazza, "Antimicrobial Activity of Individual and Mixed Fractions of Dill, Cilantro, Coriander, and Eucalyptus Essential Oils," *International Journal of Food Microbiology* 74 (March 2002): 101–9.

40. Gil Bar-Sela, Miri Cohen, Eran Ben-Arye, and Ron Epelbaum, "The Medical Uses of Wheatgrass: Review of the Gap Between Basic and Clinical Applications," *Mini-Reviews in Medicinal Chemistry* 15 (2015): 1002–10.

41. Sadaharu Miyazono, Tomoki Isayama, Francois C. Delori, and Clint L. Makino, "Vitamin A Activates Rhodopsin and Sensitizes it to Ultraviolet Light," *Visual Neuroscience* 28 (November 2011): 485–97.

42. Balu Muthaiyah, Musthafa M. Essa, Moon Lee, et al., "Dietary Supplementation of Walnuts Improves Memory Deficits and Learning Skills in Transgenic Mouse Model of Alzheimer's Disease," *Journal of Alzheimer's Disease* 42 (2014): 1397–405.

43. Shibu M. Poulose, Marshall G. Miller, and Barbara Shukitt-Hale, "Role of Walnuts in Maintaining Brain Health with Age," *Journal of Nutrition* 144 (April 2014): 561S–66S.

44. Lee J. Wylie, James Kelly, Stephen J. Bailey, et al., "Beetroot Juice and Exercise: Pharmacodynamic and Dose-Response Relationships," *Journal of Applied Physiology* 115 (May 2013): 325–36.

45. Daniel Collado Mateo, Francesco Pazzi, Francisco J. Dominguez Munoz, et al., "Ganoderma lucidum Improves Physical Fitness in Women with Fibromyalgia," *Nutricion Hospitalaria* 32 (2015): 2126–35.

46. Majid Naghdi, Maryam Maghbool, Morteza Seifalah-Zade, et al., "Effects of Common Fig (Ficus carica) Leaf Extracts on Sperm Parameters and Testis of Mice Intoxicated with Formaldehyde," *Evidence-Based and Complementary Medicine* (January 2016): 1–9.

47. Mark A. Reger, Samuel T. Henderson, Cathy Hale, et al., "Effects of Beta-Hydroxybutyrate on Cognition in Memory-Impaired Adults," *Neurobiological Aging* 25 (March 2004): 311–14.

Chapter 6: The Healing Value of Herbs, Spices, and Mushrooms

1. Alena G. Guggenheim, Kirsten M. Wright, and Heather L. Zwickey, "Immune Modulation from Five Major Mushrooms: Application to Integrative Oncology," *Integrative Medicine* 13 (February 2014): 32–44.

2. Yihuai Gao, Shufeng Zhou, Wenqi Jiang, et al., "Effects of Ganopoly (A Ganoderma Lucidum Polysaccharide Extract) on the Immune Functions in Advanced-Stage Cancer Patients," *Immunological Investigations* 32 (August 2003): 201–15.

3. Yun Zhang, Zhi-chun Lin, Ying Hu, and Fu-zhe Wang, "Effect of Ganoderma Lucidum Capsules on T Lymphocyte Subsets in Football Players 'Living High-Training Low,'" *British Journal of Sports Medicine* 42 (October 2008): 819–22.

4. Zichria Zakay-Rones, Erling Thom, T. Wollan, and J. Wadstein, "Randomized Study of the Efficacy and Safety of Oral Elderberry Extract in the Treatment of Influenza A and B Virus Infections," *The Journal of International Medical Research* 32 (April 2004): 132–40.

5. Evelin Tiralongo, Shirley S. Wee, and Rodney A. Lea, "Elderberry Supplementation Reduces Cold Duration and Symptoms in Air Travellers: A Randomized, Double-Blind Placebo-Controlled Clinical Trial," *Nutrients* 8 (April 2016).

6. Jorg Melzer, Reinhard Saller, Andreas Schapowal, and Reto Brignoli, "Systematic Review of Clinical Data with BNO-101 (Sinupret) in the Treatment of Sinusitis," *Forsch Komplementemed* 13 (April 2006): 78–87.

7. Sachin A. Shah, Stephen Sander, C. Michael White, et al., "Evaluation of Echinacea for the Prevention and Treatment of the Common Cold: A Meta-Analysis," *The Lancet Infectious Diseases* 7 (July 2007): 473–80.

8. M. Jawad, R. Schoop, A. Suter, et al., "Safety and Efficacy Profile of Echinacea purpurea to Prevent Common Cold Episodes: A Randomized, Double-Blind, Placebo-Controlled Trial," *Evidence-Based Complementary and Alternative Medicine* (September 2012).

9. Karel Raus, Stephan Pleschka, Peter Klein, et al., "Effect of an Echinacea-Based Hot Drink Versus Oseltamivir in Influenza Treatment: A Randomized, Double-Blind, Double Dummy, Multicenter, Noninferiority Clinical Trial," *Current Therapeutic Research, Clinical and Experimental* 77 (December 2015): 66–72.

10. R. C. Saxena, Ramlala Singh, P. Kumar, and S. C. Yadav, "A Randomized Double Blind Placebo Controlled Clinical Evaluation of Extract of Andrographis paniculata (KalmCold) in Patients with Uncomplicated Upper Respiratory Tract Infection," *Phytomedicine* 17 (March 2010): 178–85.

11. Swati Gupta, K. P. Mishra, and Lilly Ganju, "Broad-Spectrum Antiviral Properties of Andrographis," *Archives of Virology* 162 (March 2017): 611–23.

12. Kojo Agyemang, Lifeng Han, Erwei Liu, et al., "Recent Advances in Astragalus membranaceus Anti-Diabetic Research: Pharmacological Effects of Its Phytochemical Constituents," *Evidence Based Complementary and Alternative Medicine* (November 2013).

13. Ping Liu, Haiping Zhao, and Yumin Luo, "Anti-Aging Implications of Astragalus membranaceus (Huangqi): A Well-Known Chinese Tonic," *Aging and Disease* 8 (December 2017): 868–86.

14. Ibid.

15. Estelle Viljoen, Janicke Visser, Nelene Koen, and Alfred Musekiwa, "A Systematic Review and Meta-Analysis of the Effect and Safety of Ginger in the Treatment of Pregnancy-Associated Nausea and Vomiting," *Nutrition Journal* 19 (March 2014): 13–20.

16. Julie L. Ryan, Charles E. Heckler, Joseph A. Roscoe, et al., "Ginger (Zingiber offi-cinale) Reduces Acute Chemotherapy-Induced Nausea: A URCC CCOP Study of 576 Patients," *Supportive Care in Cancer* 20 (July 2012): 1479–89.

17. Zhongzhi Wang, Junichi Hasegawa, Xinhui Wang, et al., "Protective Effects of Ginger against Aspirin-Induced Gastric Ulcers in Rats," *Yonaga Acta Medica* 54 (March 2011): 11–19.

18. Ming-Luen Hu, Christophan K. Rayner, Keng-Liang Wu, et al., "Effect of Ginger on Gastric Motility and Symptoms of Functional Dyspepsia," *World Journal of Gastroenterology* 17 (January 2011): 105–10.

19. Vinay Rayudu and Akondi B. Raju, "Effect of Triphala on Dextran Sulphate Sodium-Induced Colitis in Rats," *Ayu* 35 (July–September 2014): 333–38.

20. Nguyen Dinh Thang, Pham Ngoc Diep, Pham Thi-Huong Lien, and Le Thi Lien, "Polygonum multiflorum Root Extract as a Potential Candidate for Treatment of Early Graying Hair," *Journal of Advanced Pharmaceutical Technology and Research* 8 (January–March 2017): 8–13.

21. Alexander Panossian and Georg Wikman, "Pharmacology of Schisandra chinensis Bail.: An Overview of Russian Research and Uses in Medicine," *Journal of Ethnopharmacology* 118 (2008): 183–212.

22. Alexander Panossian and Georg Wikman, "Evidence-Based Efficacy of Adaptogens in Fatigue, and Molecular Mechanisms Related to Their Stress-Protective Activity," *Current Clinical Pharmacology* 4 (September 2009): 198–219.

23. Sae Kwang Ku, Hyemee Kim, Joo Wan Kim, et al. "Ameliorating Effects of Herbal Formula Hemonine on Experimental Subacute Hemorrhagic Anemia in Rats," *Journal of Ethnopharmacology* 198 (February 2017): 205–13.

24. Noel M. Arring, Denise Millstine, Lisa A. Marks, and Lillian M. Nail, "Ginseng as a Treatment for Fatigue: A Systematic Review," *Journal of Alternative and Complementary Medicine* 24 (July 2018): 624–33.

25. Bao-qin Lin and Shao-ping Li, "Chapter 5: Cordyceps as an Herbal Drug," *Herbal Medicine: Biomolecular and Clinical Aspects*, 2nd ed. (Boca Raton, Florida: CRC Press/Taylor & Francis, 2011).

26. Steve Chen, Zhaoping Li, Robert Krochmal, et al., "Effect of CS-4 (Cordyceps sinensis) on Exercise Performance in Healthy Older Subjects: A Double-Blind, Placebo-Controlled Trial," *Journal of Alternative and Complementary Medicine* 16 (May 2010): 585–90.

27. Federico Brandalise, Valentina Cesaroni, Andrej Gregori, et al., "Dietary Supplementation of Hericium erinaceus Increases Mossy Fiber-CA3 Hippocampal Neurotransmission and Recognition Memory in Wild-Type Mice," *Evidence-Based Complementary and Alternative Medicine* (January 2017).

28. Koichiro Mori, Satoshi Inatomi, Kenzi Ouchi, and Yoshihito Azumi, "Improving Effects of the Mushroom Yamabushitake (Hericium erinaceus) on Mild Cognitive Impairment: A Double-Blind Placebo-Controlled Clinical Trial," *Phytotherapy Research* 23 (March 2009): 367–72.

29. Hsing-Chun Kuo, Bruce Lu, Chien-Heng Shen, and Shui-Yi Tung, "Hericium erinaceus Myecelium and Its Isolated Erinacine a Protection from MPTP-Induced Neurotoxicity through the ER Stress, Triggering an Apoptosis Cascade," *Journal of Translational Medicine* 18 (March 2016).

30. Con Stough, J. Lloyd, L. A. Downey, et al., "The Chronic Effects of an Extract of Bacopa Monniera (Brahmi) on Cognitive Function in Healthy Human Subjects," *Psychopharmacology* 156 (August 2001): 481–84.

31. Chuenjid Kongkeaw, Piyameth Dilokthornsakul, Phurit Thanarangsarit, et al., "Meta-Analysis of Randomized Controlled Trials on Cognitive Effects of Bacopa monnieri Extract," *Journal of Ethnopharmacology* 151 (November 2013): 528–35.

32. Marco Canevelli, Nawal Adali, Eirini Keaiditi, et al., "Effects of Ginkgo Biloba Supplementation in Alzheimer's Disease Patients Receiving Cholinesterase Inhibitors: Data from the ICTUS Study," *Phytomedicine* 15 (May 2014): 888–92.

33. Julia Berger, Beth Burgwyn Fuchs, George Aperis, et al., "Antifungal Chemical Compounds Identified Using a C. elegans Pathogenicity Assay," *PLOS Pathogens* 3 (February 2007): 3833–41.

34. Bin Shan, Yizhong Z. Cai, Mei Sun, and Harold Corke, "Antioxidant Capacity of 26 Spice Extracts and Characterization of Their Phenolic Constituents," *Journal of Agricultural and Food* Chemistry 53 (September 2005): 747–59.

35. Gang-sheng Wang, Jie-hua Deng, Yao-hui Ma, et al., "Mechanisms, Clinically Curative Effects, and Antifungal Activities of Cinnamon Oil and Pogostemon Oil Complex against Three Species of Candida," *Journal of Traditional Chinese Medicine* 32 (March 2012): 19–24.

36. Katey M. Lemar, Michael Patrick Turner, and David Lloyd, "Garlic (Allium sativum) as an Anti-Candida Agent: A Comparison of the Efficacy of Fresh Garlic and Freeze-Dried Extracts," *Journal of Applied Microbiology* 93 (February 2002): 398–405.

37. Leyla Bayan, Peir Hossain Koulivand, and Ali Gorji, "Garlic: A Review of Potential Therapeutic Effects," *Avicenna Journal of Phytomedicine* 4 (January–February 2014): 1–14.

38. Yasunari Takada, Anjana Bhardwaj, Pravin D. Potdar, and Bharat Aggarwal, "Nonsteroidal Anti-Inflammatory Agents Differ in Their Ability to Suppress NF-kappaB Activation, Inhibition of Expression of Cyclooxygenase-2 and Cyclin D1, and Abrogation of Tumor Cell Proliferation," *Oncogene* 23 (January 2005): 9247–58.

39. Kaiping Wang, Peng Cao, Weizhi Shui, et al., "Angelica sinensis Polysaccharide Regulates Glucose and Lipid Metabolism Disorder in Prediabetic and Streptozotocin-Induced Diabetic Mice through the Elevation of Glycogen Levels and Reduction of Inflammatory Markers," *Food and Function* 6 (March 2015): 902–9.

40. Adriene Fugh-Berman, "Herbs and Dietary Supplements in the Prevention and Treatment of Cardiovascular Disease," *Preventive Cardiology* 3 (Winter 2000): 24–32.

41. Ernst-Gerhard Loch, Hartmut Selle, and Normann Boblitz, "Treatment of Premenstrual Syndrome with a Phytopharmaceutical Formulation Containing Vitex agnus castus," *Journal of Women's Health and Gender-Based Medicine* 9 (April 2000): 315–20.

42. Lynn M. Westphal, M. L. Polan, and A. Sontag Trant, "Double-Blind, Placebo-Controlled Study of Fertilityblend: A Nutritional Supplement for Improving Fertility in Women," *Clinical and Experimental Obstetrics and Gynecology* 33 (January 2006): 205–8.

43. Elizabeth Steels, Amanda Rao, and Luis Vitetta, "Physiological Aspects of Male Libido Enhanced by Standardized Trigonella foenum-graecum Extract and Mineral Formulation," *Phytotherapy Research* 25 (February 2011): 1294–300.

44. Maryam Mehrpooya, Soghra Rabiee, Amir Larki-Harchegani, et al., "A Comparative Study on the Effect of 'Black Cohosh' and 'Evening Primrose Oil' on Menopausal Hot Flashes," *Journal of Education and Health Promotion* 7 (March 2018).

45. K. Jiang, Y. Jin, L. Huang, et al., "Black Cohosh Improves Objective Sleep in Postmenopausal Women with Sleep Disturbances," *Climacteric* 18 (2015): 559–67.

46. Ludovico Abenavoli, Raffaele Capasso, Natasa Milic, and Francesco Capasso, "Milk Thistle in Liver Diseases: Past, Present, Future," *Phytotherapy Research* 24 (October 2010): 1423–32.

47. Erica S. Lovelace, Jessica Wagoner, James MacDonald, et al., "Silymarin Suppresses Cellular Inflammation by Inducing Reparative Stress Signaling," *Journal of Natural Products* 78 (August 2015): 1990–2000.

48. Reneta Gevrenova, Magdalena Kondeva-Burdina, Nikolay Denkov, and Dimitrina Zheleva-Dimitrova, "Flavonoid Profiles of Three Bupleurum Species and In Vitro Hepatoprotective Activity of Bupleurum flavum Forsk," *Pharmacognosy Magazine* 11 (January–March 2015): 14–23.

49. Liangliang Cai, Dongwei Wan, Fanglian Yi, and Libiao Luan, "Purification, Preliminary Characterization and Hepatoprotective Effects of Polysaccharides from Dandelion Root," *Molecules* 22 (August 2017).

50. Olov Lindahl and Lars Lindwall, "Double Blind Study of Valerian Preparation," *Pharmacology Biochemistry and Behavior* 32 (April 1989): 1065–66.

51. Simin Taavoni, Neda Ekbatani, Maryam Kashaniyan, and Hamid Haghani, "Effect of Valerian on Sleep Quality in Postmenopausal Women: A Randomized Placebo-Controlled Clinical Trial," *Menopause* 18 (September 2011): 951–55.

52. John R. Keefe, Jun J. Mao, Irene Soeller, et al., "Short-Term Open-Label Chamomile (Matricaria chamomilla L.) Therapy of Moderate to Severe Generalized Anxiety Disorder," *Phytomedicine* 23 (December 2015): 1699–705.

53. Scott Shannon, Nicole Lewis, Heather Lee, and Shannon Hughes, "Cannabidiol in Anxiety and Sleep: A Large Case Series," *Permanente Journal* 23 (2019).

Chapter 7: Cannabis: The Forbidden Herb

1. A. E. Munson, L. S. Harris, M. A. Friedman, et al., "Antineoplastic Activity of Cannabinoids," *Journal of the National Cancer Institute* 55 (September 1975): 597–602.

2. Pawel Sledzinski, Joanna Zeyland, Ryszard Slomski, and Agnieszka Nowak, "The Current State and Future Perspectives of Cannabinoids in Cancer Biology," *Cancer Medicine* 7 (March 2018): 765–75.

3. Antonio Currais, Oswald Quehenberger, Aaron M. Armondo, et al., "Amyloid Proteotoxicity Initiates an Inflammatory Response Blocked by Cannabinoids," *Aging and Mechanisms of Disease* 2 (June 2016).

4. Ethan B. Russo, "Cannabis Therapeutics and the Future of Neurology," *Frontiers in Integrative Neuroscience* 18 (October 2018).

5. Marcia Frellick, "Medical, Recreational Marijuana Should Be Legal, Most Clinicians Say," *Medscape*, January 8, 2020. https://www.medscape.com/viewarticle/901761

6. Sanjay Gupta, "Dr. Sanjay Gupta to Jeff Sessions: Medical Marijuana Could Save Many Addicted to Opioids," CNN.com, April 24, 2018. https://www.cnn.com/2018/04/24/health/medical-marijuana-opioid-epidemic-sanjay-gupta/index.html

7. Suzanne Ryan-Ibarra, Marta Induni, and Danielle Ewing, "Prevalence of Medical Marijuana Use in California, 2012," *Drug and Alcohol Review* 34 (October 2014): 141–46.

8. Ethan B. Russo, "Taming THC: Potential Cannabis Synergy and Phytocannabinoid-Terpenoid Entourage Effects," *British Journal of Pharmacology* 163 (August 2011): 1344–64.

9. Esther M. Blessing, Maria M. Steenkamp, Jorge Manzanares, and Charles R. Marmar, "Cannabidiol as a Potential Treatment for Anxiety Disorders," *Neurotherapeutics* 12 (September 2015): 825–36.

10. Linda A. Parker, Erin M. Rock, and Cheryl L. Limebeer, "Regulation of Nausea and Vomiting by Cannabinoids," *British Journal of Pharmacology* 163 (August 2011): 1411–22.

11. Emilio Perucca, "Cannabinoids in the Treatment of Epilepsy: Hard Evidence at Last?" *Journal of Epilepsy Research* 7 (December 2017): 61–76.

12. Arthritis Foundation, "Arthritis Foundation CBD Guidance for Adults with Arthritis," 2019. https://www.arthritis.org/living-with-arthritis/pain-management/chronic-pain/arthritis-foundation-cbd-guidance-for-adults.php

13. Benjamin J. Whalley, Royston A. Gray, Colin G. Scott, and Nicholas A. Jones, "Antiseizure Properties of Cannabidiol (CBD) Are Attenuated in the Absence of Receptor Potential Vanilloid 1 (TRPV1) Receptors," *Neurology* 90 (April 2018).

14. Ethan B. Russo, "Clinical Endocannabinoid Deficiency Reconsidered: Current Research Supports the Theory in Migraine, Fibromyalgia, Irritable Bowel, and Other Treatment-Resistant Syndromes," *Cannabis and Cannabinoid Research* 1 (July 2016): 154–65.

15. Danielle N. Rhyne, Sarah L. Anderson, Margaret Gedde, and Laura M. Borgelt, "Effects of Medical Marijuana on Migraine Headache Frequency in an Adult Population," *Pharmacotherapy* 36 (May 2016): 505–10.

16. M. G. Gascio, L. A. Guason, L. A. Stevenson, and R. A. Ross, "Evidence That the Plant Cannabinoid Cannabigerol Is a Highly Potent a2-adrenoceptor Agonist and Moderately Potent 5HT1A Receptor Antagonist," *British Journal of Pharmacology* 158 (December 2009): 129–41.

17. Giovanni Appendino, Simon Gibbons, Anna Giana, et al., "Antibacterial Cannabinoids from Cannabis sativa: A Structure-Activity Study," *Journal of Natural Products* 71 (August 2008): 1427–30.

18. Hayes Wong and Brian E. Cairns, "Cannabidiol, Cannabinol and Their Combinations Act as Peripheral Analgesics in a Rat Model of Myofascial Pain," *Archives of Oral Biology*, 104 (August 2019): 33–39.

19. Jonathon A. Farrimond, Benjamin J. Whalley, and Claire M. Williams, "Cannabinol and Cannabidiol Exert Opposing Effects on Rat Feeding Patterns," *Psychopharmacology* 223 (April 2012): 117–29.

20. Noriyuki Usami, Takeshi Okuda, Histoshi Yoshida, et al., "Synthesis and Pharmacological Evaluation in Mice of Halogenated Cannabidiol Derivatives," *Chemical and Pharmaceutical Bulletin* 47 (November 1999): 1641–45.

21. Radu Tanasescu and Cris S. Constantinescu, "Cannabinoids and the Immune System: An Overview," *Immunobiology* 215 (August 2010): 588–97.

22. Cristina A. J. Stern, Lucas Gazarini, Ana C. Vanvossen, et al., "Tetrahydrocannabinol Alone and Combined with Cannabidiol Mitigate Fear Memory through Reconsolidation Disruption," *European Neuropsychopharmacology* 25 (February 2015): 958–65.

23. William Notcutt, Mario Price, Roy Miller, et al., "Initial Experiences with Medicine Extracts of Cannabis for Chronic Pain: Results from 34 'N of 1' Studies," *Anaesthesia* 59 (2004): 440–52.

24. Mary E. Lynch and Fiona Campbell, "Cannabinoids for Treatment of Chronic Non-Cancer Pain; A Systematic Review of Randomized Trials," *British Journal of Clinical Pharmacology* 72 (November 2011): 735–44.

25. Siri Helle, Petter Andreas Ringen, Ingrid Melle, et al., "Cannabis Use Is Associated with 3 Years Earlier Onset of Schizophrenia Spectrum Disorder in a Naturalistic, Multi-Site Sample (N=1,119)," *Schizophrenia Research* 170 (January 2016): 217–21.

26. Reto Auer, Eric Vittinghoff, Kristine Yaffe, et al., "Association between Lifetime Marijuana Use and Cognitive Function in Middle Age: The Coronary Artery Risk Development in Young Adults (CARDIA) Study," *JAMA Internal Medicine* 176 (March 2016): 352–61.

27. Silvia Rigucci, Tiago Reis Marques, M. Di Forti, et al., "Effect of High-Potency Cannabis on Corpus Callosum Microstructure," *Psychological Medicine* 46 (March 2016): 841–54.

28. Ethan B. Russo, "Taming THC: Potential Cannabis Synergy and Phytocannabinoid-Terpenoid Entourage Effects," *British Journal of Pharmacology* 163 (August 2011): 1344–64.

29. Ibid.

30. Ibid.

31. Ibid.

32. Antonio W. Zuardi, Luis C. Pereira, Regina H. Queiroz, et al., "Cannabidiol Presents and Inverted U-Shaped Dose Response Curve in a Simulated Public Speaking Test," *Brazilian Journal of Psychiatry* 41 (January–February 2019): 9–14.

33. Esther M. Blessing, Maria M. Steenkamp, Jorge Manzanares, and Charles R. Marmar, "Cannabidiol as a Potential Treatment for Anxiety Disorders," *Neurotherapeutics* 12 (September 2015): 825–36.

34. Carrie Cuttler, Alexander Spradlin, and Ryan J. McLaughlin, "A Naturalistic Examination of the Perceived Effects of Cannabis on Negative Affect," *Journal of Affective Disorders* 1 (August 2018): 198–205.

35. Karan Mathur, Vahin Vuppalanchi, Kayla Gelow, et al., "Cannabidiol (CBD) Consumption and Perceived Impact on Extrahepatic Symptoms in Patients with Autoimmune Hepatitis," *Digestive Diseases and Sciences* 65 (January 2020): 322–28.

36. Hefei Wen and Jason M. Hockenberry, "Association of Medical and Adult-Use Marijuana Laws with Opioid Prescribing for Medicaid Enrollees," *JAMA Internal Medicine* 178 (May 2018): 673–79.

37. Marcus A. Bachhuber, Brendan Saloner, Chinzano O. Cunningham, et al., "Medical Cannabis Laws and Opioid Analgesic Overdose Mortality in the United States, 1999–2010," *JAMA Internal Medicine* 174 (October 2014): 1668–73.

38. Ibid.

39. Prakash Nagarkatti, Rupal Pandey, Sadiye Amcaoglu Rieder, et al., "Cannabinoids as Novel Anti-Inflammatory Drugs," *Future Medicinal Chemistry* 1 (October 2009): 1333–49.

40. David Cheng, Adena S. Spiro, Andrew Jenner, and Brett Garner, "Long-Term Cannabidiol Treatment Prevents the Development of Social Recognition Memory Deficits in Alzheimer's Disease Transgenic Mice," *Journal of Alzheimer's Disease* 42 (July 2014): 1383–96.

41. Carina Hasenoehrl, Martin Storr, and Rudolf Schicho, "Cannabinoids for Treating Inflammatory Bowel Disease: Where Are We and Where Do We Go?" *Expert Review of Gastroenterology and Hepatology* 11 (April 2017): 329–37.

42. Timna Naftali, Lihi Bar-Lev Schleider, Iris Dotan, et al., "Cannabis Induces a Clinical Response in Patients with Crohn's Disease: A Prospective Placebo-Controlled Trial," *Clinical Gastroenterology and Hepatology* 11 (October 2013): 1276–80.

43. Daniel Couch, Hollie Cook, Catherine Ortori, et al., "Palmitoylethanolamide and Cannabidiol Prevent Inflammation Induced Hyperpermeability of the Human Gut In Vitro and In Vivo: A Randomized, Placebo-Controlled, Double-Blind Controlled Trial," *Inflammatory Bowel Diseases* 25 (May 2019): 1006–18.

44. Ester Pagano, Raffaele Capasso, Fabiana Piscitelli, et al. "An Orally Active Cannabis Extract with High Content Cannabidiol Attenuates Chemically Induced Intestinal Inflammation and Hypermotility in the Mouse," *Frontiers in Pharmacology* 4 (October 2016).

45. Sean D. McAllister, Liliana Soroceanu, and Pierre-Yves Desprez, "The Antitumor Activity of Plant-Derived Non-Psychoactive Cannabinoids," *Journal of Immune Pharmacology* 10 (June 2015): 255–67.

46. Attila Olah, Arnold Markovics, Judit Szabo-Papp, et al., "Differential Effectiveness of Selected Non-Psychotropic Phytocannabinoids on Human Sebocyte Functions

Implicates Their Introduction in Dry/Seborrhoeic Skin and Acne Treatment," *Experimental Dermatology* 25 (September 2016): 701–7.

47. Michael Har-Noy, Raphael Mechoulam, Shimon Slavin, and Ruth Gallily, "Cannabidiol Lowers Incidence of Diabetes in Non-Obese Diabetic Mice," *Autoimmunity* 39 (March 2006): 143–51.

48. Khalid A. Jadoon, Garry D. Tan, and Saoirse E. O'Sullivan, "A Single Dose of Cannabidiol Reduces Blood Pressure in Healthy Volunteers in a Randomized Crossover Study," *JCI Insight* 15 (June 2017).

49. Christopher P. Stanley, William H. Hind, and Saoirse E. O'Sullivan, "Is the Cardiovascular System a Therapeutic Target for Cannabidiol?" *British Journal of Clinical Pharmacology* 75 (February 2013): 313–22.

50. David M. Elliott, Narendra Singh, Mitzi Nagarkatti, and Prakash S. Nagarkatti, "Cannabidiol Attenuates Experimental Autoimmune Encephalomyelitis Model of Multiple Sclerosis Induction of Myeloid-Derived Suppressor Cells," *Frontiers in Immunology* 9 (August 2018).

Chapter 8: The Power of Essential Oils

1. Mahmoud M. Suhail, Weijuan Wu, Amy Cao, et al., "Boswellia Sacra Essential Oil Induces Tumor Cell-Specific Apoptosis and Suppresses Tumor Aggressiveness in Cultured Human Breast Cancer Cells," *BMC Complementary and Alternative Medicine* 11 (December 2011).

2. Xiao-ling Wang, Feng Kong, Tao Shen, et al., "Sesquiterpenoids from Myrrh Inhibit Androgen Receptor Expression and Function in Human Prostate Cancer Cells," *Acta Pharmaceutica Sinica* 32 (March 2011): 338–44.

3. Hiroki Harada, Hideki Kashiwanadi, Yuichi Kanmura, and Tomoyuki Kuwaki, "Linalool Odor-Induced Anxiolytic Effects in Mice," *Frontiers in Behavioral Neuroscience* 12 (October 2018).

4. Marlete Brum Cleff, Ana Raquel Meinerz, Melissa Xavier, et al., "In Vitro Activity of Origanum Vulgare Essential Oil against Candida Species," *Brazilian Journal of Microbiology* 41 (January–March 2010): 116–23.

5. Giorgio Capello, M. Spezzaferro, L. Grossi, et al., "Peppermint Oil (Mintoil) in the Treatment of Irritable Bowel Syndrome: A Prospective Double-Blind Placebo-Controlled Randomized Trial," *Digestive and Liver Disease* 39 (June 2007): 530–36.

6. Shahla Enshaieh, Abolfazl Jooya, Amier Hossen Siadat, and Fariba Iraji, "The Efficacy of 5% Topical Tea Tree Oil Gel in Mild to Moderate Acne Vulgaris: A Randomized, Double-Blind Placebo-Controlled Study," *Indian Journal of Dermatology, Venereology and Leprology* 73 (January–February 2007): 22–25.

7. Roza Haghgoo and Farid Abbasi, "Evaluation of the Use of a Peppermint Mouth Rinse for Halitosis by Girls Studying in Tehran High Schools," *Journal of International Society of Preventive and Community Dentistry* 3 (January–June 2013): 29–31.

8. Eun Hee Cho, Mi-Young Lee, and Myung-Haeng Hur, "The Effects of Aromatherapy on Intensive Care Unit Patients' Stress and Sleep Quality: A Nonrandomised

Controlled Trial," *Evidence-Based Complementary and Alternative Medicine* (December 2017): 1–10.

9. Siegried Kasper, Markus Gastpar, Walter E. Muller, et al., "Lavender Oil Preparation Silexan Is Effective in Generalized Anxiety Disorder: A Randomized, Double-Blind Comparison to Placebo and Paroxetine," *International Journal of Neuropsychopharmacology* 17 (June 2014): 859–69.

10. Payam Sasannejad, Morteza Saeedi, Ali Shoeibi, et al., "Lavender Essential Oil in the Treatment of Migraine Headache: A Placebo-Controlled Clinical Trial," *European Neurology* 67 (May 2012): 288–91.

11. Mahnaz Keshavarz Afshar, Sahra Behboodi Moghadam, Ziba Taghizadeh, et al., "Lavender Fragrance Essential Oil and the Quality of Sleep in Postpartum Women," *Iranian Red Crescent Medical Journal* 17 (April 2015).

12. Monica Hancianu, Oana Cioanca, Marius Mihasan, and Lucian Hritcu, "Neuroprotective Effects of Inhaled Lavender Oil on Scopolamine-Induced Dementia Via Anti-Oxidative Activities in Rats," *Phytomedicine* 20 (March 2013): 446–52.

13. Botros R. Mikhaeil, Galal T. Maatooq, Farid A. Badria, Mohamed M. A. Amer, et al., "Chemistry and Immunomodulatory Activity of Frankincense Oil," *Zeitschrift fur Naturforschung C, Journal of Biosciences* 58 (March–April 2003): 230–38.

14. Mahmoud M. Suhail, Weijuan Wu, Amy Cao, et al., "Boswellia Sacra Essential Oil Induces Tumor Cell-Specific Apoptosis and Suppresses Tumor Aggressiveness in Cultured Human Breast Cancer Cells," *BMC Complementary and Alternative Medicine* 11 (December 2015).

15. Mark Barton Frank, Qing Yang, Jeanette Osban, et al., "Frankincense Oil Derived from Boswellia carteri Induces Tumor Cell Specific Cytotoxicity," *BMC Complementary and Alternative Medicine* 9 (March 2009).

16. Yingli Chen, Chunlan Zhou, Zhendan Ge, et al., "Composition and Potential Anticancer Activities of Essential Oils Obtained from Myrrh and Frankincense," *Oncology Letters* 6 (August 2013): 1140–46.

17. Siamak Beheshti and Rezvan Aghaie, "Therapeutic Effect of Frankincense in a Rat Model of Alzheimer's Disease," *Avicenna Journal of Phytomedicine* 6 (July–August 2016): 488–475.

18. Hermann P. T. Ammon, "Boswellic Acids (Components of Frankincense) as the Active Principle in Treatment of Chronic Inflammatory Diseases," *Wiener Mdizinische Wochenschrift* 152 (February 2002): 373–78.

19. Marciele Ribas Pilau, Sydney Hartz Alves, Rudi Weiblen, et al., "Antiviral Activity of the Lippia graveiolens (Mexican oregano) Essential Oil and Its Main Compound Carvacrol against Human and Animal Viruses," *Brazilian Journal of Microbiology* 42 (October 2011): 1616–24.

20. Mark Force, William Sidney Sparks, and Robert A. Ronzio, "Inhibition of Enteric Parasites by Emulsified Oil of Oregano in Vivo," *Phytotherapy Research* 14 (May 2000): 213–14.

21. Eunkyung Kim, Youngshim Choi, Jihee Jang, and Taesum Park, "Carvacrol Protects against Hepatic Steatosis in Mice Fed a High-Fat Diet by Enhancing

SIRT1-AMPK Signaling," *Evidence-Based Complementary and Alternative Medicine* (February 2013).

22. Shigeharu Inouye, Katsuhisa Uchida, Yayoi Nishiyama, et al., "Combined Effect of Heat, Essential Oils and Salt on Fungicidal Activity against Trichophyton Mentagrophytes in a Foot Bath," *Nihon Ishinkin Gakkai Zasshi* 48 (February 2007): 27–36.

23. Sibel Karakaya, Sedef Nehir El, Nural Karagozlu, and Serpil Sahin, "Antioxidant and Antimicrobial Activities of Essential Oils Obtained from Oregano (Origanum vulgare ssp. hirtum) by Using Different Extraction Methods," *Journal of Medicinal Food* 14 (May 2011): 645–52.

24. Christine F. Carson, Katherine A. Hammer, and Thomas V. Riley, "Melaleuca alternifolia (Tea Tree) Oil: A Review of Antimicrobial and Other Medicine Properties," *Clinical Microbiology Reviews* 19 (January 2006): 50–62.

25. Oleg V. Pyankov, Evgeny V. Usachev, Olga Pyankova, and Igor E. Agranovski, "Inactivation of Airborne Influenza Virus by Eucalyptus Oils," *Aerosol Science and Technology* 46 (December 2012).

26. Andrew C. Satchell, Anne Saurajen, Craig Bell, and Ross St. C. Barnetson, "Treatment of Interdigital Tinea Pedis with 25% and 50% Tea Tree Oil Solution: A Randomized, Placebo-Controlled, Blinded Study," *Australasian Journal of Dermatology* 43 (August 2002): 175–80.

27. Harsimran Kaur Malhi, Jenny Tu, Thomas V. Riley, et al., "Tea Tree Oil Gel for Mild to Moderate Acne: A 12-Week Uncontrolled, Open-Label Phase II Pilot Study," *Australasian Journal of Dermatology* 58 (August 2017): 205–10.

28. Andrew C. Satchell, Anne Saurajen, Craig Bell, and Ross St. C. Barnetson, "Treatment of Dandruff with 5% Tea Tree Oil Shampoo," *Journal of the American Academy of Dermatology* 47 (December 2002): 852–55.

29. Diane L. McKay and Jeffrey B. Blumberg, "A Review of the Bioactivity and Potential Benefits of Peppermint Tea (Mentha Piperita L.)," *Phytotherapy Research* 20 (August 2006): 619–33.

30. Afshin Borhani Haghighi, S. Motazedian, Farshid Mohammadi, et al., "Cutaneous Application of Menthol 10% Solution as an Abortive Treatment of Migraine without Aura: A Randomized, Double-Blind, Placebo-Controlled, Crossed-Over Study," *International Journal of Clinical Practice* 64 (March 2010): 451–56.

31. Jacquelyn A. Reed, Jude Almeida, Ben Wershing, and Bryan Raudenbush, "Effects of Peppermint Scent on Appetite Control and Caloric Intake," *Appetite* 51 (September 2008): 393.

32. Parisa Yavari Kia, Farzaneh Safajou, Mahnaz Shahnazi, and Hossein Nazemiyeh, "The Effect of Lemon Inhalation Aromatherapy on Nausea and Vomiting in Pregnancy: A Double-Blinded, Randomized, Controlled Clinical Trial," *Iranian Red Crescent Medical Journal* 16 (March 2014).

33. Myung-Ae Kim, Jung-Kyu Sakong, Eun-Jin Kim, et al., "Effect of Aromatherapy Massage for the Relief of Constipation in the Elderly," *Taehan Hanho Hakhoe Chi* (February 2005): 56–64.

34. Migiwa Komiya, Takashi Takeuchi, and Etsumori Harada, "Lemon Oil Vapor Causes an Anti-Stress Effect Via Modulating the 5-HT and DA Activities in Mice," *Behavioural Brain Research* 172 (September 2006): 240–49.

35. Kamrani Farhad, Nazari Mahboubeh, Sahebalzamani Mohammed, et al., "Effect of Aromatherapy with Lemon Essential Oil on Anxiety after Orthopedic Surgery," *Iranian Journal of Rehabilitation Research in Nursing* 2 (Summer 2016): 26–31.

36. Hafsia Bouzenna, Sabah Dhibi, Noura Samout, et al., "The Protective Effect of Citrus Limon Essential Oil on Hepatotoxicity and Nephrotoxicity Induced by Aspirin in Rats," *Biomedical Pharmacotherapy* 83 (October 2016): 1327–34.

37. Ane Orchard and Sandy van Vuuren, "Commercial Essential Oils as Potential Antimicrobials to Treat Skin Disease," *Evidence-Based Complementary and Alternative Medicine* (January 2017): 1–92.

38. Mark Moss, Jenny Cook, Keith Wesness, and Paul Duckett, "Aromas of Rosemary and Lavender Essential Oils Differentially Affect Cognition and Mood in Healthy Adults," *International Journal of Neuroscience* 113 (January 2003): 15–38.

39. Daiki Jimbo, Yuki Kumura, Miyako Taniguchi, et al., "Effect of Aromatherapy on Patients with Alzheimer's Disease," *Psychogeriatrics* 9 (December 2009): 173–79.

40. Toshiko Atsumi and Keiichi Tonosaki, "Smelling Lavender and Rosemary Increases Free Radical Scavenging Activity and Decreases Cortisol Level in Saliva," *Psychiatry Research* 150 (February 2007): 89–96.

41. Jeremy J. Johnson, "Carnosol: A Promising Anti-Cancer and Anti-Inflammatory Agent," *Cancer Letters* 305 (June 2011): 1–7.

42. Yunes Panahi, Mohsen Taghizadeh, Eisa Tahmasbpour Marzony, and Amirhossein Sahebkar, "Rosemary Oil vs. Minoxidil 2% for the Treatment of Adrogenetic Alopecia: A Randomized Comparative Trial," *SKINmed* 13 (January–February 2015): 15–21.

43. Ethel Burns, C. Blamey, Steven J. Ersser, and Andrew Lloyd, "The Use of Aromatherapy in Intrapartum Midwifery Practice: An Observational Study," *Complementary Therapies in Nursing and Midwifery* 6 (March 2000): 33–34.

44. Kyung-Bok Lee, Eun Cho, and Young-Sook Kang, "Changes in 5-Hydroxytryptamine and Cortisol Plasma Levels in Menopausal Women after Inhalation of Clary Sage Oil," *Phytotherapy Research* 28 (November 2014): 1599–605.

45. Geun Hee Seol, Yun Hee Lee, Purum Kang, et al., "Randomized Controlled Trial for Salvia sclarea or Lavendula angustifolia: Differential Effects on Blood Pressure in Female Patients with Urinary Incontinence Undergoing Urodynamic Examination," *Journal of Alternative and Complementary Medicine* 19 (July 2013): 664–70.

46. Prasoon Gupta, Dinesh Kumar Yadav, Kiran Babu Siripurapu, et al., "Constituents of Ocimum Sanctum with Antistress Activity," *Journal of Natural Products* 70 (September 2007): 1410–16.

47. Marc Maurice Cohen, "Tulsi–Ocinum sanctum: A Herb for All Reasons," *Journal of Ayurveda and Integrative Medicine* 5 (October–December 2014): 251–59.

48. Puja Agrawal, V. Rai, and Ram B. Singh, "Randomized, Placebo-Controlled, Single Blind Trial of Holy Basil Leaves in Patients with Noninsulin-Dependent

Diabetes Mellitus," *International Journal of Clinical Pharmacology and Therapeutics* 31 (August 1996): 4069.

49. Manjeshwar Shrinath Baliga, Rosmy Jimmy, Karadka Ramdas Thilakchand, et al., "Ocimum Sanctum L (Holy Basil or Tulsi) and Its Phytochemicals in the Prevention and Treatment of Cancer," *Nutrition and Cancer* 65 (May 2013): 26–35.

50. Shuhua Wu, Krupa B. Patel, Leland J. Booth, et al., "Protective Essential Oil Attenuates Influenza Virus Infection: An in Vitro Study in MDCK Cells," *BMC Complementary and Alternative Medicine* 10 (November 2010).

51. Nada Chami, Sanae Bennis, Fouzia Chami, et al., "Study of Anticandidal Activity of Carvacrol and Eugenol in Vitro and in Vivo," *Oral Microbiology and Immunology* 20 (April 2005): 106–11.

52. Yang Suk Jun, Purum Kang, Sun Seek Min, et al., "Effect of Eucalyptus Oil Inhalation on Pain and Inflammatory Responses after Total Knee Replacement: A Randomized Clinical Trial," *Evidence-Based Complementary and Alternative Medicine* (June 2013).

53. Juergen Fischer and Uwe Dethlefsen, "Efficacy of Ceneole in Patients Suffering from Acute Bronchitis: A Placebo-Controlled, Double-Blind Trial," *Cough* 9 (November 2013).

54. Daiji Kagawa, Hiroko Jokura, Ryuji Ochiai, et al., "The Sedative Effects and Mechanism of Action of Cedrol Inhalation with Behavioral Pharmacological Evaluation," *Planta Medica* 69 (June 2003): 637–41.

55. Isabelle C. Hay, Margaret Jamieson, and Anthony D. Ormerod, "Randomized Trial of Aromatherapy Successful Treatment for Alopecia Areata," *JAMA Dermatology* 134 (November 1998): 1349–52.

Chapter 9: Emotional and Spiritual Secrets for Breakthrough Healing

1. Aditi Nerurkar, Asaf Bitton, and Roger B. Davis, "When Physicians Counsel about Stress: Results of a National Study," *JAMA Internal Medicine* 173 (January 2013): 76–77.

2. Heath Resources and Services Administration, "The Loneliness Epidemic," last reviewed January 2019. https://www.hrsa.gov/enews/past-issues/2019/january-17/loneliness-epidemic

3. United States Congress Joint Economic Committee, "Long-Term Trends in Deaths of Despair," September 5, 2019. https://www.jec.senate.gov/public/index.cfm/republicans/2019/9/long-term-trends-in-deaths-of-despair

4. Centers for Disease Control and Prevention, "Adverse Childhood Experiences Journal Articles by Topic Area," last reviewed April 15, 2019. https://www.cdc.gov/violenceprevention/childabuseandneglect/acestudy/journal.html?CDC_AA_refVal=https%3A%2F%2Fwww.cdc.gov%2Fviolenceprevention%2Facestudy%2Fjournal.html

5. Lewina O. Lee, Peter James, Emily S. Zevon, et al., "Optimism Is Associated with Exceptional Longevity in Two Epidemiological Cohorts of Men and Women," *PNAS* 37 (September 2019): 18357–62.

6. Benjamin P. Chapman, Kevin Fiscella, Ichiro Kawachi, et al., "Emotion Suppression and Mortality Risk over a 12-Year Follow-Up," *Journal of Psychosomatic Research* 75 (October 2013): 381–85.

7. Matthew D. Lieberman, Naomi I. Eisenberger, Molly J. Crockett, et al., "Putting Feelings into Words: Affective Labeling Disrupts Amygdala Activity in Response to Affective Stimuli," *Psychological Science* 18 (2005): 421–28.

8. Barbara L. Fredrickson, Michael A. Cohn, Kimberly A. Coffey, et al., "Open Hearts Build Lives: Positive Emotions, Induced through Loving-Kindness Meditation, Build Consequential Personal Resources," *Journal of Personality and Social Psychology* 95 (November 2008): 1045–62.

9. Helen Y. Weng, Andrew S. Fox, Alexander J. Shackman, et al., "Compassion Training Alters Altruism and Neural Responses to Suffering," *Psychological Science* 24 (July 2013): 1171–80.

10. Summer Allen, "The Science of Gratitude," Greater Good Science Center, May 2018. https://ggsc.berkeley.edu/images/uploads/GGSC-JTF_White_Paper-Gratitude -FINAL.pdf

11. Aliya Alimujiang, Ashley Wiensch, Jonathan Boss, et al., "Association between Life Purpose and Mortality among U.S. Adults Older Than 50 Years," *Journal of the American Medical Association Network* Open 2 (May 2019).

12. Jane K. Ferguson, Eleanor W. Willemsen, and MayLynn V. Castaneto, "Centering Prayer as a Healing Response to Stress: A Psychological and Spiritual Practice," *Pastoral Psychology* 59 (June 2009): 305–29.

13. Christopher G. Ellison, Matt Bradshaw, Kevin J. Flannelly, and Kathleen C. Galek, "Prayer, Attachment to God, and Symptoms of Anxiety-Related Disorders Among U.S. Adults," *Sociology of Religion* 75 (February 2014): 208–33.

14. Cheryl J. Wakslak and Yaacov Trope, "Cognitive Consequences of Affirming the Self: The Relationship between Self-Affirmation and Object Construal," *Journal of Experimental Social Psychology* 45 (July 2009): 927–32.

15. Christopher N. Cascio, Matthew Brook O'Donnel, Francis J. Tinney, et al., "Self-Affirmation Activates Brain Systems Associated with Self-Related Processing and Reward and Is Reinforced by Future Orientation," *Social Cognitive and Affective Neuroscience* 11 (April 2016): 621–29.

16. Lee Rowland and Oliver Scott Curry, "A Range of Kindness Activities Boost Happiness," *Journal of Social Psychology* 159 (May 2018): 340–43.

Chapter 10: Ancient Therapies and Lifestyle

1. Paul F. Engelhardt, L. K. Daha, T. Zils, et al., "Acupuncture in the Treatment of Psychogenic Erectile Dysfunction: First Results of a Prospective Randomized Placebo-Controlled Study," *International Journal of Impotence Research* 15 (November 2003): 343–46.

2. Centers for Disease Control and Prevention, "Therapeutic Drug Use," last reviewed January 19, 2017. https://www.cdc.gov/nchs/fastats/drug-use-therapeutic.htm

3. Centers for Disease Control and Prevention, "Trends in Adults Receiving a Recommendation for Exercise of Other Physical Activity from a Physician or Other Health Professional," NCHS Data Brief No. 86, February 2012. https://www.cdc.gov/nchs/products/databriefs/db86.htm

4. Arthur Yin Fan and Sarah Faggert, "Distribution of Licensed Acupuncturists and Educational Institutions in the United States in Early 2015," *Journal of Integrative Medicine* 16 (January 2018): 1–5.

5. Yan Zhang, Lixing Lao, Haiyan Chen, and Rodrigo Ceballos, "Acupuncture Use among American Adults: What Acupuncture Practitioners Can Learn from National Health Interview Survey 2007," *Evidence-Based Complementary and Alternative Medicine* (February 2012).

6. Klaus Linde, Gianni Allais, Benno Brinkhaus, et al., "Acupuncture for the Prevention of Episodic Migraine," *Cochrane Database of Systematic Reviews* 2016 (June 2016).

7. Yu-Jeong Cho, Yun-Kyung Song, Yun-Yeop Cha, et al., "Acupuncture for Chronic Low Back Pain: A Multicenter, Randomized, Patient-Assessor Blind, Sham-Controlled Clinical Trial," *Spine* 38 (April 2013): 549–57.

8. Andrew J. Vickers, Angel M. Cronin, Alexandra C. Maschino, et al., "Acupuncture for Chronic Pain: Individual Patient Data Meta-Analysis," *Archives of Internal Medicine* 172 (October 2012): 1444–53.

9. Andrew J. Vickers, Emily A. Vertosick, George Lewith, et al., "Acupuncture for Chronic Pain: Update of an Individual Patient Data Meta-Analysis," *Journal of Pain* 19 (May 2018): 455–74.

10. Huijuan Cao, Xingfang Pan, Hua Li, and Jianping Liu, "Acupuncture for Treatment of Insomnia: A Systematic Review of Randomized Controlled Trials," *Journal of Alternative and Complementary Medicine* 15 (November 2009): 1171–86.

11. National Cancer Institute, "Acupuncture (PDQ)-Health Professional Version," updated January 17, 2020. https://www.cancer.gov/about-cancer/treatment/cam/hp/acupuncture-pdq#cit/section_2.6

12. Wei Li, Ping Yin, Lixing Lao, and Shifen Xu, "Effectiveness of Acupuncture Used for the Management of Postpartum Depression: A Systematic Review and Meta-Analysis," *BioMed Research International* 2019 (March 2019).

13. Huijuan Cao, Xun Li, and Jianping Liu, "An Updated Review of the Efficacy of Cupping Therapy," *PLOS One* 7 (February 2012).

14. Maximilian Braum, Miriam Schwickert, Arya Nielsen, et al., "Effectiveness of Traditional Chinese 'Gua Sha' Therapy in Patients with Chronic Neck Pain: A Randomized Controlled Trial," *Pain Medicine* 12 (March 2011): 362–69.

15. Qing Ren, Xinyu Yu, Fujiu Liao, et al., "Effects of Gua Sha Therapy on Perimenopausal Syndrome: A Systematic Review and Meta-Analysis of Randomized Controlled Trials," *Complementary Therapies in Clinical Practice* 31 (May 2018): 268–77.

16. Xiaolan Xie, Liqiong Lu, Xiaoping Zhou, et al., "Effect of Gua Sha Therapy on Patients with Diabetic Peripheral Neuropathy: A Randomized Controlled Trial," *Complementary Therapies in Clinical Practice* 35 (May 2019): 348–52.

17. Felix J. Saha, Gianna Brummer, Romy Lauche, et al., "Gua Sha Therapy for Chronic Low Back Pain: A Randomized Controlled Trial," *Complementary Therapies in Clinical Practice* 34 (February 2019): 64–69.

18. Erland Pettman, "A History of Manipulative Therapy," *Journal of Manipulative Therapy* 15 (2007): 165–74.

19. Ibid.

20. Pamela M. Rist, Audrey Hernandez, Carolyn Bernstein, et al., "The Impact of Spinal Manipulation on Migraine Pain and Disability: A Systematic Review and Meta-Analysis," *Headache* 59 (April 2019): 532–42.

21. Jessica J. Wong, Heather M. Shearer, Sivano Mior, et al., "Are Manual Therapies, Passive Physical Modalities or Acupuncture Effect for the Management of Patients with Whiplash-Associated Disorders or Neck Pain and Associated Disorders? An Update of the Bone and Joint Decade Task Force on Neck Pain and Its Associated Disorders by the OPTIMa Collaboration," *Spine Journal* 16 (December 2016): 1598–630.

22. Valter Santilli, Ettore Beghi, and Stefano Finucci, "Chiropractic Manipulation in the Treatment of Acute Back Pain and Sciatica with Disc Protrusion: A Randomized Double-Blind Clinical Trial of Active and Simulated Spinal Manipulations," *Spine Journal* 6 (March–April 2006): 131–37.

23. Madhu Mia Iyer, Evangelia Skokos, and Denise Piombo, "Chiropractic Management Using Multimodal Therapies on Two Pediatric Patients with Constipation," *Journal of Chiropractic Medicine* 16 (December 2017): 340–45.

24. N.H. Nielsen, G. Bronfort, T. Bendix, et al., "Chronic Asthma and Chiropractic Spinal Manipulation: A Randomized Clinical Trial," *Clinical and Experimental Allergy* 25 (January 1995): 80–88.

25. Denise M. Goodman, Alison E. Burke, Edward H. Livingston, "Low Back Pain," *JAMA Patient Page* 309 (2013).

26. Hoon Chung, Tianong Dai, Sulbha K. Sharma, et al., "The Nuts and Bolts of Low-Level (Light) Therapy," *Annals of Biomedical Engineering* 40 (February 2012): 516–33.

27. Javad T. Hashmi, Ying-Ying Huang, Bushra Z. Osmani, et al., "Role of Low-Level Laser Therapy in Neurorehabilitation," *PM&R: The Journal of Injury, Function, and Rehabilitation* 2 (December 2010): S292–305.

28. NIH National Center for Complementary and Integrative Health, "Yoga: What You Need to Know," updated May 2019. https://nccih.nih.gov/health/yoga/introduction.htm

29. NIH National Center for Complementary and Integrative Medicine, "Tai Chi and Qi Gong: In Depth," updated October 2016. https://nccih.nih.gov/health/taichi/introduction.htm

30. Chao Suo, M. F. Singh, Nicola J. Gates, et al., "Therapeutically Relevant Structural and Functional Mechanisms Triggered by Physical and Cognitive Exercise," *Molecular Psychiatry* 21 (November 2016): 1633–42.

31. Matthew P. Herring, Marni L. Jacob, Cynthia Suveg, et al., "Feasibility of Exercise Training for the Short-Term Treatment of Generalized Anxiety Disorder: A Randomized Controlled Trial," *Psychotherapy and Psychosomatics* 81 (2011): 21–28.

32. Brett R. Gordon, Cillian P. McDowell, Mats Hallgren, et al., "Association of Efficacy of Resistance Exercise Training with Depressive Symptoms: Meta-Analysis and Meta-Regression Analysis of Randomized Clinical Trials," *JAMA Psychiatry* 75 (June 2018) 566–76.

33. Bum Jin Park, Yuko Tsunetsugu, Tamami Kasetani, et al., "The Physiological Effects of Shinrin-Yoku (Taking in the Forest Atmosphere or Forest Bathing): Evidence from Field Experiments in 24 Forests across Japan," *Environmental Health and Preventive Medicine* 15 (January 2010): 18–26.

34. Paul K. Piff, Pia Dietze, Matthew Feinberg, et al., "Awe, the Small Self, and Prosocial Behavior," *Journal of Personality and Social Psychology* 108 (2015): 883–99.

35. Ben Wigert and Sangeeta Agrawal, "Employee Burnout, Part 1: The 5 Main Causes," Gallup, July 12, 2018. https://www.gallup.com/workplace/237059/employee-burnout-part-main-causes.aspx

36. Ibid.

37. Denise Albieri, Jodas Salvagioni, Francine Nesello Melanda, et al., "Physical, Psychological and Occupations Consequences of Job Burnout: A Systematic Review of Prospective Studies," *PLOS One* 12 (October 2017).

38. Benjamin Baird, Jonathon Smallwood, Michael D. Mrazek, et al., "Inspired by Distraction: Mind Wandering Facilitates Creative Incubation," *Psychological Science* 23 (August 2012): 1117–22.

39. Nielsen Insights, "Time Flies: U.S. Adults Now Spend Nearly Half a Day Interacting with Media," July 31, 2018. https://www.nielsen.com/us/en/insights/article/2018/time-flies-us-adults-now-spend-nearly-half-a-day-interacting-with-media/

40. American Psychological Association, "Stress in America: Coping with Change," February 23, 2017. https://www.apa.org/news/press/releases/stress/2017/technology-social-media.pdf

41. Clare Anderson and Charlotte R. Platten, "Sleep Deprivation Lowers Inhibition and Enhances Impulsivity to Negative Stimuli," *Behavioural Brain Research* 217 (March 2011): 463–66.

42. Gaetan Chevalier, Stephen T. Sinatra, James L. Oschman, and Richard M. Delany, "Earthing (Grounding) the Human Body Reduces Blood Viscosity: A Major Factor in Cardiovascular Disease," *Journal of Alternative and Complementary Medicine* 19 (February 2013): 102–10.

43. Richard Brown, Gaetan Chevalier, and Michael Hill, "Grounding after Moderate Eccentric Contractions Reduces Muscle Damage," *Open Access Journal of Sports Medicine* 6 (2015): 305–17.

44. Gaetan Chevalier, Sheila Patel, Lizabeth Weiss, et al., "The Effects of Grounding (Earthing) on Bodyworkers' Pain and Overall Quality of Life: A Randomized Controlled Trial," *Explore (NY)* 15 (May–June 2019): 181–90.

45. James L. Oschman, Gaetan Chevalier, and Richard Brown, "The Effects of Grounding (Earthing) on Inflammation, the Immune Response, Wound Healing, and Prevention and Treatment of Chronic and Inflammatory and Autoimmune Diseases," *Journal of Inflammation Research* 8 (2015): 83–96.

46. Shan Shu and Hui Ma, "Restorative Effects of Classroom Soundscapes on Children's Cognitive Performance," *International Journal of Environmental Research and Public Health*," 16 (January 2019): 293.
47. Cassandra D. Gould van Praag, Sarah N. Garfinkle, Oliver Sparasci, et al., "Mind-Wandering and Alterations to Default Mode Network Connectivity When Listening to Naturalistic Versus Artificial Sounds," *Scientific Reports* 7 (March 2017).

Chapter 11: Understanding the Five Organ Systems of TCM

1. Eric S. Kim, Kaitlin A. Hagan, Francine Grodstein, et al., "Optimism and Cause-Specific Mortality: A Prospective Cohort Study," *American Journal of Epidemiology* 185 (January 2017): 21–29.

Chapter 12: Prescriptions for 70+ Conditions

1. Chao-xian Zhang, Yong-mei Qin, and Bao-rui Guo, "Clinical Study on the Treatment of Gastroesophageal Reflux by Acupuncture," *Chinese Journal of Integrative Medicine* 16 (August 2010): 298–303.
2. Inger M. Janssen, Sibylle Sturtz, Guido Skipka, et al., "Ginkgo Biloba in Alzheimer's Disease: A Systematic Review," *Wiener Medizinische Wochenschrift* 160 (December 2010): 539–46.
3. Ruth E. Cooper, Emma Williams, Seth Seegobin, et al., "Cannabinoids in Attention-Deficit/Hyperactivity Disorder: A Randomised-Controlled Trial," *European Neuropsychopharmacology* 27 (August 2017): 795–808.
4. Dana Barchel, Orit Stolar, Tal D-Haan, et al., "Oral Cannabidiol Use in Children with Autism Spectrum Disorder to Treat Related Symptoms and Comorbidities," *Frontiers in Pharmacology* 9 (January 2019).
5. Noriko Kodama, Kiyoshi Komuta, and Hiroaki Nanba, "Can Maitake MD-Fraction Aid Cancer Patients?" *Alternative Medicine Review* 7 (June 2002): 236–39.
6. Suresh Kumar, Arun Bansal, Arunloke Chakrabarti, and Sunit C. Singhi, "Evaluation of Efficacy of Probiotics in Prevention of Candida Colonization in a PICU: A Randomized Controlled Trial," *Critical Care Medicine* 41 (February 2013): 565–72.
7. Jennifer A. Shuford, James M. Steckelbert, and Robin Patel, "Effects of Fresh Garlic Extract on Candida Albicans Biofilms," *Antimicrobial Agents and Chemotherapy* 49 (January 2005): 473.
8. Thivanka Muthumalage and Irfan Rahman, "Cannabidiol Differentially Regulates Basal and LPS-Induced Inflammatory Responses in Macrophages, Lung Epithelial Cells, and Fibroblasts," *Toxicology and Applied Pharmacology* 382 (November 2019).
9. Alexandre R. de Mello Schier, Natalia P de Oliveira Ribeiro, Danielle S. Coutinho, et al., "Antidepressant-like and Anxiolytic-like Effects of Cannabidiol: A Chemical Compound of Cannabis Sativa," *CNS & Neurological Disorders: Drug Targets* 13 (2014): 953–60.

10. Paul Crawford, "Effectiveness of Cinnamon for Lowering Hemoglobin A1C in Patients with Type 2 Diabetes: A Randomized, Controlled Trial," *Journal of the American Board of Family Medicine* 22 (September–October 2009): 507–12.

11. Institute for Quality and Efficiency in HealthCare, "Can Probiotics Help against Diarrhea?" updated December 19, 2019. https://www.ncbi.nlm.nih.gov/books/NBK373095/

12. Yuqing Zhang, Tuhina Neogi, Clara Chen, et al., "Cherry Consumption and Decreased Risk of Recurrent Gout Attacks," *Arthritis and Rheumatology* 64 (December 2012): 4004–11.

13. Khalid A. Jadoon, Garry D. Tan, and Saoirse E. O'Sullivan, "A Single Dose of Cannabidiol Reduces Blood Pressure in Healthy Volunteers in a Randomized Crossover Study," *JCI Insight* 2 (June 2017).

14. Tina Didari, Shilan Mozaffari, Shekoufeh Nikfar, and Mohammad Abdollahi, "Effectiveness of Probiotics in Irritable Bowel Syndrome: A Systematic Review with Meta-Analysis," *World Journal of Gastroenterology* 21 (March 2015): 3072–84.

15. Hoseein Kehdmat, Ashraf Karbasi, Mohsen Amini, et al., "Aloe Vera in Treatment of Refractory Irritable Bowel Syndrome: Trial on Iranian Patients," *Journal of Research in Medical Sciences* 18 (August 2013).

16. R. K. Rao and Geetha Samak, "Protection and Restitution of Gut Barrier by Probiotics: Nutritional and Clinical Implications," *Current Nutrition and Food Science* 9 (May 2013): 99–107.

17. Itamar Yehuda, Zecharia Madar, Alicia Isabel Leikin-Frenkel, and Snait Tamir, "Glabridin, an Isoflavan from Licorice Root, Down-Regulates Expression and Activity under High Glucose Stress and Inflammation," *Molecular Nutrition and Food Research* 59 (June 2015): 1041–52.

18. Sina Mojaverrostami, Maryam Nazm Bojnordi, Maryam Ghasemi-Kasman, et al., "A Review of Herbal Therapy in Multiple Sclerosis," *Advanced Pharmaceutical Bulletin* 8 (November 2018): 575–90.

19. Ibid.

20. Inaki Lete and Jose Allue, "The Effectiveness of Ginger in the Prevention of Nausea and Vomiting during Pregnancy and Chemotherapy," *Integrative Medicine Insights* 11 (2016): 11–17.

21. Engy Victor Beshay, "Therapeutic Efficacy of Artemisia Absinthium against Hymenolepsis Nana: In Vitro and in Vivo Studies in Comparison with the Anthelmintic Praziquantel," *Journal of Helminthology* 92 (June 2017): 1–11.

22. Hsing-Chun Kuo, Bruce Lu, Chien-Heng Shen, and Shui-Yi Tung, "Hericium erinaceus Myecelium and Its Isolated Erinacine a Protection from MPTP-Induced Neurotoxicity through the ER Stress, Triggering an Apoptosis Cascade," *Journal of Translational Medicine* 18 (March 2016).

23. Deborah J. Cook, Jennie Johnstone, John C. Marshall, et al., "Probiotics: Prevention of Severe Pneumonia and Endotracheal Colonization Trial—PROSPECT: A Pilot Trial," *Trials* 17 (2016).

24. Ernst-Gerhard Loch, Hartmut Selle, and Normann Boblitz, "Treatment of Premenstrual Syndrome with a Phytopharmaceutical Formulation Containing Vitex agnus castus," *Journal of Women's Health and Gender-Based Medicine* 9 (April 2000): 315–20.

25. B. Palmieri, C. Laurino, M. Vadala, "A Therapeutic Effect of CBD-Enriched Ointment in Inflammatory Skin Diseases and Cutaneous Scars," *Clinical Therapeutics* 170 (March–April 2019): e93–99.

Index

Page numbers in *italics* indicate illustrations or charts.